Neuroplasticity-based Neurorehabilitation

Jens Bo Nielsen
Rasmus Feld Frisk
Jakob Lorentzen
Lisbeth Højkjær Larsen
Editors

Neuroplasticity-based Neurorehabilitation

Springer

Editors
Jens Bo Nielsen
Department of Neuroscience
University of Copenhagen
Copenhagen, Denmark

Rasmus Feld Frisk
Department of Neuroscience
University of Copenhagen
Copenhagen, Denmark

Jakob Lorentzen
Department of Neuroscience
University of Copenhagen
Copenhagen, Denmark

Lisbeth Højkjær Larsen
Department of Neuroscience
University of Copenhagen
Copenhagen, Denmark

ISBN 978-3-031-81119-7 ISBN 978-3-031-81120-3 (eBook)
https://doi.org/10.1007/978-3-031-81120-3

This Springer imprint is published by the registered company Springer Nature Switzerland AG
The registered company address is: Gewerbestrasse 11, 6330 Cham, Switzerland

Preface

Purpose of Book and Target Group

Our knowledge of how the brain works has increased dramatically within the past 15–20 years. New optogenetic techniques and multisite recordings in animal experiments have provided information about the interaction between brain areas. Non-invasive imaging and electrophysiological techniques have allowed us to study related patterns of activity in the human brain. The combination of these new sources of information has had a huge impact on our understanding of the brain both during healthy development and ageing as well as in the response to injury, disease and rehabilitation. Importantly, we now have an emerging understanding of plasticity of the brain at the molecular, cellular and network level as a basis for recovery of function. This understanding provides a powerful framework for the development of general guidelines for practical neurorehabilitation.

Despite the importance in communicating this new knowledge to pre- and post-graduate students of neurorehabilitation, neuroscience, biology, physiology, medicine and physiotherapy, there is at present no textbook, which covers this research field in its entirety from basic neurobiology to practical neurorehabilitation. This is the purpose of this book.

The central theme will be to link neurobiology to normal and impaired function and to provide a fundamental understanding of the link between neuroplasticity and improved function in relation to neurorehabilitation.

The book is primarily written for pre- and post-graduate students in neurorehabilitation, but students of neuroscience, medicine, physiology, biology, exercise physiology and physiotherapy may also benefit from the book.

Book Structure

The book includes an introduction to research-based neurorehabilitation and is subsequently divided into three sections. Part I covers basic neurobiology and its practical applications. In Part II, neuroplasticity is defined and described, starting from its origins in neurodevelopmental plasticity and progressing to ways in which science-based knowledge and advances in technologies can promote neuroplasticity and improve neurorehabilitation. In Part III, different neurological disorders are highlighted to exemplify condition-specific challenges and opportunities. The book concludes with a chapter on future directions. To optimally link basic neurobiological theory to practical neurorehabilitation, each chapter starts by introducing a descriptive case story.

This book benefits from the diverse perspectives of its contributors, who represent various fields. Each author contributes with a unique background, introducing varied perspectives. This diversity provides readers with a comprehensive understanding of neuroplasticity-based neurorehabilitation from a range of experts.

Copenhagen, Denmark — Jens Bo Nielsen
Copenhagen, Denmark — Rasmus Feld Frisk
Copenhagen, Denmark — Jakob Lorentzen
Copenhagen, Denmark — Lisbeth Højkjær Larsen

Contents

1 Towards Science-Based Neurorehabilitation

Jens Bo Nielsen, Christina Rostrup Kruuse, Jakob Lorentzen, Rasmus Feld Frisk, and Lisbeth Højkjær Larsen

Abstract

This chapter will introduce the book and explain the mission of the book. Current neurorehabilitation is to some extent based on theoretical concepts with little scientific evidence. Not all existing interventions, procedures, and techniques have sufficient scientific evidence to demonstrate that they work, and the experience of individual therapists and traditional approaches in local rehabilitation units are often the main reason for using specific interventions. Providing solid scientific evidence of each rehabilitation procedure is costly and will take decades to achieve. It may also be questioned whether it is necessary to demonstrate the efficiency of all existing rehabilitation techniques and procedures in expensive randomized clinical studies, since many of the techniques that are used in routine clinical practice are unlikely to have any effect with our current understanding of how the nervous system and the human body function. It is possible to save time, money, resources, and probably also lives if knowledge from human neurobiology is used to focus on therapies and procedures that are the most likely to work in practice. This will simplify the efforts that need to be put into providing evidence of which therapies and procedures work the best. The book is based on this fundamental idea.

Keywords

Neurorehabilitation · Plasticity · Clinical trials · Adaptive designs · Neuroplasticity-based therapy · Evidence-based practice

1.1 Defining the Terms

Neurorehabilitation is defined by WHO as a set of interventions designed to optimize functioning and reduce disability in individuals with health conditions in interaction with their environment. In its most comprehensive scope, neurorehabilitation includes the complete restoration or construction of function after a nervous system injury and the prevention of functional decline after a neurological diagnosis (see Box 1.1). The aim is to enable individuals to resume or maintain an independent and meaningful daily life. This is a long, complex process, which involves numerous factors, spanning from acute surgical interventions at the time of diagnosis to workplace adjustments to

J. B. Nielsen (✉) · J. Lorentzen · R. F. Frisk · L. H. Larsen
Department of Neuroscience, University of Copenhagen, Copenhagen, Denmark
e-mail: jbnielsen@sund.ku.dk; jlorentzen@sund.ku.dk; frisk@sund.ku.dk; lihl@sund.ku.dk

C. R. Kruuse
University of Copenhagen, Rigshospitalet, Copenhagen, Denmark
e-mail: christina.kruuse@regionh.dk

J. B. Nielsen et al. (eds.), *Neuroplasticity-based Neurorehabilitation*, https://doi.org/10.1007/978-3-031-81120-3_1

accommodate any lingering disability. It is not the purpose of this book to cover all these steps, but to focus specifically on the core of any neurorehabilitation program: how people with brain injury can be helped to obtain/maintain and optimize function. With this focus, the importance of practice and (re)learning following damage to the nervous system will be emphasized. Within the framework of the International Classification of Functioning, Disability and Health (ICF) (WHO, 2013), the emphasis is on impairments and activities/limitations, whereas participation in society, such as maintaining a social network or the process of resuming work duties, largely falls outside the scope of the book (Fig. 1.1). The significance of environmental and personal factors for recovery of function will be an integrated part of Sect. 1.2, where the practical challenges in promoting recovery of function will be discussed.

Box 1.1 Habilitation or Rehabilitation

The development of the nervous system, plasticity of the nervous system during development, neurodevelopmental disorders, and interventions early in life have been given special attention. Lesions to the nervous system early in life differ from lesions later in life in at least two major ways: Firstly, the nervous system is more plastic and may therefore, to some extent, repair itself early in life so that the functional consequences of a lesion may be less than what is seen later in life. Secondly, persons who are born with a neurodevelopmental disorder have no personal experience of a life without the disorder and may experience it as an integrated part of them as an individual. These two factors are of fundamental importance for the very different approach that needs to be adopted in a training or learning program for people with early rather than late lesions to the nervous system. However, the comparison of the different approaches that need to be adopted helps to illustrate many of the key points that are of importance in any training and learning program for people with late lesions, and although there is no "re" before the habilitation of children and adults with early brain lesions, it makes sense to include both as they help to enlighten each other. The term "neuro**re**habilitation" has been kept rather than having to add the strictly speaking more correct term "neurohabilitation" for this same reason.

Degenerative disorders such as Parkinson's disease, multiple sclerosis, and dementia have been included, although these disorders are by definition not caused by an event confined in time such as a traumatic incidence or a stroke but involve a continuous degenerative process, for which there at present is no cure, but for which the physical and cognitive consequences to some extent may be alleviated or postponed.

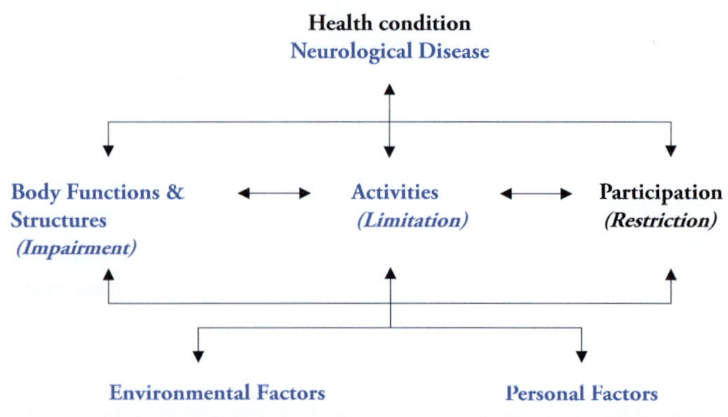

Fig. 1.1 International Classification of Functioning, Disability, and Health (ICF). The blue color presents aspects covered in this book. Reprinted with permission of the World Health Organization (WHO), and all rights are reserved by the organization

The core issue that the book aims to tackle is the challenge of substantiating with convincing scientific evidence the efficiency of any therapeutic intervention in facilitating the recovery of function following central nervous system lesions. Neurorehabilitation is a complex and prolonged process that currently demands substantial human resources. With global healthcare systems facing escalating demands due to shifts in population demographics, advances in medical care, and associated rising costs, there exists a limit to the investment each country can make in promoting the recovery of function after central nervous system damage.

Neurorehabilitation encounters difficulty in gaining public support as it lacks dramatic cures, and its patients are often elderly and frail for other reasons. Therefore, it becomes imperative to assess the cost-effectiveness of rehabilitation. In this context, the paramount consideration is to discontinue therapies that prove ineffective and employ those that demonstrate efficiency in large, conclusive, well-controlled studies. The challenge, naturally, lies in determining which therapies are effective and which are not.

1.2 How to Determine the Effectiveness of Therapy

Humans possess an inherent inclination to identify patterns and seek explanations for phenomena in the surroundings. Even when there is no logical or scientific foundation for a cause-and-effect relationship between two events, the brain strives to find coherence in the coincidence, suspecting that one event led to the other. This adaptive ability serves a practical purpose of significant evolutionary importance, as it lies at the heart of food avoidance when experiencing illness following food consumption. Though challenging to prove, it wouldn't be surprising if evolution has hardwired the brain to make causal inferences based on correlations between events, even when these events are purely coincidental. This cognitive ability is instrumental for navigation and comprehension of a complex and unpredictable world.

However, the inclination to identify patterns and infer causal connections from coincidences also leads to potential errors in judgment. Without an innate statistical acumen, humans are not good at calculating the frequency of occurrence of two events together to dismiss mere chance. Consequently, when witnessing a patient spontaneously recovering after a specific intervention, there's a risk of mistakenly attributing the recovery to the intervention. Personal experience, bolstered by the conviction of having "seen it with my own eyes," often holds such sway that even robust scientific evidence, supported by sophisticated statistics, demonstrating the contrary, may struggle to dislodge the belief in the intervention's efficacy.

The observation of recovery following an intervention cannot and should not be used to infer a causal relationship—even with repeated observations. Regardless of the frequency of these instances, there might be no genuine causal link. Spontaneous recovery without intervention remains a valid possibility.

Only a meticulously designed, controlled scientific study with adequate statistical power can conclusively determine the efficiency of an intervention. It necessitates a conscious and deliberate departure from the instinctive reliance on personal experience and the belief in what "we see with our own eyes."

1.3 The RCT Study

The universally accepted gold standard for providing evidence of the clinical efficiency of a therapy is the randomized controlled clinical trial (RCT). The first RCT study in medicine was published by Austin Bradford Hill and colleagues in 1948, and the RCT standard has been developed and refined since then to allow conclusive evidence to be reached with as few confounders as possible (Anon, 1948). Central is the random assignment of patients to an intervention or a control group, which allows comparison of the intervention to existing therapy (or no therapy/placebo). The random assignment of patients to the two groups should make the two groups comparable with respect to important confounders, which might influence the outcome (sex, age, socio-economic status, etc.). This is not always achieved, especially in smaller RCT studies, and unbalanced groups are often why conclusions from RCT studies must be moderated. Central is also the selection of a specific primary outcome measure prior to the study's initiation so that an adequate statistical model, including a power analysis of the required number of subjects, may be established. Depending on the primary outcome measure, it is usually required to perform the study with a blinded analysis of outcome measures so that neither the researchers nor the participants know which group the individual participant has been assigned to. This is required in drug trials since the knowledge of treatment greatly influences the outcome and may also bias the evaluation of results, especially if measures are not objective and validated in relation to the patient population. However, because of the nature of most neurorehabilitation interventions, it is seldom possible to achieve proper blinding—at least of the patient—and it is a general challenge that most RCT studies in neurorehabilitation end up as single-blinded rather than double-blinded. It is simply not possible to train patients without their knowledge. It is also not possible to blind the therapists who are responsible for the therapy. However, this is usually solved by blinding the researchers, who perform tests and measurements, and preventing communication between the therapists and researchers during the study period as much as possible. Adequately powered RCT studies are thus currently the best way of providing solid scientific evidence of the effect of treatment—also in the field of neurorehabilitation.

1.4 The Problem with RCTs

Unfortunately, only a few therapies in the field of neurorehabilitation have been found to have sufficient evidence from RCT studies to be recommended as part of routine clinical practice (Novak et al., 2013). Most systematic reviews of RCT studies in the field end with some version of the statement that "more high-quality studies with sufficient power are necessary before any firm conclusions can be made." To take a few randomly selected examples:

Campbell et al. (2016) reviewed 13 RCT studies on physiotherapy in multiple sclerosis patients. Of these, only one study had made appropriate power calculations and turned out to be underpowered due to dropouts. The review concludes that "physiotherapy may be effective" but that "appropriately powered studies are required." As of 2024, such studies have not been conducted.

Roeder et al. (2015) reviewed 9 RCT studies on strength training in Parkinson's disease patients. Although they observed that strength training may increase muscle strength in PD patients as compared to no exercise, they were unable to conclude whether strength training had any advantages over other forms of exercise and ended stating that "Findings should be interpreted with caution due to the relatively high risk of bias of most studies" (Roeder et al., 2015).

Katalinic et al. (2011) reviewed 25 RCT studies on the effect of passive stretching on joint mobility in neurological populations and found high-quality evidence that stretching had no or only little short-term or long-term effect on joint mobility but could not exclude immediate effects or that stretching for more than the 3–4 months, which was the maximal intervention period investigated in the studies, would have an effect (Katalinic et al., 2011).

Chen et al. (2023) reviewed 14 RCT studies on the effect of non-invasive brain stimulation on motor outcomes in spinal cord injured subjects, and although they found a positive effect, the p-value was marginal and the studies too heterogeneous to conclude anything but that "Further high-quality clinical trials are needed to support or refute the use and optimize the stimulation parameters of NIBS in clinical practice" (Chen et al., 2023).

The scientific literature is full of examples like this, which can be confirmed by a quick Medline database search. Systematic reviews with strict Cochrane criteria for how to conduct the search and subsequent analysis of studies are convenient to get an overview of the RCT studies on specific interventions, but they do not solve the problem that the RCT studies are very seldom sufficiently strong to make any firm conclusions. They only pinpoint the problem—they do not solve it. The suggestion to introduce systematic reviews of systematic reviews also only helps to point out that there are not only too many low-quality RCT studies published but also too many systematic reviews summarizing those RCT studies. This is a structural problem. Researchers need to publish to get funded, and journals are, to an increasing extent, happy to comply since for most journals, more published papers equals more money earned. The increasing number of open journals, which rely on a business model where the authors pay to get their work published, is an important part of this problem, as also illustrated by the high number of journals willing to publish fake scientific papers with little or no peer reviewing (Hawkes, 2013).

The deficiency of RCT studies is also clear from an extensive review of 166 RCT studies evaluating the efficiency of 64 interventions used to treat children with cerebral palsy (Novak et al., 2013). Only 16% of the 131 outcome measures in the studies showed convincing evidence of a treatment effect. Another 6% showed convincing lack of evidence. This means that in almost 80% of the cases, the studies were of too low power to provide any conclusive evidence and fell in the categories "probably effective" or "probably not effective." This is a lot of work, money, and time invested in obtaining a question mark.

Even when successful, there are two interrelated phenomena that may diminish the value of an RCT study: One is "the infinite space of variables," and the other is "the curse of the negative finding."

The infinite space of variables refers to the many variables that may limit how far the findings in any single study can be generalized. If the study was performed in patients with multiple sclerosis, it may be questioned if the intervention would also be efficient in other neurological patients or in MS patients at a different stage of their disease or different age. If the intervention consisted of 10 weeks of exercise every two days, it may be questioned if exercise every three days or four days would also have worked. Would 20 weeks have worked better, or would five weeks have been enough? Which kind of exercise works better—running, bicycling, or? How many minutes per day is required, and how intensive should the exercise be? All these questions may guarantee work for many researchers for decades.

Negative findings have the inherent problem that absence of evidence is not evidence of absence. This is the reason negative findings are likely underrepresented in the scientific literature and thereby a main cause of bias in systematic reviews. This inherent problem with negative findings is also the reason why treatments that have made it into clinical practice are difficult to get out again. One single positive finding may outweigh 10 or more negative findings.

It should also be considered that the RCT design relies on comparison of two groups: an intervention and an often poorly defined control group using traditional frequency statistics. This means that it is necessary to decide the size of the two populations before the start of the study based on power calculations and continue the study until all subjects have been recruited before revealing whether the intervention worked or not. In either case, the researchers are likely to consider whether changes to the intervention might give a different result (different dose, different frequency of dose, etc.—i.e., explore the infinite space of variables). In this case they will have to start all over again with a completely new RCT study. These inherent problems in the RCT study explain why implementation of new treatment often takes decades (Flores-Mateo & Argimon, 2007).

So, to sum up: RCT studies are expensive, they take up a lot of human resources, and they take a very long time to complete. Despite this, they seldom provide the conclusive evidence needed in neurorehabilitation.

1.5 What Can Be Done in the Future?

1.5.1 Multi-Center International Networks and Adaptive Clinical Trials

First, badly designed and underpowered RCT studies should be abandoned. They are a waste of time and resources. Clinical studies require large numbers, and the only way to obtain sufficiently large numbers is through multi-center collaboration—at a national and preferably an international level. This requires agreement on outcome measures and sharing of data, which is a challenge, but, nevertheless, the only way forward. It calls for collaboration rather than competition.

Creating international collaboration between multiple centers is only part of the solution. Recent developments in the theoretical and statistical framework of clinical studies have pointed to the many advantages of conducting adaptive clinical studies in which Bayesian statistics rather than traditional frequency statistics are applied to the data (Pallmann et al., 2018).

Studies have documented that adaptive designs increase the efficiency of clinical trials while reducing costs and enhancing the likelihood of detecting the true benefit of a new treatment (Bhatt & Mehta, 2016).

Adaptive designs in clinical trials involve using accumulating data to decide whether and how to modify an ongoing trial without compromising research integrity (Morgan et al., 2014). The primary goal is to enhance the flexibility, efficiency, and speed of clinical trials (Mahajan & Gupta, 2010). In an adaptive trial, adjustments can be made to the study's design, the number of participants enrolled, and the allocation of individuals to different treatments while the trial is still in progress (see Fig. 1.2). These modifications are guided by predefined rules based on data collected from patients already in the study, assessing their responses to various treatments. Adaptive designs also offer more flexibility than traditional clinical studies, allowing researchers to allocate more participants to treatments showing better performance and fewer to those demonstrating poorer results. Also, ineffective treatments can be promptly eliminated, making room for new treatments as they become available. This dynamic approach enables researchers to optimize trial outcomes in real-time based on emerging data.

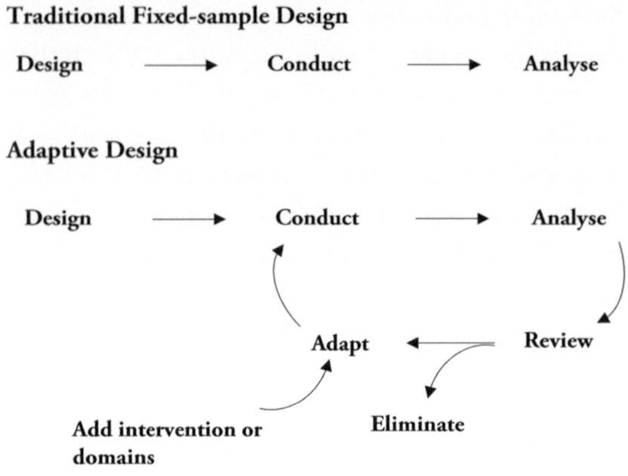

Fig. 1.2 Schematic presentation of traditional clinical trial design with fixed sample size (top row) and adaptive clinical design with predefined review(s) and adaptation(s) (bottom row)

1.5.2 Neuroplasticity-Based Neurorehabilitation

While waiting for sufficient evidence from large-scale, multicenter, adaptive clinical trials, patients still need the best possible treatment that can be provided. A common framework for deciding which therapies are the most likely to work based on the available knowledge is therefore necessary. This should not be based on prior experience and tradition ("because I have seen it with my own eyes"), but rather on what has the best chance of working based on current scientific understanding of how the body and the nervous system function. There are unfortunately still many therapies and procedures that are used in neurorehabilitation centers globally and are being promoted in "scientific" papers, but which have very little likelihood of helping the patients in the most efficient way based on the current understanding of how the body and especially the nervous system works.

This understanding has increased rapidly in the last few years, and therapies that were developed many decades ago need to be changed accordingly or, alternatively, abandoned when they turn out not to comply with the current understanding.

This book's ambition is to give the reader in the beginning of the twenty-first century an idea of the current knowledge of neurobiology as a basis for deciding how best to help patients recover function after brain and spinal cord injuries. The ambition is not to develop a new concept or a new therapy that provides strict rules of how recovery of function is promoted in the best possible way. The knowledge of today may be outdated tomorrow, and anyone with a keen ambition to help people recover function following brain and spinal cord injury needs to be fully aware of that fact. This is a daunting task that requires constant updating. Daily practice needs to be flexibly adjusted to the latest scientific knowledge. The ambition of this book is to mediate some of that knowledge and give the reader an idea of the current knowledge of how the nervous system works and how it changes function with experience (neuroplasticity). Crucially, this knowledge has to be translated into sensible interventions that can be evaluated scientifically so that practical neurorehabilitation can be improved globally.

References

Anon. (1948). STREPTOMYCIN treatment of pulmonary tuberculosis. *British Medical Journal, 2*(4582), 769–782.

Bhatt, D. L., & Mehta, C. (2016). Adaptive designs for clinical trials. *The New England Journal of Medicine, 375*(1), 65–74. https://doi.org/10.1056/NEJMra1510061

Campbell, E., Coulter, E. H., Mattison, P. G., Miller, L., McFadyen, A., & Paul, L. (2016). Physiotherapy rehabilitation for people with progressive multiple sclerosis: A systematic review. *Archives of Physical Medicine and Rehabilitation, 97*(1), 141–151 e143. https://doi.org/10.1016/j.apmr.2015.07.022

Chen, J. M., Li, X. L., Pan, Q. H., Yang, Y., Xu, S. M., & Xu, J. W. (2023). Effects of non-invasive brain stimulation on motor function after spinal cord injury: A systematic review and meta-analysis. *Journal of Neuroengineering and Rehabilitation, 20*(1), 3. https://doi.org/10.1186/s12984-023-01129-4

Flores-Mateo, G., & Argimon, J. M. (2007). Evidence based practice in postgraduate healthcare education: A systematic review. *BMC Health Services Research, 7*, 119. https://doi.org/10.1186/1472-6963-7-119

Hawkes, N. (2013). Spoof research paper is accepted by 157 journals. *British Medical Journal, 347*, f5975. https://doi.org/10.1136/bmj.f5975

Katalinic, O. M., Harvey, L. A., & Herbert, R. D. (2011). Effectiveness of stretch for the treatment and prevention of contractures in people with neurological conditions: A systematic review. *Physical Therapy, 91*(1), 11–24. https://doi.org/10.2522/ptj.20100265

Mahajan, R., & Gupta, K. (2010). Adaptive design clinical trials: Methodology, challenges and prospect. *Indian Journal of Pharmacology, 42*(4), 201–207. https://doi.org/10.4103/0253-7613.68417

Morgan, C. C., Huyck, S., Jenkins, M., Chen, L., Bedding, A., Coffey, C. S., et al. (2014). Adaptive design: Results of 2012 survey on perception and use. *Therapeutic Innovation & Regulatory Science, 48*(4), 473–481. https://doi.org/10.1177/2168479014522468

Novak, I., McIntyre, S., Morgan, C., Campbell, L., Dark, L., Morton, N., et al. (2013). A systematic review of interventions for children with cerebral palsy: State of the evidence. *Developmental Medicine and Child Neurology, 55*(10), 885–910. https://doi.org/10.1111/dmcn.12246

Pallmann, P., Bedding, A. W., Choodari-Oskooei, B., Dimairo, M., Flight, L., Hampson, L. V., et al. (2018). Adaptive designs in clinical trials: Why use them, and how to run and report them. *BMC Medicine, 16*(1), 29. https://doi.org/10.1186/s12916-018-1017-7

Roeder, L., Costello, J. T., Smith, S. S., Stewart, I. B., & Kerr, G. K. (2015). Effects of resistance training on measures of muscular strength in people with Parkinson's disease: A systematic review and meta-analysis. *PLoS One, 10*(7), e0132135. https://doi.org/10.1371/journal.pone.0132135

WHO. (2013). *How to use the ICF: T A practical manual for using the International Classification of Functioning, Disability and Health (ICF)*. Available via WHO. Retrieved 24 May, 2024, from https://www.who.int/publications/m/item/how-to-use-the-icf%2D%2D-a-practical-manual-for-using-the-international-classification-of-functioning-disability-and-health.

Part I

Neurobiological Basis of Neurorehabilitation

2 Touch and Proprioception

Jean-marc Aimonetti and Yoh'i Zennou-Azogui

Abstract

Somesthesis is the ability to detect internal or external stimuli of mechanical or thermal nature. This relies upon activation of receptors located in skin and deeper tissues such as muscles. Information from the body reaches different somatosensory brain structures, giving rise to tactile, affective, and kinesthetic sensations that guide our interactions with the environment. Although the chapter will refer to tactile and proprioceptive modalities, things are more complicated; all these receptors have several functions. The integration of their input into the somatosensory and motor cortices contributes to the perception of touch and limb movements and positions. Finally, numerous methods of rehabilitation have been proposed based on the activation of touch and proprioceptive receptors, notably in the case of stroke or cerebral palsy.

Keywords

Somesthesis · Touch · Proprioception · Somatosensory pathways · Rehabilitation

Box 2.1 Case Story

In 1985, Oliver Sacks published his best-seller, The Man Who Mistook His Wife for a Hat and Other Clinical Tales (Sacks, 1985). The chapter entitled "The Disembodied Lady" concerned the patient, Ginette. She was 30 years old when she lost her sense of touch, i.e., sensitivity to pressure and vibrations, and proprioception, the sense of position and movements of our limbs, following a Guillain-Barré syndrome and a second episode of polyneuropathy. The face and part of the trunk were preserved, and so were temperature and pain senses, which suggests that the large myelinated sensory fibers were selectively affected. Her neurologist, Yves Lamarre, looked after her. He taught her how to compensate for the loss of touch with visual compensation. She had to watch everything she did. In Sacks' book, she says that sometimes she loses her arms; she thinks they are in one place but finds them somewhere else. Ginette recently passed away. She has been the subject of numerous important scientific publications, including the confirmation of an affective touch, distinct from discriminative touch.

J.-m. Aimonetti (✉) · Y. Zennou-Azogui
Aix Marseille Univ, CNRS, CRPN
(Centre de Recherche en Psychologie et Neurosciences—UMR 7077), Marseille, France
e-mail: jean-marc.aimonetti@univ-amu.fr; yohi.zennou-azogui@univ-amu.fr

J. B. Nielsen et al. (eds.), *Neuroplasticity-based Neurorehabilitation*,
https://doi.org/10.1007/978-3-031-81120-3_2

2.1 Tactile Sensitivity, Discriminative Touch

With a surface area of almost 2 m^2 in adults, skin is the body's largest sensory organ. Skin and brain originate from the same embryonic tissue, ectoderm. From an early age, touch is an essential sense for cognitive development. Little David Vetter, an immunocompromised child who spent his short life in a sterile bubble, was unfortunately witness to the consequences of a lack of emotional touch in humans. Intelligent and curious for his first 10 years, David became depressed and developed autistic syndrome as he neared puberty.

Tactile sensitivity relies on receptors sensitive to low-threshold mechanical stimuli like pressure or vibration. Hand glabrous skin contains the highest concentration of mechanoreceptors, with nearly 17,000 units in each hand. There are at least four types of low-threshold mechanoreceptors with different properties that enable them to provide information of different qualities and temporal and spatial aspects of touch: Meissner's corpuscles, Pacinian corpuscles, Merkel's discs, and Ruffini's endings. All these receptors have myelinated innervation of the Aβ type, providing rapid conduction of nerve impulses in humans (see Table 2.1). In both hairy and glabrous skin, free nerve endings encode temperature and nociceptive information. These fibers are unmyelinated with slow velocity conduction (see Fig. 2.1).

Box 2.2 Skin mechanoreceptors in humans

Low-threshold mechanoreceptors are distinguished primarily by their properties of adaptation to maintenance of stimulus application. Rapidly adapting receptors, Meissner and Pacinian, respond in irregular bursts to the application of the stimulus and to its withdrawal but stop discharging while pressure is maintained. The slowly adapting receptors, Merkel and Ruffini, also encode stimulus application but discharge during pressure maintenance, at least for a certain time. These adaptive properties do not explain why clothing is not felt when worn. Any limb movement causes skin stroking from clothing, which excites most of the tactile receptors. As they are not relevant, these messages are attenuated in cortical areas and do not induce conscious sensation.

These receptors are also distinguished by the size and shape of their receptive field, i.e., the area of the skin subjected to mechanical deformation. Type I units, the most superficial, are Meissner's corpuscles and Merkel's discs, with small receptive fields with well-defined edges and several hot spots, the areas of greatest sensitivity. Type II units, located deeper in the dermis, are Ruffini's endings and Pacinian corpuscles, with diffuse, broad receptive fields and a single hot spot (Johnson, 2001).

(continued)

Table 2.1 Classification of sensory fibers in peripheral nerves

Fiber diameter (μm)	Axon number	Fiber group	Conduction velocity (m/s)	Sensory function	Receptor type (examples)
Myelinated					
12–20	Ia/Ib	Aα	72–120	Proprioception	Muscle spindle/Golgi tendon organ
6–12	II	Aβ	36–72	Touch, proprioception	Mechanoreceptors
1–6	III	Aδ	4–36	Pain, temperature	Nociceptors, thermoreceptors
Unmyelinated					
0.2–1.5	IV	C	0.4–2.0	Pain, touch, temperature	Free nerve endings

Box 2.2 (continued)

Meissner corpuscles are in the dermal papillae, and their density is highest at the fingertips, with almost two units per mm^2, where tactile acuity is also highest. While their spatial resolution is fairly low, their temporal resolution is high, and they encode local deformations produced when exploring fine textures such as satin. Their frequency composition response reflects oscillations of skin induced by texture exploration. These mechanoreceptors are also essential for regulating grip force: when manipulating an object, there are often micro-slides between the skin and the object that help to identify the object's shape. These tiny deformations of skin activate Meissner's corpuscles, and the resulting nerve signals regulate the grip force via reflex loops (Johnson, 2001).

Pacinian corpuscles are the largest mechanoreceptors in humans at around 3–4 mm in length; they are encapsulated in an onion-like structure acting as a high-pass filter with a time constant of around 4 ms. With very large receptive fields, sometimes the whole hand, Pacinian corpuscles have very low spatial resolution. It has long been thought that their main function was to code distant events when an object is handled. Johnson (2001) gives a nice example that illustrates their functional role: When we make cement, we perceive the texture of the sand at the end of the shovel as well as if we were touching the sand with our fingers. Another example is the blind man's white cane. This long-distance transmission function would be impossible without the high-pass filter; all the intense low-frequency vibrations resulting from manual activities would contaminate the response of Pacinian corpuscles. They may encode small vibrations around 10–15 nm at the ideal frequency of around 500 Hz (Skedung et al., 2013).

Located in the basal layer of the epidermis, Merkel discs account for 25% of mechanoreceptors in the human hand and are also present in hairy skin, particularly in the most sensitive areas. In the glabrous skin, Merkel discs, often grouped in tens at the papillary ridges of opposite fingerprints, form veritable tactile domes. They are particularly sensitive to relief and edges, whatever the force of application, and encode fine pressure best. Their spatial resolution is close to a millimeter, while their receptive field is between 2 and 3 mm^2. This fine resolution relies upon the presence of several hot spots in the receptive field. These probably correspond to individual branches of the axon. Merkel discs are essential players in haptic touch; their activation threshold is ten times lower when pressure is applied dynamically. Their slowly adapting afferents respond in dynamic bursts to stimulus application but encode indentation maintained with irregular tonic discharge; this suggested early on the possibility of a synapse between Merkel cells and their afferent terminals. In rat vibrissae follicles, Ikeda and colleagues showed that Merkel cells, specifically Piezo two ion channels and not the sensory endings of SA I fibers, are indeed the origin of mechanical pressure transduction (Ikeda et al., 2014). Merkel cells also sense cooling with TRMP8 channels (Bouvier et al., 2018). Similarly, Ikeda and colleagues succeeded in inducing allodynia by applying capsaicin, the active ingredient in chili peppers, which normally targets TRPV1 channels sensitive to nociceptive stimuli. This study raises the question of the role of Merkel discs in chronic pain, notably about itch (Bataille-Savattier et al., 2023).

Ruffini endings constitute the last type of low-threshold mechanoreceptors linked to fibers Aβ. Located deep in the dermis, in the longitudinal axis of muscles, the tactile function of these mechanoreceptors was recognized only recently. When Ruffini discovered them on a biopsy of his own index finger, he thought they were heat receptors;

(continued)

Box 2.2 (continued)
however, they are absent from the foreskin, where heat sensation is felt. There has also long been debate about their tactile function, as they have never been found in the glabrous skin of monkeys. In humans, these afferents, whose sensory endings have the highest activation thresholds, are particularly sensitive to skin stretching. Johnson and colleagues proposed that differences in manual dexterity between monkeys and humans may be partly due to the lack of Ruffini endings in monkeys (Johnson, 2001). Indeed, Ruffini endings could provide information on the exact position of the fingers and hand when handling objects, in addition to proprioceptive information from the muscles. In addition to this proprioceptive function, Ruffini endings could complement information from Meissner's corpuscles about the movement direction of objects being handled.

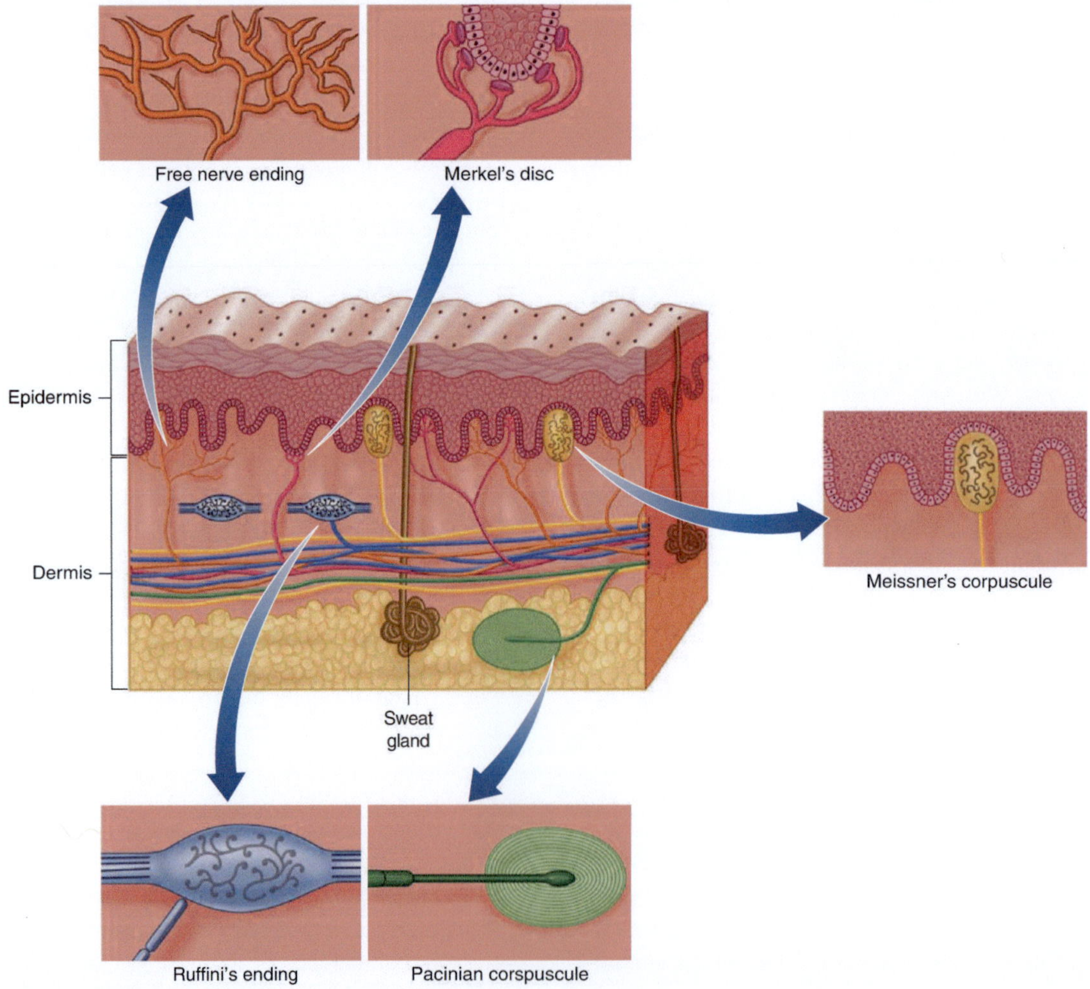

Fig. 2.1 Section of hairless skin. Starting with the epidermis, which is poorly innervated only by free endings, the dermis contains most of the low-threshold tactile mechanoreceptors. Adipocytes provide thermal and physical protection for the deepest organs

2.2 Tactile Sensitivity, Affective Touch

In addition to this fast conduction system, hairy and less glabrous skin have free endings in the epidermis that respond specifically to light and slow stroking, preferentially applied at a neutral temperature, i.e., close to that of human skin (Schirmer et al., 2023). The maximum response of these tactile C fibers is observed for stimuli applied around 3 cm per second, which correlates with psychophysical evaluation of pleasantness. The tactile C system suggests the existence of a duality in touch: alongside the sensory discrimination system provided by the mechanoreceptors seen above, mammals also have an affective and motivational system supported by C-tactile fibers, which are by far the most represented and probably spared by aging.

Historically, C-tactile fibers were discovered in cats at the beginning of electrophysiology. Zotterman thought they were tickle receptors. They were then forgotten before being recorded in humans by Nordin. Later experiments by Olausson and colleagues on the deafferented patient Ginette confirmed their primary function related to affective touch. This affective and motivational system may reinforce intimate social relationships by promoting the release of oxytocin and endorphins. However, it would be simplistic to ignore the contribution of Aβ fibers to affective touch and, above all, the notion of context. Touch can only be affective if it is given by someone who has a reason to do so (Schirmer et al., 2023).

2.3 Proprioception

Skeletal muscles possess a large amount of sensory innervation in their fleshy parts. Muscle spindles are receptors sensitive to stretching of the homonymous muscle. Their density varies with muscle function, with up to a hundred receptors per gram of muscle tissue in the fine muscles of the finger.

Muscle spindles are made of specific contractile muscle fibers, the intrafusal fibers (Fig. 2.2). Their central part is encapsulated in connective tissue, and nuclei are grouped there in the form of a chain or sack, giving rise to different types of fibers. This central part constitutes the sensory organ with two types of mechanosensitive endings: the primary endings give rise to the Ia afferences, myelinated fibers with rapid conduction velocity; the secondary endings branch into a bunch in the para-equatorial regions and give rise to the secondary afferences with slower conduction. Primary endings have a dynamic sensitivity, meaning that they rather encode the time of muscle stretching, while secondary endings encode rather the sustained stretching of skeletal muscles, i.e., they exhibit mostly a static sensitivity. The static or dynamic sensitivity of muscle spindles is modulated by the central nervous system thanks to gamma motor (γ) neurons (see Chap. 5). It has been shown in humans that this γ system may adjust the proprioceptive feedback depending on task requests or emotions (Ackerley et al., 2017). Finally, muscle spindles express ASIC3, a dual-function protein, and they may have a role in the development of the pain associated with tissue acidosis, which means that proprioception training may be beneficial for pain relief (Lee & Chen, 2023). Muscles also contain Golgi tendon organs at their extremities. They give rise to Ib afferents (Table 2.1) and encode mainly the force produced during contraction (see also Chap. 5). The nerve signals carried by Ib afferents are also integrated with information from muscle spindles to improve proprioceptive information.

All these afferents provide sensory feedback about muscle stretching, limb position, and force. They contribute to spinal reflexes (see further in Chap. 5), but also to kinesthesia, and *in fine* to maintain and adjust the homunculus both in motor and somatosensory cortices.

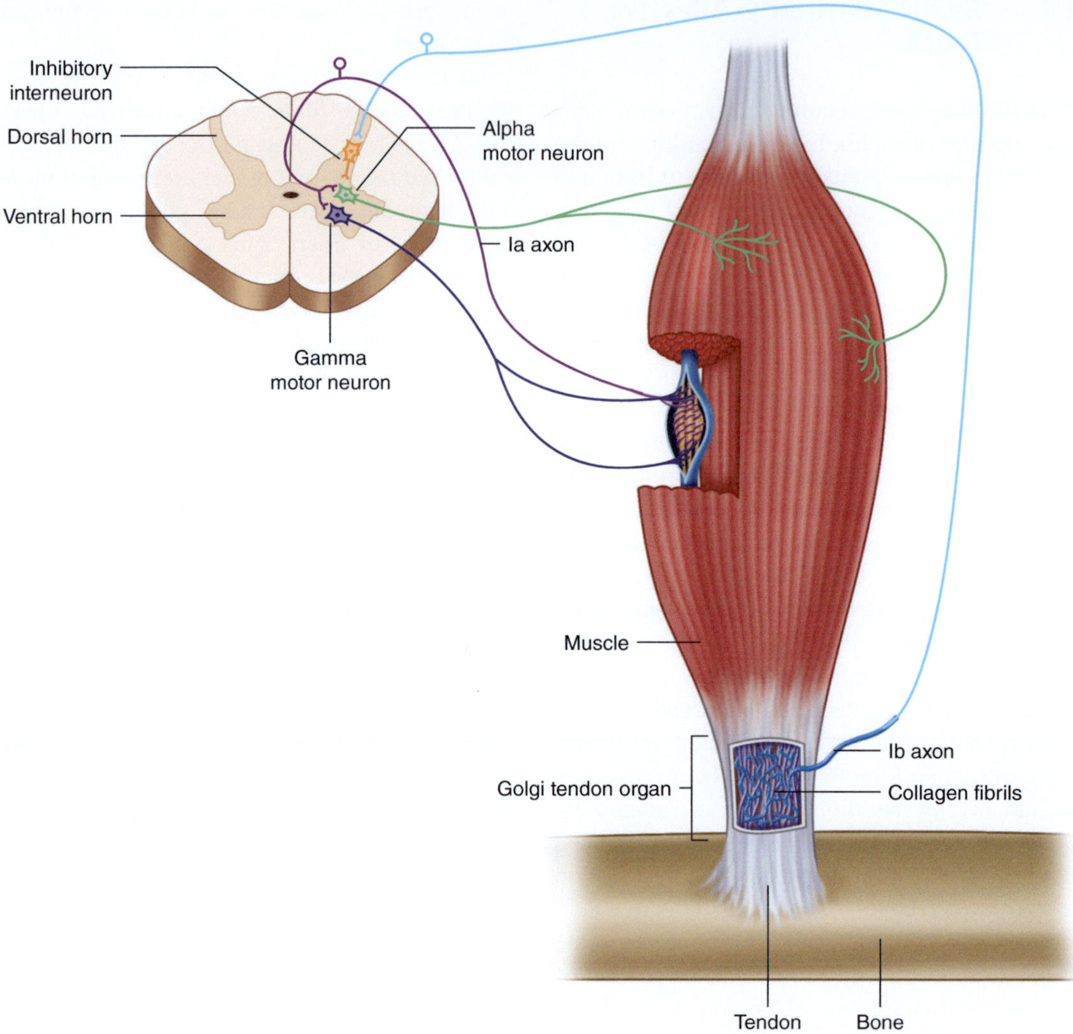

Fig. 2.2 Schematic representation of a muscle spindle and a Golgi tendon organ. The muscle spindles are located in the muscle in parallel or in series with the muscle fibers. Two different sensory afferents originate from the muscle spindles: gr. Ia afferents (purple) and gr. II afferents (not illustrated). The Ia afferents enter the spinal cord through the dorsal horn and have direct monosynaptic connections with the alpha (green) and gamma (deep blue) motor neurons in the ventral horn. The alpha motor neurons innervate the muscle fibers, and the gamma motor neurons innervate the muscle spindles. The Golgi tendon organs are located in the tendons and give rise to gr. Ib sensory afferents (light blue). The Ib afferents have indirect connections to the alpha motor neurons through sets of inhibitory and excitatory interneurons. An example of the most direct pathway through inhibitory interneurons is illustrated (orange)

2.4 Central Nervous Pathways and Somatosensory Input Processing

Two major ascending pathways convey somatosensory information from the limbs and trunk to the brain: the dorsal column system (also referred to as the lemniscal system) and the spinothalamic system (also called the anterolateral system). Body proprioceptive and discriminative touch sensations are transmitted by the dorsal column system mainly to the primary somatosensory cortex in the postcentral gyrus of the parietal lobe of the brain (see Fig. 2.3), while affective touch,

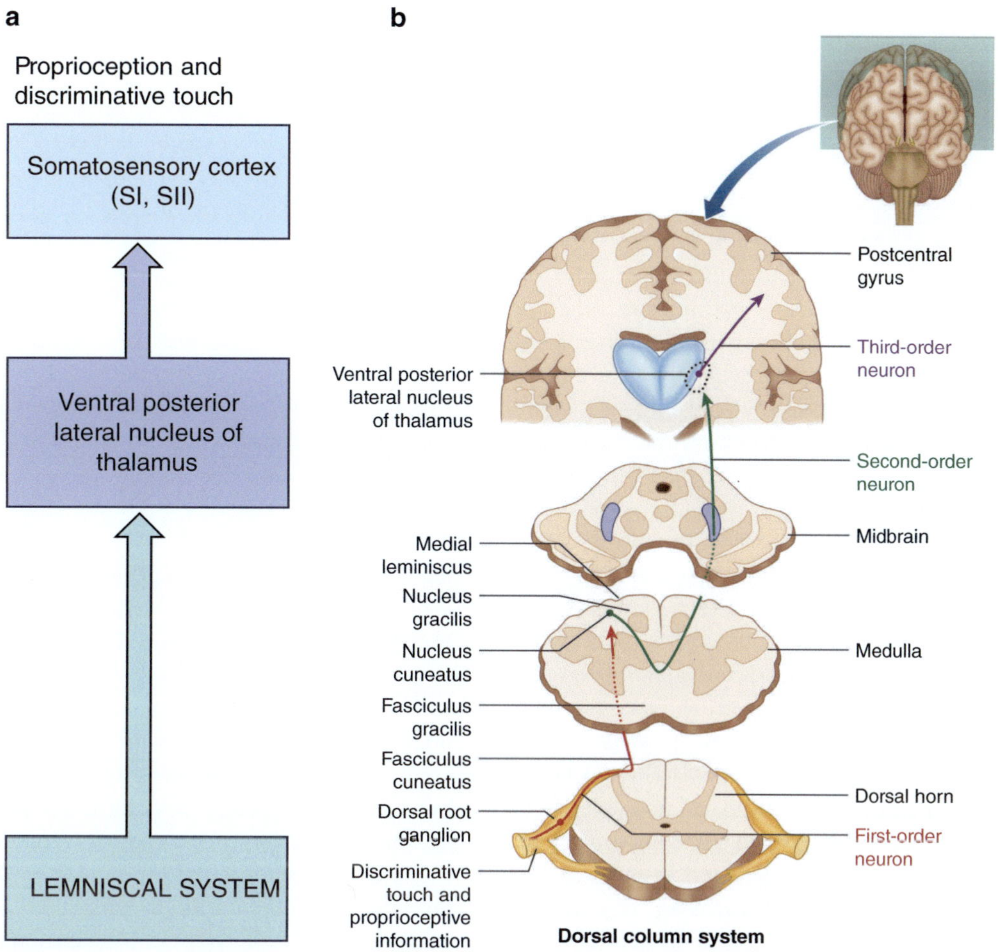

Fig. 2.3 Ascending pathways for proprioception and discriminative touch—the dorsal column or lemniscal system—are depicted (**a**) schematically and (**b**) in anatomical slices at different levels of the nervous system. The cell bodies for somatosensory afferents (including those involved in proprioception and discriminative touch) are located in the dorsal root ganglions (first-order neurons). The axons are bipolar, with one end coming from the sensory organs (muscle spindles or touch receptors in the skin) and the other end entering the spinal cord through the dorsal horn and ascending in the dorsal columns. At the rostral end of the spinal cord, the axons make synaptic contact with the second-order neurons located in the nucleus Cuneatus and nucleus Gracilis. The second-order neurons cross the midline in the medulla and ascend in the medial lemniscus to the ventral posterior lateral nucleus of the thalamus, where they make synaptic contact with the third-order neurons. These ascend to the postcentral gyrus of the cortex—the somatosensory cortex (SI and SII)—where they make synaptic contact with the fourth-order neurons

pain, and thermal information are transmitted to the somatosensory cortex by the spinothalamic system (see Box 2.3 and Chap. 3).

Box 2.3 The major somatosensory ascending pathways

The lemniscal system, responsible for transmitting proprioceptive and discriminative touch information, enters the spinal cord via the first-order neuron in the dorsal root ganglion (see Fig. 2.3). Information is then transmitted to the spinal cord via the dorsal root to the dorsal column and back to the caudal part of the medulla oblongata and passed on to the second-order neurons within the gracilis and cuneiform nuclei. Fibers from the dorsal column are organized somatotopically, with the gracilis nucleus coming from lower limbs and the cuneiform nucleus from upper limbs. Once past these nuclei, fibers cross the median line of the spinal cord. They then form the medial lemniscus and project to ventroposterolateral (VPL) neurons of the thalamus, which are third-order neurons, and finally project to the primary and secondary somesthetic cortices.

The anterolateral (spinothalamic) system transmits affective touch, pain, and thermal information. This pathway is described in detail in Chap. 3 (Fig. 3.1). Both fibers from the lemniscal and anterolateral pathways project to the primary somatosensory cortex located in the postcentral gyrus of the parietal lobe. Neurons processing cutaneous stimuli form a somatotopic layout (Al-Chalabi et al., 2023), known as Penfield's homunculus in humans, representing the cutaneous body parts. These topographically organized, i.e., somatotopic maps, are characterized by an anisomorphic representation of cutaneous regions: those of functional importance to species (hands, face, and tongue in monkeys and humans; snout in rodents, etc.) occupy larger cortical territories. The largest cortical territories also represent skin territories with a high density of mechanoreceptors (see Fig. 2.4).

It seems, however, that reality is more complex. For instance, the famous discontinuity of genitals under feet has been challenged. Recently, it has even been proposed that the whole body is mapped onto much larger areas than just the primary somatosensory cortex, including parietal cortex but also insula (Saadon-Grosman et al., 2020). These results expand Penfield's initial data to a higher level of somatosensory processing probably contributing to human cognition.

VPL nuclei in the thalamus project to two cortical areas, the primary somesthetic cortex (S1) in the anterior parietal cortex and the secondary somesthetic cortex (S2) in the lateral sulcus. In primates, at least ten cortical areas processing somatosensory information have been found, each with their own properties. These areas can be subdivided into two: the posterior system includes areas 5 and 7, which manage somatosensory functions such as object recognition and knowledge of limb position and movement.

Somatosensory (mechanosensory and nociceptive) information from the face is conveyed from the periphery to the thalamus via the trigeminal somatic sensory system. The sensory fibers coming from the trigeminal ganglion enter the brainstem at the pons and relay on the trigeminal complex, mainly on the principal nucleus and the spinal nucleus, which process mechanosensory information and thermal/pain stimuli, respectively. Axons from the second neuron trigeminal brainstem nuclei decussate and reach the ventral posterior medial (VPM) nucleus of the thalamus via the trigeminothalamic tract. Then, third-order neurons of the thalamus send their axons mainly to primary somatosensory cortex.

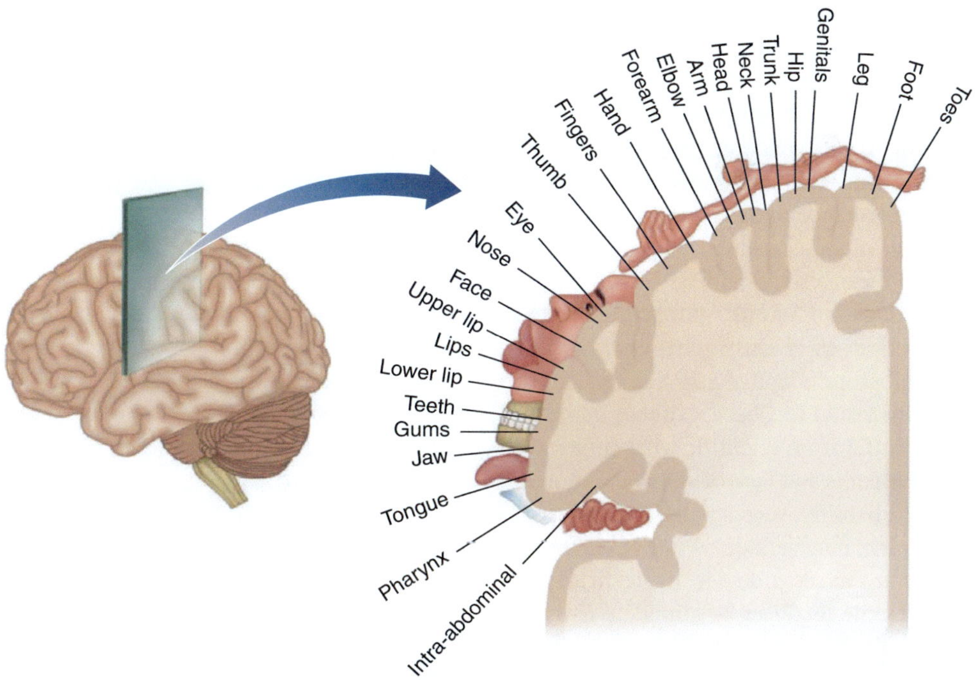

Fig 2.4 The representation of different parts of the body in the somatosensory cortex according to Penfield is shown for the left hemisphere in the sagittal plane (as illustrated from the whole brain 3-D view to the left)

Cutaneous and proprioceptive inputs are conveyed in a topographic order through the sensory fibers to the cortex, where they constitute somatotopically organized representational maps, i.e., they respect the topological arrangement of peripheral receptors. These maps constitute the so-called sensory homunculus, in which the relative cortical representation of each body part is different (see Fig. 2.4). For example, the areas processing tactile information from the hand are much larger than those processing information from the back skin. This is linked to the density of receptors in the different skin territories, but also to their functional role: the hand is strongly involved in tactile exploration and discrimination, which is not the case for the back skin.

Although the general organization of these cortical representations is topographically invariant from one subject to another, they have idiosyncratic organizational specificities. Indeed, numerous studies in animals (Recanzone et al., 1992; Rosselet et al., 2006) and humans (Pascual-Leone & Torres, 1993) support the idea that somatotopic S1 maps are substantially remodeled by new sensory experiences throughout life. This experience-dependent plasticity, which is closely dependent on the nature of behavioral activities, includes modifications of the map resolution, as receptive fields are sharpened or expanded. It may also involve changes in the spatial domain of neuronal receptive fields, which can also shift to nearby or distant peripheral skin territories, leading to changes of the overall cortical representation of stimulated body parts. The representational somatosensory maps also remodel after cortical damage or peripheral denervation.

2.5 Touch and Proprioception in Rehabilitation

Stroke is a significant cause of disability worldwide. Most stroke patients experience upper extremity motor impairments, resulting in reduced performance of activities in their natural environment, often associated with central post-stroke pain (see also Chap. 3). Over the last twenty years, numerous publications have claimed the virtues of early rehabilitation based on tactile or proprioceptive stimulation, or even coupled with visual feedback. Although many of the studies suffer from scientific weaknesses such as few participants and lack of statistical or methodological reliability, sensory therapy appears to be a low-risk intervention with positive outcomes. For instance, a device liable to provide visual and tactile feedback to stimulate daily life upper extremity activity in stroke patients is efficient at small but significantly increasing the activity of paretic muscles (Langerak et al., 2023). In animals, sensorimotor training promotes functional recovery and somatosensory cortical map reactivation following cervical spinal cord injury (Martinez et al., 2009). After focal ischemic damage to the somatosensory cortex, early and moderate sensory stimulation limits expansion of electrophysiological dysfunction and cortical tissue loss and exerts a protective effect on perilesion representations (Xerri & Zennou-Azogui, 2014).

Training based on muscle tendon vibration, liable to induce kinesthetic illusions, has also been found to improve proprioceptive integration in patients with Parkinson's disease (Ribot-Ciscar et al., 2017). Similarly, proprioceptive training significantly increases the amplitude of voluntary shoulder flexion in patients suffering from facioscapulohumeral muscular dystrophy (Ribot-Ciscar et al., 2015). In these and other studies, the sensory, perceptual, and motor components induced by muscle tendon vibration may contribute to reducing the deleterious effects of gradual motor impairments. When movement is reduced, the central representation of the limbs is impaired, which in turn affects the ability to command the muscles. Clearly, kinesthetic illusions may interrupt this vicious circle, as also shown in individuals suffering from cerebral palsy (Smorenburg et al., 2011). Last but not least, the pleasurable aspects that characterize treatments based on kinesthetic illusions compared with other treatments should be emphasized, as this aspect would enhance patient compliance with the rehabilitation program and enhance commitment.

Review Questions

- What type of information do proprioceptors provide?
- What could be the functional interests of specifically sparing affective touch with aging?

References

Ackerley, R., Aimonetti, J.-M., & Ribot-Ciscar, E. (2017). Emotions alter muscle proprioceptive coding of movements in humans. *Scientific Reports, 7*, 8465. https://doi.org/10.1038/s41598-017-08721-4

Al-Chalabi, M., Reddy, V., & Alsalman, I. (2023). Neuroanatomy, posterior column (dorsal column). In *StatPearls*. StatPearls Publishing.

Bataille-Savattier, A., Le Gall-Ianotto, C., Lebonvallet, N., et al. (2023). Do Merkel complexes initiate mechanical itch? *Experimental Dermatology, 32*, 226–234. https://doi.org/10.1111/exd.14685

Bouvier, V., Roudaut, Y., Osorio, N., et al. (2018). Merkel cells sense cooling with TRPM8 channels. *The Journal of Investigative Dermatology, 138*, 946–956. https://doi.org/10.1016/j.jid.2017.11.004

Ikeda, R., Cha, M., Ling, J., et al. (2014). Merkel cells transduce and encode tactile stimuli to drive aβ-afferent impulses. *Cell, 157*, 664–675. https://doi.org/10.1016/j.cell.2014.02.026

Johnson, K. O. (2001). The roles and functions of cutaneous mechanoreceptors. *Current Opinion in Neurobiology, 11*, 455–461.

Langerak, A. J., Regterschot, G. R. H., Evers, M., et al. (2023). A sensor-based feedback device stimulating daily life upper extremity activity in stroke patients: A feasibility study. *Sensors, 23*, 5868. https://doi.org/10.3390/s23135868

Lee, C., & Chen, C. (2023). Role of proprioceptors in chronic musculoskeletal pain. *Experimental Physiology*, EP090989. https://doi.org/10.1113/EP090989

Martinez, M., Brezun, J.-M., Zennou-Azogui, Y., et al. (2009). Sensorimotor training promotes functional recovery and somatosensory cortical map reactivation following cervical spinal cord injury: Recovery and cortical plasticity after spinal cord injury. *The European Journal of Neuroscience, 30*, 2356–2367. https://doi.org/10.1111/j.1460-9568.2009.07019.x

Pascual-Leone, A., & Torres, F. (1993). Plasticity of the sensorimotor cortex representation of the reading finger in Braille readers. *Brain, 116*, 39–52. https://doi.org/10.1093/brain/116.1.39

Recanzone, G. H., Merzenich, M. M., & Jenkins, W. M. (1992). Frequency discrimination training engaging a restricted skin surface results in an emergence of a cutaneous response zone in cortical area 3a. *Journal of Neurophysiology, 67*, 1057–1070. https://doi.org/10.1152/jn.1992.67.5.1057

Ribot-Ciscar, E., Milhe-De Bovis, V., Aimonetti, J.-M., et al. (2015). Functional impact of vibratory proprioceptive assistance in patients with facioscapulohumeral muscular dystrophy. *Muscle & Nerve, 52*, 780–787. https://doi.org/10.1002/mus.24605

Ribot-Ciscar, E., Aimonetti, J.-M., & Azulay, J.-P. (2017). Sensory training with vibration-induced kinesthetic illusions improves proprioceptive integration in patients with Parkinson's disease. *Journal of the Neurological Sciences, 383*, 161–165. https://doi.org/10.1016/j.jns.2017.11.016

Rosselet, C., Zennou-Azogui, Y., & Xerri, C. (2006). Nursing-induced somatosensory cortex plasticity: temporally decoupled changes in neuronal receptive field properties are accompanied by modifications in activity-dependent protein expression. *The Journal of Neuroscience, 26*, 10667–10676. https://doi.org/10.1523/JNEUROSCI.3253-06.2006

Saadon-Grosman, N., Loewenstein, Y., & Arzy, S. (2020). The 'creatures' of the human cortical somatosensory system. *Brain Communicaitons, 2*, fcaa003. https://doi.org/10.1093/braincomms/fcaa003

Sacks, O. (1985). *The man who mistook his wife for a hat and other clinical tales*. Summit Books.

Schirmer, A., Croy, I., & Ackerley, R. (2023). What are C-tactile afferents and how do they relate to "affective touch"? *Neuroscience and Biobehavioral Reviews, 151*, 105236. https://doi.org/10.1016/j.neubiorev.2023.105236

Skedung, L., Arvidsson, M., Chung, J. Y., et al. (2013). Feeling small: Exploring the tactile perception limits. *Scientific Reports, 3*, 2617. https://doi.org/10.1038/srep02617

Smorenburg, A. R. P., Ledebt, A., Feltham, M. G., et al. (2011). The positive effect of mirror visual feedback on arm control in children with spastic hemiparetic cerebral palsy is dependent on which arm is viewed. *Experimental Brain Research, 213*, 393–402. https://doi.org/10.1007/s00221-011-2789-6

Xerri, C., & Zennou-Azogui, Y. (2014). Early and moderate sensory stimulation exerts a protective effect on perilesion representations of somatosensory cortex after focal ischemic damage. *PLoS One, 9*, e99767. https://doi.org/10.1371/journal.pone.0099767

Pain

3

Hugo Massé-Alarie, Jason Bouffard, and Laurent J. Bouyer

Abstract

Pain is an output of the brain and a complex subjective experience. In this chapter, we describe the neuroanatomy and neural mechanisms underlying nociception and pain perception, from the transduction mechanisms in nociceptors through the description of the neural pathways conveying nociceptive information to the brain and its modulation at various neural levels to post-injury sensitization mechanisms. The chapter emphasizes the significance of understanding the neurophysiology and the different types of pain to tailor interventions for individuals dealing with pain. The importance of a comprehensive approach to pain evaluation, going beyond intensity, is underscored with six core outcome domains. These domains, including emotional functioning and global improvement perception, are important in evaluating clinical outcomes for patients with chronic pain. The chapter also guides the reader through the management of chronic pain, describing non-pharmacological and non-invasive interventions. Finally, two adjunct therapies, transcutaneous electrical nerve stimulation and non-invasive brain stimulation, are presented as means to target neural plasticity for enhanced pain management. With strong neurophysiological mechanistic examples and references, this chapter provides students of neuroscience and neurorehabilitation with a comprehensive understanding of pain, guiding them toward nuanced strategies in assessing and rehabilitating individuals living with pain.

Keywords

Nociception · Nociceptive pain · Nociplastic pain · Neuropathic pain · Pain neurophysiology · Sensitization · Pain assessment · Pain management

> **Box 3.1 Case Story**
> Mr. Tremblay had a farming accident 2 years ago. His hand got stuck in his lawn mower while performing repairs and got seriously injured. At the time of the injury,

(continued)

H. Massé-Alarie · L. J. Bouyer (✉)
Center for Interdisciplinary Research in Rehabilitation and Social Integration (CIRRIS), NeuroQuebec Research Center, and School of Rehabilitation Sciences, Faculty of Medicine, Université Laval, Quebec City, QC, Canada
e-mail: hugo.masse-alarie@fmed.ulaval.ca; laurent.bouyer@rea.ulaval.ca

J. Bouffard
Center for Interdisciplinary Research in Rehabilitation and Social Integration (CIRRIS), NeuroQuebec Research Center, and School of Rehabilitation Sciences, Faculty of Medicine, Université Laval, Quebec City, QC, Canada

Department of Kinesiology, Faculty of Medicine, Université Laval, Quebec City, QC, Canada
e-mail: jason.bouffard@kin.ulaval.ca

J. B. Nielsen et al. (eds.), *Neuroplasticity-based Neurorehabilitation*,
https://doi.org/10.1007/978-3-031-81120-3_3

Box 3.1 (continued)
Mr. Tremblay experienced immediate severe pain that provided him information that he needed to remove his hand from the lawn mower (nociceptive pain). Despite his rapid reflex withdrawal, his arm was severely injured. However, his pain modulation mechanisms allowed him to get back home and seek help.

Once at the hospital, the medical team could not save his hand and had to amputate the hand at the wrist. When he woke up, Mr. Tremblay immediately experienced stump pain that was manageable with medication. He also experienced the feeling that his hand was still present but that he could not move it (i.e., phantom sensations). He also experienced a crushing type of pain in his phantom hand that was not controlled by the medication.

In the following weeks, his stump healed, and stump pain mostly disappeared. The phantom limb pain, however, was still present, intense, and unpredictable. At the beginning of his rehabilitation, Mr. Tremblay did not talk about his phantom limb pain to his therapists because he was afraid that he would not be believed or taken seriously. How can someone experience pain in a limb that does not exist? When therapists asked him to rate his pain intensity, he focused on stump pain, which was now absent. Therapists therefore focused on other aspects of rehabilitation and did not offer pain management interventions, as they believed this was not an issue. He was able to learn to use his prosthesis, went back home, and was able to get back to work on his farm. Still, his remaining phantom limb pain caused him significant distress, which was amplified by his fear of being considered crazy if he talked about it. It also greatly interfered with his sleep, his activities of daily living, and his social interactions.

During a follow-up assessment with his psychologist several months after the accident, he "accidently" mentioned the distress caused by his phantom pain. When he told his psychologist about his fear of not being believed, the therapist immediately responded that phantom limb pain was very common after an amputation and explained the causes of the sensation and pain in the phantom limb. She also referred him to an occupational therapist to explore potential solutions to help with this pain. Mr. Tremblay immediately felt a huge relief. He still experienced pain, but the fact that he felt believed significantly reduced his distress.

Mr. Tremblay subsequently told his occupational therapist about his pain experience and the impact it had on his life. She explained that residual representation of the amputated hand in his brain was the reason that he could still feel it. She also explained that a potential cause of phantom limb pain was a maladaptive reorganization within the brain and that a way to reverse such reorganization is to "use the phantom hand." However, since his amputation, Mr. Tremblay was not able to move his phantom hand, and any attempt to move it increased the pain. His therapist taught him a method called mirror therapy, during which he moved both his intact and phantom hands while looking at the intact hand's reflection within a mirror. Following 4 weeks of this intervention, his phantom limb pain decreased significantly. Encouraged by his therapist, he continued to voluntarily move his phantom hand during his daily life.

3.1 Definition and Prevalence of Pain

Pain is defined as "an unpleasant sensory and emotional experience associated with, or resembling that associated with, actual or potential tissue damage" (IASP, 2021). It is a subjective construct influenced by a person's life experiences, genetics, and social environment. It is not only a sensory but also an emotional experience. Due to its aversiveness, pain is unpleasant, can be debilitating, and produces a state of suffering. Pain is often comorbid with emotional and cognitive factors such as fear, avoidance, anxiety, and catastrophizing, both in its acute and chronic states.

Pain results from the modulation, processing, and integration of nociception within the central nervous system (CNS). Nociception is defined as "*the neural process of encoding a stimulus that is damaging or threatens damage to normal tissues*" (IASP, 2021). It is important to note that, although often concomitantly present, nociception is not sufficient nor necessary to produce pain. In fact, nociception can occur in the absence of pain and pain in the absence of nociception. For example, the activation of nociceptors can result in a motor withdrawal response with an absence of painful sensation. It is therefore critical to emphasize that pain and nociception are distinct, yet related phenomena.

Pain is a teaching signal that motivates the avoidance of behaviors that may compromise tissue integrity. Some children are born without the ability to experience pain due to a genetic disorder. They have a shorter life expectancy than typically developing children, supporting the idea that pain may act as a primary punishment signal to negatively reinforce the avoidance of behaviors that may threaten survival. However, this adaptive role of pain is lost when pain becomes chronic.

While acute pain is a normal phenomenon that every person will experience during their lifetime, chronic pain is a pathological response that results from maladaptive plasticity in the neural circuitry normally responsible for pain. Internationally, chronic pain is the leading cause of disability, and its prevalence in the adult population ranges from 13% to 50% (Fayaz et al., 2016). In neurological populations, pain is a highly prevalent symptom in various health conditions such as stroke (11–50%), spinal cord injury (68%), and limb amputation (59%). It is therefore extremely important to address pain management during neurorehabilitation.

Understanding the mechanisms underlying pain modulation and chronic pain development allows clinicians and researchers to develop targeted interventions for neurological populations, thereby optimizing rehabilitation outcomes and overall quality of life.

3.2 From Potential Tissue Damage to the Perception of Pain

Pain is an "output" of the CNS. This "output" is shaped by the processing, modulation, and integration of multiple sources of information originating from several regions of the brain, spinal cord, and specialized peripheral sensory receptors.

Nociceptors are at the core of pain perception. They are specialized sensory receptors distinct from regular mechanoreceptors and thermoceptors, as they only respond to noxious stimuli, i.e., stimuli leading to potential or actual tissue damage. Nociceptors comprise various subtypes detecting different categories of noxious stimuli: **thermal nociceptors** respond to extreme temperatures; **mechanical nociceptors** are activated by intense physical pressure or deformation; and **chemical nociceptors** are sensitive to specific substances released during tissue injury or inflammation. **Polymodal nociceptors** respond to a combination of thermal, mechanical, and chemical factors. Nociceptors are distributed throughout the body's tissues, including the skin, muscles, and visceral organs.

Upon activation by noxious stimuli, nociceptors generate action potentials in Aδ and C afferent nerve fibers (ref to Table 2.1). These primary afferent fibers convey the nociceptive signals to the dorsal horn of the spinal cord. Within the dorsal horn gray matter, primary afferents synapse with second-order neurons. This is the first level of nociceptive signal processing and integration.

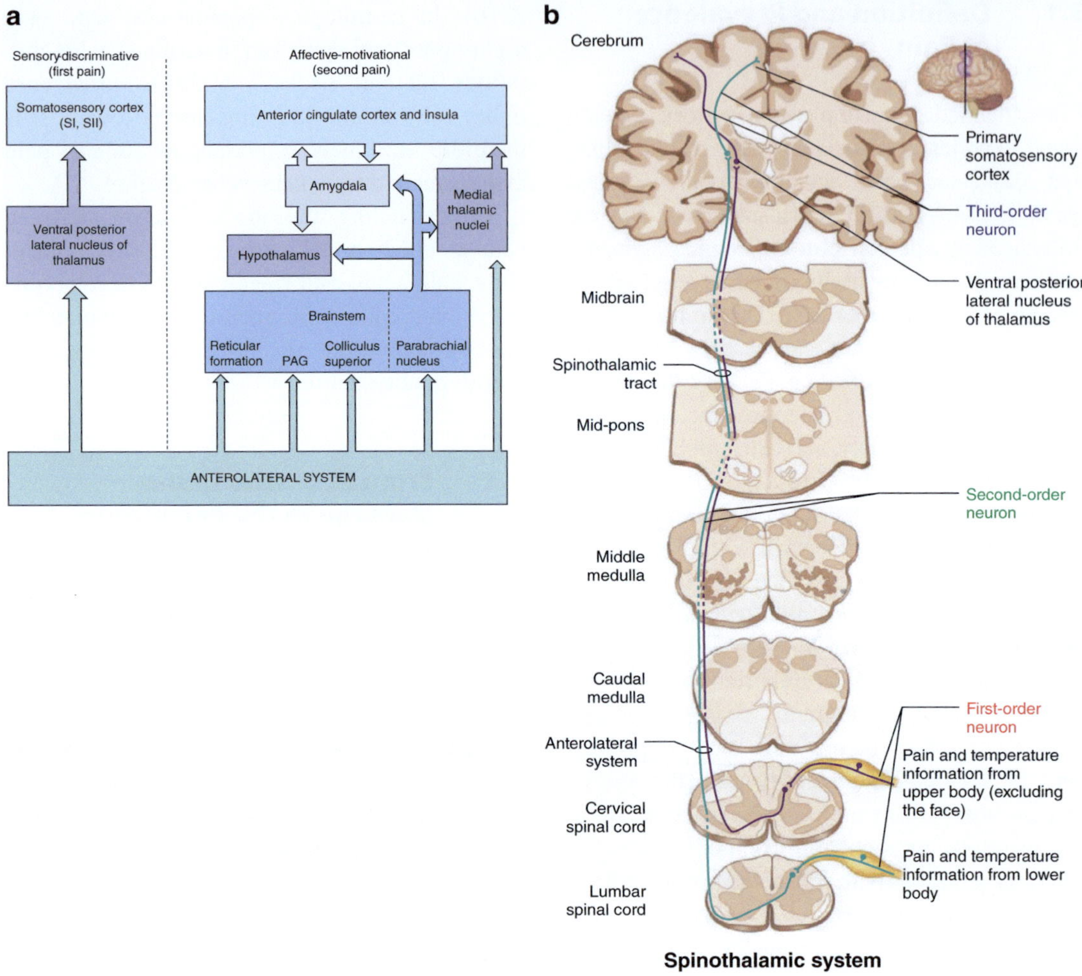

Fig. 3.1 Ascending pathways for pain and temperature sensation—the spinothalamic or anterolateral system—are illustrated (**a**) schematically and (**b**) in anatomical slices at different levels of the nervous system. Similar to other somatosensory senses, the cell bodies are located in the dorsal root ganglions (first-order neurons). The axons are bipolar, with one end coming from the sensory organs (free nerve endings) and the other end entering the spinal cord through the dorsal horn, where they make synaptic contact with the second-order neurons. The axons of the second-order neurons cross the midline and ascend in the anterior-lateral part of the spinal cord (therefore, the anterolateral system) until they reach the ventral posterior lateral nucleus of the thalamus, where they make synaptic contact with the third-order neurons. These ascend to the postcentral gyrus of the cortex—the somatosensory cortex (SI and SII)—where they make synaptic contact with the fourth-order neurons. In addition to this, there are projections to the superior colliculus, the periaqueductal gray, the reticular formation, the parabrachial nucleus, and the medial thalamic nuclei as part of affective-motivational pain processing (depicted in **a**). Either directly or indirectly through the hypothalamus and the amygdala, pain information reaches the cingulate and insula cerebral cortex

From the dorsal horn grey matter, second-order sensory neurons cross the midline to ascend in the anterolateral white matter of the spinal cord via the spinothalamic tract to the ventral posterior lateral nucleus of the thalamus. The thalamus serves as a crucial relay station, distributing nociceptive information to various brain regions, including the somatosensory cortex (S1) for processing sensory aspects of pain (location and discrimination) and the limbic system for emotional and affective dimensions (Fig. 3.1). Details of brain areas involved in pain perception are described in Box 3.2.

On their way to the cortex, nociceptive information can be modulated at each synapse, from the first synapse in the dorsal horn of the spinal cord, all the way up to the brain. Therefore, pain perception can be quite different (smaller or larger) from the actual peripheral noxious stimuli. Descending pathways consisting of a complex network of neural connections involving several brain regions play a pivotal role in this modulation of nociceptive inputs and in the regulation of pain perception. Their function is discussed in more detail below.

3.3 Mechanisms of Pain Modulation

Pain modulation involves an intricate interplay of spinal and descending mechanisms within the CNS (Fig. 3.2). The presence of these distributed

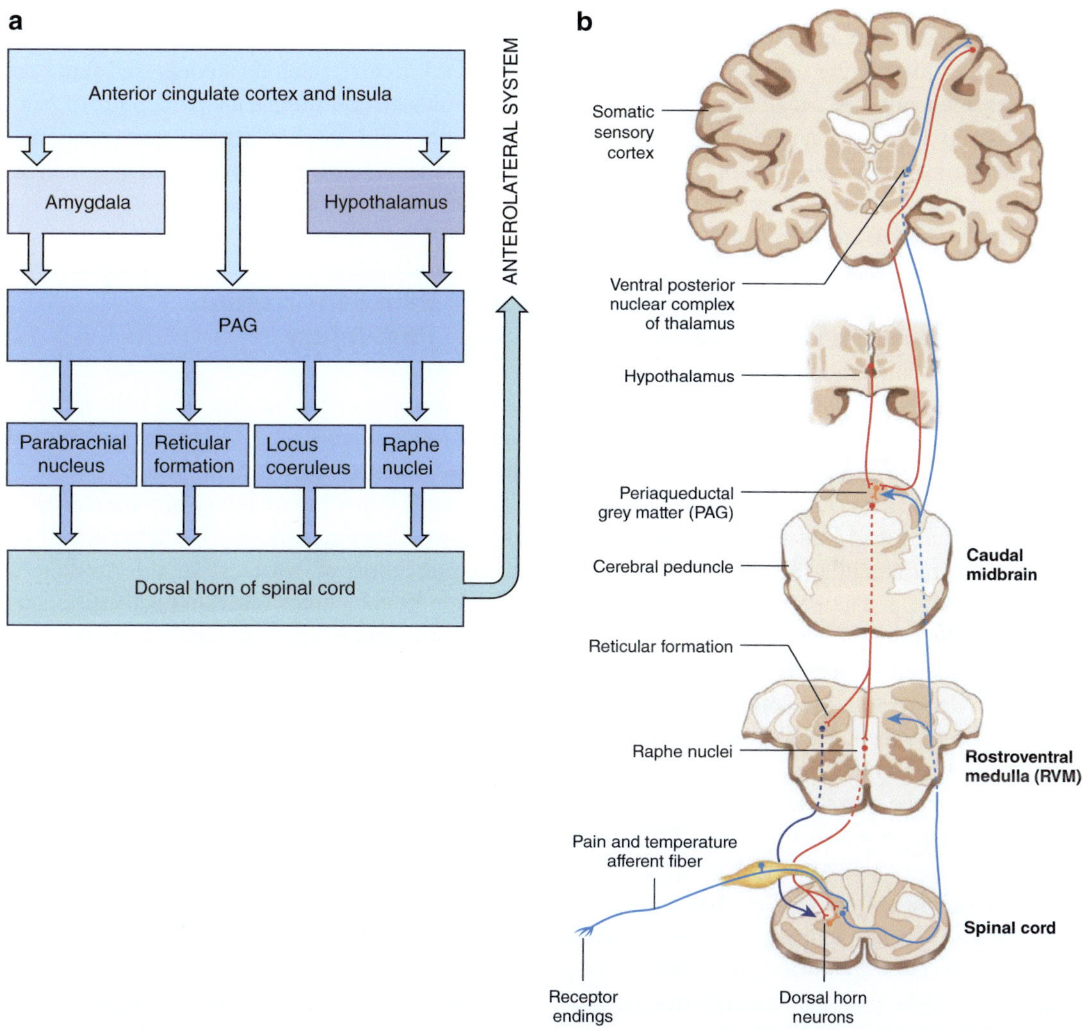

Fig. 3.2 Pathways and neural structures involved in descending modulation of pain are depicted (**a**) schematically and (**b**) in anatomical slices at different levels of the nervous system. The connection between the primary and secondary neurons in the dorsal horn is an important site for descending modulation of pain. Nuclei in the medulla (the parabrachial nucleus, the reticular formation, the locus coeruleus, and the raphe nuclei) control local interneurons that release endorphins and enkephalins, which efficiently modulate transmission from the first to the second order neurons. The medullary nuclei are in turn controlled by the midbrain periaqueductal gray matter, which is controlled by the hypothalamus, amygdala, and cingulate and insula cerebral cortex

mechanisms highlights the dynamic nature of pain modulation within the CNS. It also emphasizes the brain's capacity to exert control over the processing and perception of pain.

At the spinal level, the **gate control theory** proposed by Melzack and Wall in 1965 suggests that non-noxious inputs, such as touch or pressure mechanoreceptors and associated large fibers (e.g., Aβ), can inhibit the transmission of nociceptive signals in the dorsal horn of the spinal cord. This inhibition occurs through the activation of inhibitory interneurons, effectively "closing the gate" to pain transmission. This theory underlies in part the efficacy of techniques like transcutaneous electrical nerve stimulation (TENS) used in pain management. In parallel with this spinal inhibitory control, excitatory neurotransmitters such as glutamate can enhance the activity of spinal nociceptive circuits, amplifying the perception of pain.

Located *in the midbrain*, a key structure in descending pain modulation is the periaqueductal grey (PAG), an integration center for pain processing and regulation. It receives input from various brain regions, including the cortex, amygdala, and hypothalamus, in response to emotional and cognitive factors, stress, and endogenous opioids. The PAG, in turn, sends descending projections to the rostroventral medulla (RVM), a region in the medulla oblongata. The RVM contains a heterogeneous population of neurons that can either facilitate or inhibit nociceptive pain transmission, called the ON–OFF cells, which are modulated through opioid receptors. This dualistic role is crucial for fine modulation of the nociceptive inputs entering the dorsal horn of the spinal cord. The descending projections from the PAG to the RVM, and from the RVM to the spinal cord, release serotonin and norepinephrine onto spinal interneurons. These neurotransmitters activate receptors on nociception-transmitting neurons, reducing or augmenting their excitability and thus modulating nociceptive signal transmission. In addition, the brain also releases endogenous opioids (endorphins and enkephalins), which act as powerful analgesics. These opioids bind to specific receptors in the spinal cord and in multiple brain areas, inhibiting nociceptive transmission and reducing pain perception. Together these mechanisms are referred to as descending inhibition for the inhibitory circuits and descending excitation for the facilitating ones. The duality between descending and spinal inhibition and excitation allows for fine-tuning pain responses depending on the context.

In addition to these mechanisms, higher brain regions, including the prefrontal cortex and limbic system, play a significant role in modulating pain perception by projecting to the brainstem areas involved in pain modulation. *Cognitive factors*, like distraction and attention, as well as *emotional factors*, such as anxiety and fear, can either enhance or diminish the perception of pain. Identifying and intervening on emotional and cognitive factors are now considered as a mandatory part of pain management.

3.4 Pain Sensitization Post-Injury

Pain sensitization post-injury is a neurophysiological process where the peripheral and central nervous systems become hypersensitive to noxious stimuli following an injury or a pathological condition. This phenomenon is characterized by an amplification of nociceptive information, a reduction in nociceptor threshold activation, and the development of allodynia (pain in response to normally non-noxious stimuli). It occurs primarily in response to tissue damage, inflammation, or nerve injury, and it can persist long after the initial injury has healed.

3.4.1 Peripheral Sensitization

Peripheral sensitization involves heightened sensitivity of nociceptors at the injury site, often due to inflammatory processes and the release of substances like prostaglandins and substance P. These changes significantly contribute to the amplification of nociceptive signals and maintenance of pain. Key neuroplastic changes associated with peripheral sensitization include: (1) Nociceptor Sensitization: nociceptors become more sensitive to noxious stimuli due to increased responsiveness to inflammatory mediators and sensitizing substances and reduction in activation threshold. (2) Enhanced Neurotransmitter Release: Sensitized nociceptors release neurotransmitters like substance P and glutamate more readily, intensifying the signaling of nociceptive messages to spinal cord neurons. (3) Inflammatory Response: Peripheral sensitization is closely tied to the ongoing inflammatory response at the injury site. Inflammatory mediators sensitize nociceptors and contribute to tissue swelling and increased blood flow, which further enhance the pain experience. (4) Long-Lasting Effects: Peripheral sensitization can persist as long as the inflammatory process continues, even after the initial injury has healed. Some patients suffering from chronic pain can present with peripheral sensitization. These neuroplastic changes may explain why injuries and inflammatory conditions can lead to heightened pain sensitivity and prolonged pain experiences in some patients.

Allodynia is characterized by perception of pain in response to typically non-painful stimuli. This condition arises when mild sensory inputs like light touch or gentle pressure are interpreted as painful sensations. Allodynia reflects a maladaptive response in the nervous system and is often associated with various pain conditions, particularly neuropathic pain (see Sect. 3.5).

3.4.2 Central Sensitization

Central sensitization involves neuroplastic changes in the CNS in response to body injuries or persistent pain. These neuroplastic changes amplify nociception and may result in augmented and maintained pain experience. Key neuroplastic changes associated with central sensitization include: (1) Increased Synaptic Efficacy: Synaptic transmission between neurons in the spinal cord becomes more efficient, intensifying the transmission of nociceptive signals. (2) NMDA Receptor Sensitization: N-Methyl-D-Aspartate (NMDA) receptors, typically after strong stimulation, become more sensitive. Weaker stimuli can then activate them, amplifying nociceptive signals. (3) Wind-Up Phenomenon: Repeated or prolonged noxious stimuli lead to progressive increases in spinal cord neuron responsiveness, resulting in heightened pain sensitivity. (4) Long-Term Potentiation (LTP): Similar to mechanisms in learning and memory (see Chap. 6), central sensitization involves persistent strengthening of synapses transmitting nociceptive signals, maintaining heightened pain sensitivity. (5) Brain Function Alterations: Central sensitization can affect brain regions involved in pain processing, increasing pain perception and emotional responses. These neuroplastic changes create a state of CNS hyperexcitability, causing individuals to perceive non-noxious stimuli as painful and experience chronic, intensified pain. It is critical to highlight that central sensitization is involved in most types of pain (acute and chronic, nociceptive, neuropathic, and nociplastic). For further reading on the topic of pain neurophysiology see Marchand (2009).

Box 3.2 The Pain Matrix

The pain matrix is a term used to describe the distributed neural network that encompasses various brain regions involved in the perception, evaluation, and modulation of pain. Functional components of the pain matrix comprise multiple brain regions, each contributing to different facets of the pain experience:

Somatosensory Cortex: At the core of the pain matrix lies the somatosensory cortex. This region is responsible for decoding the sensory aspects of pain, such as its location, intensity, and quality. It provides a spatial map of the body, allowing us to pinpoint the source of pain accurately (see Fig. 2.4).

Thalamus: The thalamus serves as a central relay station within the pain matrix. It receives incoming pain signals from the

(continued)

Box 3.2 (continued)

spinal cord and other sensory pathways and further distributes this information to various cortical and subcortical regions for processing and integration.

Limbic System: Pain is not merely a sensory experience; it also carries emotional and affective dimensions and influences memories. The limbic system, including the hippocampus, amygdala, and anterior cingulate cortex, contributes to emotional responses, pain-related memories, and the evaluation of pain's unpleasantness (see Chap. 11).

Prefrontal Cortex: The prefrontal cortex plays a critical role in pain modulation and coping. It helps regulate emotional responses to pain and engages in cognitive processes that influence pain perception, such as attention and expectation (see Chap. 9).

Basal Ganglia and Cerebellum: These subcortical structures contribute to the motor and autonomic responses to pain. They are involved in reflexive movements and physiological changes that accompany painful stimuli (see Chap. 5).

Neurorehabilitation Implications

- When neurological injuries or conditions disrupt any component of the pain matrix, it can lead to pain. Neurorehabilitation strategies must consider the integrity of the pain system when addressing pain in patients with neurological deficits. Multidisciplinary approaches that encompass physical therapy, cognitive-behavioral interventions, pharmacotherapy, and neuromodulation techniques aim to restore or optimize the function of the pain matrix components.

Box 3.3 The Placebo Effect

The placebo effect is an important phenomenon in the domain of pain modulation. It is characterized by the amelioration of symptoms in response to a treatment devoid of intrinsic therapeutic efficacy, solely attributable to the subject's belief in its effectiveness and the context of care. More specifically, it is a situation where when a non-active substance is given to a patient, the latter feels a reduction in his pain intensity if he expects to have received a real medication. A placebo effect can be observed in over 50% of the population. For many years, patients responding to a placebo medication were believed not to be in real pain and sometimes considered to lie about their condition. However, studies have later shown that the placebo effect can be reversed when Naloxone, an antagonist to opioid receptors, is given to patients. Therefore, the placebo effect is a real physiological mechanism whereby patients unconsciously activate the release of endogenous opioids to modulate their pain response. The placebo effect underscores the profound impact of psychological variables on nociceptive processing and highlights the intricate interdependence between cognitive-affective factors and neural substrates governing pain perception. This nuanced understanding holds profound implications for advancing comprehensive pain management paradigms, necessitating an integrative approach that encompasses both pharmacological and psychosocial dimensions in the design of enhanced therapeutic strategies.

3.5 The Multiple Types of Pain

There are distinct pain mechanisms that may be involved in pain generation and perception. They can be described by 3 types of pain: nociceptive, neuropathic, and nociplastic pain (IASP, 2021). Identifying the predominant pain mechanism can optimize treatment effectiveness by utilizing personalized interventions for pain management. Table 3.2 summarizes the characteristics of these different types of pain.

3.5.1 Nociceptive Pain

Nociceptive pain is defined as *"Pain that arises from actual or threatened damage to non-neural tissue and is due to the activation of nociceptors"* (IASP, 2021). In other words, this means that nociceptive pain occurs following the activation of peripheral nociceptors in a normally functioning CNS. For example, nociceptors—located in peripheral tissues—can be activated secondary to external stimuli (e.g., mechanical, chemical, thermal) onto body tissues coming from the environment or by self-generated stress on body structures (e.g., in response to external perturbation or secondary to muscle contraction). Nociceptive pain can be elicited by both (i) threatening and non-damaging stimuli (Fig. 3.3a) or (ii) damaging stimuli. The former usually consists of the activation of nociceptors giving rise to a transient experience of pain without tissue damage; in this case, nociception and pain were successful in protecting tissue integrity. A stimulus provoking tissue damage activates the nociceptors and elicits nociceptive pain. In this case, the injury will produce peripheral and central sensitization in response to the resulting inflammation. A stimulus that was usually innocuous before tissue injury may now elicit pain. This adaptive response will likely limit the force transmitted to the lesioned tissue, thereby fostering healing and recovery by avoidance of potentially damaging movements/behaviors. Thus, nociceptive pain may be experienced in non-lesioned and lesioned tissues and is secondary to the activation of nociceptors.

The CNS is normally functioning in the presence of nociceptive pain, conversely to neuropathic and nociplastic pain (see below). Nociceptive pain plays the primary role of pain, which is to protect body integrity by conditioning motor behaviors.

3.5.2 Neuropathic Pain

Neuropathic is defined as *"Pain caused by a lesion or disease of the somatosensory nervous system"* (IASP, 2021). Neuropathic pain is often divided into two subclasses based on the site of the lesion or disease: peripheral and central. Peripheral neuropathic pain is caused by a lesion/disease of the peripheral somatosensory nervous system (e.g., diabetic neuropathy), whereas central neuropathic pain refers to a lesion/disease of the central somatosensory system (e.g., thalamic stroke, spinal cord injury). Neuropathic pain is often described in terms such as burning (or fire-like), electric shock-like, shooting, and stabbing. Also, it may be accompanied by other symptoms based on the site of the lesion/disease and the role of the injured nerve/root, such as sensory (e.g., hypoesthesia, allodynia) and motor deficits, paresthesia (pins and needles), and altered or absent reflexes. Sensory symptoms (e.g., pain, hypoesthesia) are usually related to the territory or dermatomes innervated by the lesioned nerves or dorsal roots.

A lesion of neural tissues causes a cascade of changes in the nervous system, eliciting peripheral and central amplification of nociceptive inputs (Fig. 3.3b). For example, ectopic action potential generation, peripheral and central sensitization, disinhibition, and facilitation of the nociceptive inputs in the CNS (dorsal horn and brain) are some of the mechanisms that are involved in the apparition and maintenance of neuropathic pain (Costigan et al., 2009). Damage or dysfunction of the nervous system can lead to the rewiring of sensory pathways, causing the brain to misinterpret innocuous stimuli as painful, which can lead to allodynia, for example. Brain plasticity in the presence of neuropathic pain has also been observed in humans. Patients with neuropathic pain secondary to lumbar radiculopathy showed larger activation of glial cells in the sensorimotor cortex and thalamus, suggesting a link with neuroinflammation.

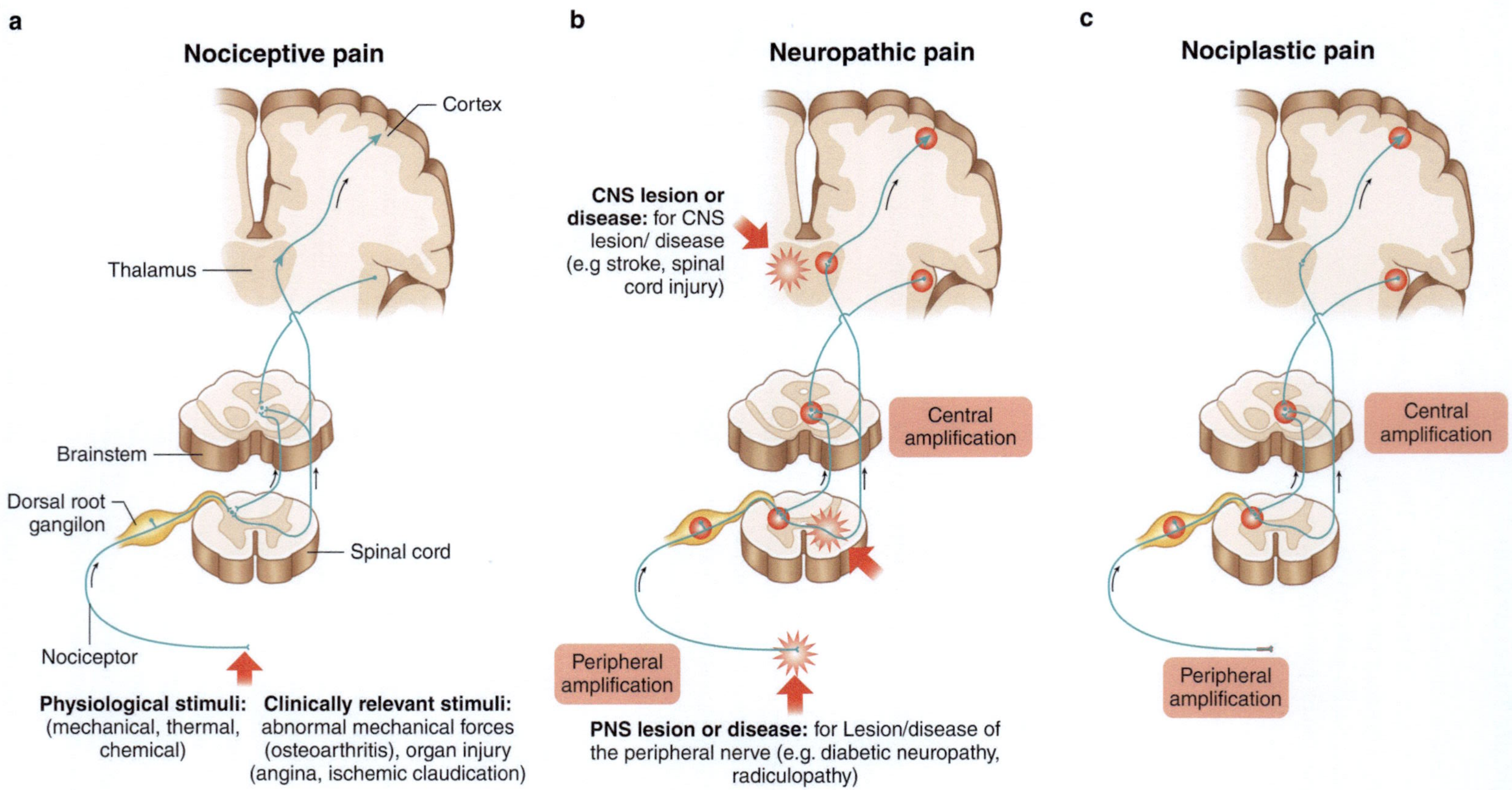

Fig. 3.3 Schemas depicting the different types of pain based on their underlying neural mechanisms: (**a**) Nociceptive pain secondary to physiological activation of nociceptors; (**b**) Neuropathic pain; and (**c**) Nociplastic pain. The red circles (neuropathic and nociplastic pain) indicate areas of the nervous system that can be modified in each type of pain. The "sun" indicates a lesion of a body structure. Note that although peripheral and central amplification occur in neuropathic and nociplastic pain, mechanisms leading to this amplification differs: neuropathic pain is secondary to a lesion or disease of the nervous system, whereas it is not the case for nociplastic pain

3.5.3 Nociplastic Pain

In 2016, the term nociplastic pain was introduced as a new pain type. This became essential as the profile of many patients with pain did not correspond to the proposed nociceptive or neuropathic pain definitions. Patients with nociplastic pain are classified by exclusion as demonstrated by its definition: *"pain arises from altered nociception despite no clear evidence of actual or threatened tissue damage causing the activation of peripheral nociceptors or evidence for disease or lesion of the somatosensory system causing the pain."* (IASP, 2021) Nociplastic is a portmanteau word created from the terms nociception and plasticity in the objective of highlighting the presence of maladaptive plasticity in the nociceptive/pain system. Patients with nociplastic pain present with an alteration in the CNS that amplifies nociception and contributes to the maintenance of pain over time (Fig. 3.3c). Nociplastic pain is predominant in specific pain conditions such as fibromyalgia, central regional painful syndrome, and whiplash (Table 3.2). Brain reorganization and malfunction have been experimentally documented in the latter conditions. For example, a lower brain volume in specific brain areas contributing to pain perception, such as the anterior cingulate cortex and the prefrontal cortex, and a lower functional connectivity in the descending modulation system were identified in participants with fibromyalgia compared to controls. These changes in brain morphometry and functional connectivity in participants with fibromyalgia can explain the presence of alterations in conditioned pain modulation (CPM) and exercise-induced hypoalgesia (EIH) that are proxies of the efficacy of the pain modulation system (see below for discussion on CPM and EIH). Although studies rarely recruit only chronic nociplastic pain patients, some brain imaging studies observed a larger contribution of brain areas involved in emotional and cognitive processing (e.g., mesolimbic systems and prefrontal cortex) in patients who developed chronic low back pain compared to patients who recovered from an acute episode. It is likely that cognitive and psychological factors such as pain catastrophizing, fear of pain/movement, anxiety, and depression are more related to nociplastic pain.

3.5.4 Mixed Pain

It is important to note that clinically, pain types are not mutually exclusive and can co-exist in a given patient (Shraim et al., 2021). If such is the case, the patient is said to have mixed pain. When possible, however, the identification of a predominant pain type (nociceptive, neuropathic, nociplastic) helps to tailor the pain rehabilitation intervention.

3.6 Assessing Pain for/during Neurorehabilitation

Evaluating pain is a complex task that should extend beyond the sole assessment of pain intensity. Best practice recommends considering six core outcome domains when evaluating clinical outcomes for individuals coping with chronic pain: pain intensity/quality, physical functioning, emotional functioning, global perception of improvement and satisfaction with the intervention, symptoms and adverse events, and compliance (Patel et al., 2021). Pain assessment is inherently multidimensional, encompassing evaluation of its intensity, sensory attributes, and affective qualities. The assessment of factors that can modulate pain is also frequently recommended. Due to the subjective nature of pain, it is predominantly evaluated through patient-reported outcome measures (PROMs). Some questionnaires are generic, suitable for assessing any pain, while others aim to isolate specific dimensions (e.g., shoulder pain induced by functional activities in wheelchair users). In some situations, such as in individuals with cognitive disorders, an external observer (e.g., a caregiver) can detect pain signs (e.g., facial expressions). Acute and chronic pain can induce physiological changes, analyzable through various neural imaging and stimulation technologies.

3.6.1 Subjective Pain Measures (PROMs)

Pain intensity represents the most frequently assessed dimension of pain, with the utilization of simple tools such as the numerical rating scale, verbal rating scale, visual analog scale, or pictorial scales (e.g., pain faces) (Patel et al., 2021). In a conventional numerical rating scale, individuals are prompted to assign a number between 0 (indicating no pain) and 10 (representing the worst imaginable pain) to quantify the intensity of their pain within a specified time frame (e.g., current pain or average pain over the past week). It is crucial to note that, given the large number of factors that can influence pain, the intensity of pain exhibits considerable variation within an individual and even more so across different individuals. To illustrate the interindividual variability in pain intensity, a study assessed pain intensity in 321 young adults subjected to a constant 48°C heat stimulation, revealing a range of pain intensity scores from 4/10 to 10/10 (Fillingim, 2017). This variability observed in a controlled laboratory setting is magnified in clinical populations experiencing pain in their daily lives.

Pain quality, through the assessment of the affective and sensory dimensions of pain, aids in understanding its impact on the individual as well as the underlying mechanisms giving rise to the painful experience (Patel et al., 2021). A simple method to distinguish between the intensity and affective components of pain (e.g., unpleasantness) involves drawing an analogy with another sensory experience. For example, one might use music as a reference. The intensity of pain could be compared to the volume of music at a concert. For the affective dimension of pain, the comparison would be more with the individual's preference or aversion to the music. The McGill Pain Questionnaire, developed by Ronald Melzack in 1975 and its subsequently updated shorter forms, serves as a comprehensive scale aimed at offering a detailed assessment of the sensory and affective attributes of pain. Using these questionnaires, participants rate the intensity of various pain forms associated with specific descriptors, some of which are affectively charged (e.g., tiring-exhausting, fearful) or linked to neuropathic pain (e.g., electric shock, caused by light touch). Certain scales, such as DN-4 and pain DETECT, were specifically designed to identify neuropathic pain using a limited number of items.

3.6.2 Objective Pain Measures

Although PROMs are essential for the assessment of pain due to its subjective nature, objective measures of pain contribute to a better understanding of neural mechanisms underlying pain experiences and intervention effectiveness. Two broad categories of objective methodologies can be identified: quantitative sensory testing (QST) and neuroimaging/neurostimulation methodologies.

Quantitative sensory testing (QST) examines sensory function through the assessment of perceptual responses to different stimuli (Table 3.1) (Backonja et al., 2013). Although QST does not

Table 3.1 The battery of quantitative sensory testing measures

Measures	Parameters
Thermal sensory acuity and pain	Warm detection threshold Cold detection threshold Number of paradoxical heat sensations Thermal sensory limen Heat pain threshold Cold pain threshold
Mechanical acuity (von Frey filaments)	Mechanical detection threshold
Mechanical pain threshold (weighted pinprick)	Mechanical pain threshold
Mechanical stimulus/response-functions (Weighted pinprick + tactile stimuli)	Mechanical pain sensitivity Tactile allodynia
Repeated pinprick stimulation	Wind-up ratio (temporal summation of pain)
Vibration acuity	Vibration detection threshold
Pressure pain threshold (Pressure gauge device)	Pressure pain threshold
Conditioned pain modulation	Pain threshold ratio (% of change from the test prior to the painful stimulus)
Exercise-induced hypoalgesia	Pain threshold ratio (% of change from test prior to exercise)

represent a direct assessment of nervous system functioning, it can help to estimate the integrity of various pain perception and modulation mechanisms. For instance, while hyperalgesia experienced at the site of an injury can result from central and peripheral sensitization, increased pain sensitivity at a remote site (e.g., hand hyperalgesia for an individual with low back pain) is most likely related to central mechanisms. Moreover, paradigms such as Conditioned Pain Modulation (CPM) or Exercise-Induced Hypoalgesia (EIH) can be used to evaluate pain modulation in humans. For both paradigms, pain sensitivity is evaluated before and after an external stimulation (CPM = intense tonic pain; EIH = exercise). If pain modulation mechanisms are normally functioning, hypoalgesia is elicited by these stimuli.

Although QST measures are psychophysical methods involving the precise control of stimuli applied to an individual, they still depend on the subjective definition of sensory/pain threshold or rating. The direct measurement of CNS functioning through neuroimaging and neurostimulation assessments does not rely on such subjective responses.

As pain experience influences and is influenced by the activity of several structures within the CNS (the pain matrix), neurostimulation and neuroimaging assessments are available to probe the spatiotemporal functioning of these structures in relation to pain. They include electroencephalography (EEG), functional magnetic resonance imaging (fMRI), positron emission tomography (PET) imaging, and transcranial magnetic stimulation (TMS) (Morton et al., 2016). A detailed description of these methods is presented in Box 3.4. Each method has its own advantages and limitations.

Imaging and stimulation techniques have been used to identify a cerebral "pain signature." However, it has faced many challenges, including (1) the wide variety of CNS structures involved in pain processing; (2) the fact that these CNS structures are also involved in non-painful phenomena (e.g., negative emotion, salience); and (3) CNS responses change according to various contextual factors. However, their combination with well-designed nociceptive and contextual stimuli (e.g., manipulating emotional response) has contributed to the development of current knowledge about the role of different CNS regions in pain processing. Neuroimaging and neurostimulation assessments in various clinical populations have demonstrated how changes in the CNS in various contexts might contribute to the development of chronic pain.

Box 3.4 Neurostimulation and Neuroimaging Techniques

Electroencephalography (EEG) has a precise temporal resolution (in milliseconds) but a limited spatial resolution. In the context of pain assessment, EEG is mainly used to quantify brain responses evoked by a brief noxious stimulus such as a laser (i.e., laser-evoked potential) or electrical shock. Brief and longer-duration noxious stimuli have also been shown to affect the time-frequency characteristics of EEG signals. EEG assessment in clinical pain populations is more limited and includes the comparison between resting-state signals and sensory-evoked potentials evoked in patients with and without pain.

Functional magnetic resonance imaging (fMRI) and positron emission tomography (PET) imaging have much better spatial resolution than EEG and can measure whole-brain metabolic activity from which one can infer synaptic activity. However, their temporal resolution is limited and requires long-duration measurements at rest (resting state) or during a task/stimuli (task-based). As for EEG, these techniques have been largely used to evaluate brain response to experimental pain stimuli and to compare brain activity and connectivity between individuals living with and without pain (Morton et al., 2016).

Neurostimulation techniques applying electric or magnetic stimuli to different levels of the nervous system (central: e.g., pri-

(continued)

Box 3.4 (continued)
mary motor cortex; peripheral: e.g., nerves) are used to probe specific neural circuits function in relation to pain. For instance, the nociceptive withdrawal (or lower limb flexion) reflex is used as a proxy of the sensitivity of the nociceptive system. During this test, a noxious electrical stimulation is applied to an afferent nerve or to the skin and leads to muscle activation consistent with a withdrawal movement strategy. Transcranial magnetic stimulation (TMS) consists of placing a magnetic coil over the skull and passing a brief electrical current through the coil, thereby generating a magnetic field that passes through the skull without attenuation. The magnetic field generates an electrical current in the brain and depolarizes cortical neurons positioned perpendicular to the electrical current. TMS applied to the primary motor cortex elicits motor-evoked potentials (MEP). Various stimulation parameters and MEP characteristics can be measured to reflect on the organization and functioning of cortical circuits projecting to the muscles studied. TMS can also be used as an intervention using repetitive stimulation that modifies cortical excitability. Low-frequency rTMS (1–5 Hz) usually reduces cortical excitability, while high-frequency increases it (10–20 Hz—see Sect. 3.9.2) (Lefaucheur et al., 2020).

3.7 Best Practices for Pain Management

Guidelines for the management of chronic musculoskeletal pain usually recommend prioritizing non-pharmacological and non-invasive interventions through active management of the condition. For example, education, physical activity using different exercises (e.g., strengthening, aerobic), psychotherapy (e.g., cognitive behavioral therapy), self-management of the condition, and some complementary alternative medicine (e.g., mindfulness) are recommended as the first line of treatment for many pain conditions (Bernstein et al., 2017). Although some overlaps are present, different types of pain may necessitate different treatments (Table 3.2). Non-pharmacological management of nociplastic pain conditions, such as fibromyalgia, using physical activity and psychotherapy is effective to improve quality of life and pain. Neuropathic pain management slightly differs, and there is less evidence for the efficacy of active management using physical activity, although psychotherapy is frequently recognized as an effective treatment. Transcutaneous Electrical Nerve Stimulation (TENS) is recommended as first-line care and repetitive TMS as second-line care for neuropathic pain (see Sect. 3.9). Importantly, as discussed in previous sections, cognitive and emotional factors are risk factors for the development of chronic pain. Identifying and targeting these factors through psychotherapy or psychologically informed approaches is encouraged for any type of pain, although they could be more prevalent in nociplastic pain.

Table 3.2 Examples of conditions, characteristics and interventions related to the different types of pain

	Nociceptive	Neuropathic	Nociplastic
Pain conditions[a]	Acute pain Osteoarthritis	Thalamic stroke Peripheral neuropathy (e.g. secondary to diabetes mellitus) Polyneuropathy Spinal cord injury	Fibromyalgia Chronic Regional Pain Syndrome Temporomandibular disorders Whiplash disorder
		Phantom pain	
	Low back pain associated with radiculopathy		
Subjective/ objective assessment	Localised pain Consistent pain patterns reproduced by tissue loading and movement Absence of remote hyperalgesia or alteration in pain modulation systems (e.g. CPM, EIH)	Neuroanatomical pain distribution Allodynia Specific subjective pain descriptors (e.g. electric shock, shooting) Consistent pain patterns reproduced by tissue loading of the nerve (for peripheral neuropathic pain) Lesion of the somatosensory nervous system (e.g. using electromyography or MRI)	Diffuse and widespread pain Variable and aberrant pattern of pain Presence of local and remote hyperalgesia (e.g. using QST) Alteration in pain modulation system (e.g. using CPM, EIH) Presence of significant and numerous emotional and cognitive factors (e.g. depressive symptoms, fear avoidance behaviors, catastrophizing)
Rehabilitation interventions[b]	Physical activity Manual therapy	Mirror therapy Central neurostimulation Psychotherapy (e.g. cognitive behavioral therapy)	Pain education Physical activity Psychotherapy (e.g. cognitive behavioral therapy) Mirror therapy Central neurostimulation Motor imagery
	Education (e.g. advice to stay active) Self-management Peripheral neurostimulation (as adjunct treatment and/or self-management strategy)		

[a]These examples are suggestions of *predominant* pain mechanisms for different conditions. For example, it is possible that various mechanisms can produce one pain condition. Also, low back pain could be the result of each of the different pain mechanisms (sole or in combination)

[b]Including nonsurgical, non-pharmacological and non-invasive interventions but excluding medical management

3.8 Physical Activity Interventions and Pain

Physical activity is associated with numerous physical and psychological benefits, and maintaining an active lifestyle is widely recommended for individuals, whether they are living with chronic pain or not. Several studies have also demonstrated that adherence to various physical activity programs can reduce pain in individuals with neurological and musculoskeletal disorders.

While most studies agree that physical activity is an effective intervention for controlling pain in these clinical populations, determining the most suitable type of physical activity for a given individual can be challenging. Common findings indicate that engaging in physical activity is more effective than no activity in managing pain. However, most physical activity interventions, such as aerobic, strengthening, and motor control exercises, yield comparable results. While this conclusion may suggest that all physical activity interventions are indeed equal, it is likely that certain individuals may obtain more benefit from specific interventions. A recent meta-analysis confirmed that individualized physical activity interventions lead to greater low back pain reduction when compared to generalized interventions, thus supporting the latter hypothesis (Fleckenstein et al., 2022).

While physical activity is often the primary intervention for recovering from motor deficits induced by neurological disorders, its role in pain management within this population is often mistakenly overlooked (Mercier et al., 2017). Recently, intensive post-stroke upper extremity training primarily targeting motor deficits led to a large decrease in pain for at least 3 months in a subgroup of participants who initially experienced severe and/or neuropathic pain. Conversely, pain intensity slightly increased with time for those who experienced mild and/or non-neuropathic pain at baseline. In addition to showing the overall beneficial effects of physical activity on pain, such studies also emphasize the fact that different types of pain might respond differently to physical activity (Aprile et al., 2021).

For patients presenting with very severe motor deficits, it might sometimes be particularly challenging to engage in physical activity involving a paralyzed (or amputated) limb. A straightforward solution to perform physical activity in such conditions and potentially benefit from its hypoalgesic effects is to move spared body segments (e.g., using a hand ergometer for an individual living with paraplegia). In addition, the sole activation of motor pathways within the CNS can influence pain, even if it does not result in an actual body movement. This forms the basis of interventions such as motor imagery and mirror therapy, which have shown some effectiveness in decreasing pain in individuals living with an amputation or complex regional pain syndrome (Flor & Diers, 2009).

3.8.1 Mechanisms Underlying the Effects of Physical Activity on Pain

Physical activity has the potential to influence most pain perception and modulation mechanisms presented in Sects. 3.2 and 3.3. Pain is often attributed to a dysfunction of the neuromusculoskeletal system, causing a mechanical activation of nociceptors. For example, ineffective sensorimotor functions of shoulder girdle muscles are believed to contribute to the risk of shoulder impingement, resulting in musculoskeletal lesions and nociceptor activation. Many researchers and clinicians argue that improved sensorimotor functions (e.g., strength, proprioception, motor control) through physical activity can reduce the risk of such mechanical stimuli activating nociceptors, thereby explaining the efficacy of physical activity interventions. Although this explanation is plausible for some individuals, physical activity can also decrease sensitivity to controlled nociceptive stimuli (as measured with QST) (Sluka et al., 2018). This decreased sensitivity may be related to changes in the balance between inhibitory and excitatory activity in PAG and RVM neurons through regular activation of the opioid system, as well as the balance between pro-inflammatory and anti-inflammatory functions of the immune system. The voluntary activation of neural pathways involved in motor control, whether through actual or imagined movements, can also contribute to shaping CNS organization and counteracting maladaptive plasticity associated with pain conditions (Flor & Diers, 2009). Finally, physical activity, especially when coupled with psychologically informed interventions, can act on psychosocial determinants of pain such as kinesiophobia and fear avoidance beliefs.

3.8.2 Movement as a Cause for Pain

While physical activity is generally considered a remedy for pain, it can sometimes be its cause (Søgaard & Sjøgaard, 2017). Acutely, fatiguing exercises can heighten the perception of pain and may increase pain sensitivity in individuals living with (nociplastic) chronic pain. Certain forms of regular physical activity can also lead to the development of musculoskeletal injuries and pain. For example, approximately half of wheelchair users will develop shoulder pain, often due in part to repetitive wheelchair propulsion. Such pain can have a profound impact on social participation and quality of life and should be taken seriously. Clinicians should therefore be aware of conditions leading to nociceptive stimuli during physical activity and find solutions to control it (e.g., wheelchair propulsion training, arm positioning for flaccid stroke, prosthesis/wheelchair adjustments). These interventions will assist individuals living with chronic pain in engaging in meaningful physical activity and benefiting from its numerous favorable effects on physical and mental health, including pain management.

3.9 Adjunct Interventions to Target Neural Plasticity and Optimize Active Pain Management: Non-Invasive Neurostimulation

3.9.1 Peripheral Stimulation

Transcutaneous Electrical Nerve Stimulation (TENS) is commonly used to reduce and manage pain. TENS consists of applying low-current electrical pulses through the skin using surface electrodes, usually at the pain site. Different modes of stimulation can be used (e.g., conventional [high-frequency, short stimulus duration] and acupuncture-like [low-frequency, long stimulus duration]). Depending on the stimulation mode, different mechanisms drive pain reduction. Conventional TENS mainly depolarizes large somatosensory fibers (Aβ) and elicits sensory perception. In contrast, acupuncture-like TENS depolarizes large and smaller somatosensory fibers (Aβ, Aδ) as well as motor fibers and elicits both sensory perception and muscle contractions. Many overlapping neurophysiological mechanisms are responsible for the pain reduction for both TENS modes as described in Table 3.3. For example, both modes activate the spinal gate control mechanism and brainstem areas (e.g., PAG, RVM) but through different types of opioid receptors (δ- vs. μ-opioid receptors) (Sluka, 2016).

TENS has been shown to be effective in reducing pain in patients with neuropathic pain and fibromyalgia. Pain reduction occurs mostly during TENS and immediately after. Once TENS is stopped, there is no long-term efficacy. Thus, the effect of TENS should be used similarly to that of pain medications, aiming to elicit pain relief that may facilitate the performance of daily living or physical activities.

3.9.2 Central Stimulation

Non-invasive brain stimulation (NIBS) refers to a group of techniques used to modulate or modify the excitability of brain areas non-invasively. Different NIBS have been tested to reduce pain. Repetitive transcranial magnetic stimulation (rTMS) and transcranial direct current stimulation (tDCS) are commonly used in research and emerging in clinical practice.

For pain relief, it is generally recognized that high-frequency rTMS over M1 provides the best effects (Lefaucheur et al., 2020). Proposed mechanisms are an opioid system and PAG activation and thalamus inactivation (see Table 3.3 for the detailed mechanisms) (Galhardoni et al., 2015). Repetitive TMS is effective in reducing central

Table 3.3 Neurophysiological mechanisms for TENS and NIBS

	TENS mode		NIBS techniques[a]	
	Conventional (high-frequency)	Acupuncture-like (low-frequency)	rTMS	tDCS
Gate control (spinal inhibition)	√	√	?	?
↓ Sensitization (e.g. reduction in pain threshold)	√	√	√	√
Change in thalamic activity	?	?	√	√
Descending inhibition (PAG, RVM)	√	√	√	?
Opioid system involved	δ	μ	μ	μ
↓ Pro-inflammatory cytokins	√	?	√	√

TENS transcranial electrical nerve stimulation, *NIBS* non-invasive brain stimulation, *PAG* periaqueductal gray, *RVM* rostro-ventro-median nucleus

[a]Mechanisms may differ depending on the site of stimulation

Table adapted from Sluka (2016)

neuropathic pain (e.g., secondary to brain lesion), immediately after a stimulation session and in the longer term. There is also emerging evidence that M1 or dorso-lateral prefrontal cortex rTMS can reduce nociplastic pain (e.g., fibromyalgia). Targeting the prefrontal cortex in nociplastic pain could influence both pain and negative emotional and cognitive factors, which are predictors of a poor prognosis.

Transcranial DCS consists of the application of low-intensity electrical direct current through the skull using superficial electrodes on the scalp. Contrary to rTMS, tDCS does not directly depolarize the neurons in the brain. Instead, it would increase (anodal tDCS) or decrease (cathodal tDCS) brain activity by subthreshold modulation of neuronal membrane excitability. Similar underlying neural mechanisms as for rTMS have been suggested (see Table 3.3). A meta-analysis reported a significant reduction in pain intensity with tDCS, and the effect was found to be meaningful in patients with chronic pain (Knotkova et al., 2013). In patients with chronic low back pain, tDCS reduced pain intensity immediately after the end of treatment, but the effect was not maintained in the long run. In fibromyalgia, a clinically and meaningfully important reduction in pain intensity was observed. For neuropathic pain, tDCS is effective in reducing pain intensity.

In conclusion, NIBS is a promising technique to manage pain, although its effects are relatively modest. Usually, when used alone, its effects do not last in the long term. NIBS should therefore be used in conjunction with active pain management strategies.

3.10 General Conclusion

In summary, this chapter presented the neural complexity of pain, encouraging the use of individually tailored interventions and a combined subjective-objective evaluation approach. Recognizing pain as a complex subjective experience explains why factors beyond its intensity alone should be considered during assessment. Regarding pain management, diversified strategies emphasizing non-pharmacological interventions and targeting specific types of pain are proposed. The inclusion of transcutaneous electrical nerve stimulation and non-invasive brain stimulation as adjunct therapies for pain management emphasizes the importance of targeting neural plasticity to enhance treatment outcomes.

Review Questions

- Describe peripheral and central mechanisms in pain modulation.
- Imagine that you accidentally put your hand on a hot stove. What is the pathway in the CNS?
- What are the challenges in pain assessment?

References[1]

Aprile, I., Germanotta, M., Cruciani, A., Pecchioli, C., Loreti, S., Papadopoulou, D., Montesano, A., Galeri, S., Diverio, M., Falsini, C., Speranza, G., Langone, E., Carrozza, M. C., & Cecchi, F. (2021). Poststroke shoulder pain in subacute patients and its correlation with upper limb recovery after robotic or conventional treatment: A secondary analysis of a multicenter randomized controlled trial. *International Journal of Stroke, 16*, 396–405. https://doi.org/10.1177/1747493020937192

Backonja, M. M., Attal, N., Baron, R., Bouhassira, D., Drangholt, M., Dyck, P. J., Edwards, R. R., Freeman, R., Gracely, R., Haanpaa, M. H., Hansson, P., Hatem, S. M., Krumova, E. K., Jensen, T. S., Maier, C., Mick, G., Rice, A. S., Rolke, R., Treede, R. D., Serra, J., Toelle, T., Tugnoli, V., Walk, D., Walalce, M. S., Ware, M., Yarnitsky, D., & Ziegler, D. (2013). Value of quantitative sensory testing in neurological and pain disorders: NeuPSIG consensus. *Pain, 154*, 1807–1819. https://doi.org/10.1016/j.pain.2013.05.047

Bernstein, I. A., Malik, Q., Carville, S., & Ward, S. (2017). Low back pain and sciatica: Summary of NICE guidance. *British Medical Journal, 356*.

Costigan, M., Scholz, J., & Woolf, C. J. (2009). Neuropathic pain: A maladaptive response of the nervous system to damage. *Annual Review of Neuroscience, 32*, 1–32. https://doi.org/10.1146/annurev.neuro.051508.135531

[1]A complete list of references supporting this chapter is available as Supplementary material (https://doi.org/10.5683/SP3/KUHY9W).

Fayaz, A., Croft, P., Langford, R. M., Donaldson, L. J., & Jones, G. T. (2016). Prevalence of chronic pain in the UK: A systematic review and meta-analysis of population studies. *BMJ Open, 6*, e010364. https://doi.org/10.1136/bmjopen-2015-010364

Fillingim, R. B. (2017). Individual differences in pain: Understanding the mosaic that makes pain personal. *Pain, 158*(Suppl. 1), S11–S18. https://doi.org/10.1097/j.pain.0000000000000775

Fleckenstein, J., Floessel, P., Engel, T., Krempel, L., Stoll, J., Behrens, M., & Niederer, D. (2022). Individualized exercise in chronic non-specific low back pain: A systematic review with meta-analysis on the effects of exercise alone or in combination with psychological interventions on pain and disability. *The Journal of Pain, 23*, 1856–1873. https://doi.org/10.1016/j.jpain.2022.07.005

Flor, H., & Diers, M. (2009). Sensorimotor training and cortical reorganization. *Neurorehabilitation, 25*, 19–27. https://doi.org/10.3233/NRE-2009-0496

Galhardoni, R., Correia, G. S., Araujo, H., Yeng, L. T., Fernandes, D. T., Kaziyama, H. H., Marcolin, M. A., Bouhassira, D., Teixeira, M. J., & de Andrade, D. C. (2015). Repetitive transcranial magnetic stimulation in chronic pain: A review of the literature. *Archives of Physical Medicine and Rehabilitation, 96*, S156–S172. https://doi.org/10.1016/j.apmr.2014.11.010

IASP (2021). *Terminology*. https://www.iasp-pain.org/resources/terminology/.

Knotkova, H., Nitsche, M. A., & Cruciani, R. A. (2013). Putative physiological mechanisms underlying tDCS analgesic effects. *Frontiers in Human Neuroscience, 7*, 628. https://doi.org/10.3389/fnhum.2013.00628

Lefaucheur, J. P., Aleman, A., Baeken, C., Benninger, D. H., Brunelin, J., Di Lazzaro, V., Filipovic, S. R., Grefkes, C., Hasan, A., Hummel, F. C., Jaaskelainen, S. K., Langguth, B., Leocani, L., Londero, A., Nardone, R., Nguyen, J. P., Nyffeler, T., Oliveira-Maia, A. J., Oliviero, A., Padberg, F., Palm, U., Paulus, W., Poulet, E., Quartarone, A., Rachid, F., Rektorova, I., Rossi, S., Sahlsten, H., Schecklmann, M., Szekely, D., & Ziemann, U. (2020). Evidence-based guidelines on the therapeutic use of repetitive transcranial magnetic stimulation (rTMS): An update (2014–2018). *Clinical Neurophysiology, 131*, 474–528. https://doi.org/10.1016/j.clinph.2019.11.002

Marchand, S. (2009). *Le phénomène de la douleur*. Masson.

Mercier, C., Roosink, M., Bouffard, J., & Bouyer, L. J. (2017). Promoting gait recovery and limiting neuropathic pain after spinal cord injury. *Neurorehabilitation and Neural Repair, 31*, 315–322. https://doi.org/10.1177/1545968316680491

Morton, D. L., Sandhu, J. S., & Jones, A. K. (2016). Brain imaging of pain: State of the art. *Journal of Pain Research, 9*, 613–624. https://doi.org/10.2147/JPR.S60433

Patel, K. V., Amtmann, D., Jensen, M. P., Smith, S. M., Veasley, C., & Turk, D. C. (2021). Clinical outcome assessment in clinical trials of chronic pain treatments. *Pain Reports, 6*, e784. https://doi.org/10.1097/PR9.0000000000000784

Shraim, M. A., Masse-Alarie, H., & Hodges, P. W. (2021). Methods to discriminate between mechanism-based categories of pain experienced in the musculoskeletal system: A systematic review. *Pain, 162*, 1007–1037. https://doi.org/10.1097/j.pain.0000000000002113

Sluka, K. A. (2016). *Mechanisms and management of pain for the physical therapist*. Lippincott Williams & Wilkins.

Sluka, K. A., Frey-Law, L., & Hoeger Bement, M. (2018). Exercise-induced pain and analgesia? Underlying mechanisms and clinical translation. *Pain, 159*(Suppl. 1), S91–S97. https://doi.org/10.1097/j.pain.0000000000001235

Søgaard, K., & Sjøgaard, G. (2017). Physical activity as cause and cure of muscular pain: evidence of underlying mechanisms. *Exercise and Sport Sciences Reviews, 45*, 136–145.

Vision and Perception

4

Ro J. Robotham, Kathleen Vancleef, and Randi Starrfelt

Abstract

Vision is the perceptual sense that is most highly developed in humans, and a large proportion of the brain is dedicated to this sense. Brain injury can lead to a wide range of visual impairments that can have important consequences for the individuals affected. To detect, understand, and provide appropriate rehabilitation for brain-based visual impairments, an understanding of the complexity of how the brain processes vision is necessary. This chapter provides a comprehensive description of how vision is processed in the brain. This includes a description of how cells in the back of the eye transform information about light coming from the surroundings into neural signals, how this information is projected to the visual cortex in the back of the brain for basic processing, and how the information is further processed into meaningful representations along a ventral and a dorsal pathway. Impairments associated with damage at different stages of visual processing are described along the way, including visual field deficits, cerebral achromatopsia, visual object agnosia, prosopagnosia, pure alexia, simultanagnosia, optic ataxia, ocular apraxia, and topographical disorientation. Recommendations related to the assessment and rehabilitation of brain-based visual impairments are also provided.

Keywords

Visual perception · Visual field impairment · Hemianopia · Agnosia · Prosopagnosia · Brain injury · Stroke

R. J. Robotham (✉) · R. Starrfelt
Department of Psychology, University of Copenhagen, Copenhagen, Denmark
e-mail: ro.robotham@psy.ku.dk; randi.starrfelt@psy.ku.dk

K. Vancleef
Department of Psychology, Durham University, Durham, UK
e-mail: kathleen.vancleef@durham.ac.uk

Box 4.1 Case Story

Peter, a 72-year-old man, was preparing dinner for guests, when he suddenly lost consciousness. The next thing he remembers is waking up in the stroke unit. Here he was surprised to find that the ward had hired nurses who seemed to be identical triplets. It was only when a stranger with a familiar voice appeared at the door that he realised that something was terribly wrong. The stranger was in fact his wife. Peter had suffered a stroke that affected his ability to recognise faces. A structural MRI scan performed a couple of months after his stroke revealed bilateral occipito-temporal damage (with more extensive damage in the right hemisphere). He was quickly discharged from the unit, as his stroke did not seem to have caused any motor or severe cognitive impairments. In the months and years following his injury, he discovered that his stroke had also affected other aspects

(continued)

J. B. Nielsen et al. (eds.), *Neuroplasticity-based Neurorehabilitation*,
https://doi.org/10.1007/978-3-031-81120-3_4

Box 4.1 (continued)

of his vision. Finally, six years after his stroke, formal assessment revealed that he had a wide range of visuo-cognitive impairments: His reading had become slower and less precise, he had total colour blindness, he had wayfinding problems, and he struggled to get a visual overview in visually complex environments. Assessment also demonstrated that he had lost parts of his left and right visual fields. Not only did his visual impairments affect his ability to perform everyday tasks, but they also affected him emotionally. He avoided social gatherings, as he often ended up introducing himself repeatedly to people that he knew well, leaving people wondering whether he had dementia. He no longer was the avid reader that he used to be, as reading was now too laborious. His interest in nature and flowers had faded, as he now perceived the world in tones of grey. The above had driven him into a depression. As Peter's visual acuity was unaffected by his stroke, many would find it difficult to understand why he had so much trouble with a range of visual tasks.

To detect, understand, and provide appropriate rehabilitation for Peter's challenges, one needs to understand the complexity of visual processing in the brain. For example, if a patient has problems reading, it might seem intuitive to make the text larger; however, in Peter's case, as the reading problems are caused by his visual field impairment and not reduced visual acuity, texts with smaller font size are in fact much easier for him to read. This chapter describes how visual input is processed in the brain and how vision can be affected by brain injury. Then, some of the methods available for assessing brain-based visual impairments are introduced, as are the types of interventions that can help.

Vision is the perceptual sense that is most highly developed in humans, and a large proportion of the brain is dedicated to this sense. The ability to perceive the world visually is often taken for granted. However, when vision is compromised through brain injury, its complexity and importance become particularly apparent. Put simply, vision involves transforming information in the form of light from the surroundings into meaningful representations that can guide behaviour when interacting with the environment. While this might sound straight forward, visual processing is in fact highly complex and involves many processes, as will become apparent throughout this chapter. First, this chapter describes how cells in the back of the eyes transform information about light coming from the surroundings into neural signals and send this information to the visual cortex in the back of the brain. Then, the basic operations that occur in the visual cortex are described and how information is further processed along two pathways. The first pathway runs from the occipital pole along the temporal lobe and enables us to recognise stimuli in the environment. The second runs from the occipital pole towards the parietal lobes and enables us to determine where stimuli are located, and to build visuospatial representations to guide motor interactions with the environment (see Box 4.2). Throughout the chapter, the consequences that brain injury can have at these different processing stages in the visual system are discussed.

Box 4.2 Anatomical Structures Involved in Vision and Perception

The lateral geniculate nucleus (LGN), located in the thalamus, receives visual information from the optic nerves and relays it to the visual cortex. The visual cortex contains the Primary Visual Cortex (V1), located in the occipital lobe. It processes basic visual information like shapes, colours, and motion. Secondary visual areas, often referred to as extrastriate areas, include regions like V2, V3, V4, and V5 (also known as MT). These areas are adjacent to V1 and are responsible for processing more complex visual information beyond the basic features detected in V1 (Figs. 4.1 and 4.2).

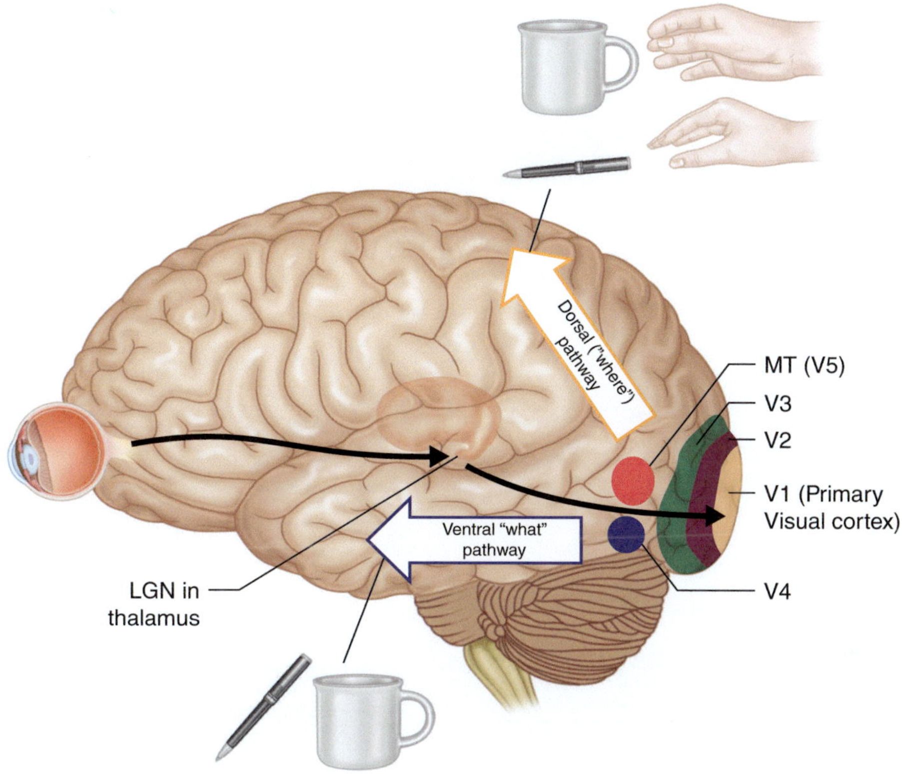

Fig. 4.1 Neural information is transferred from the retina in the eye via the Lateral Geniculate Nucleus in the thalamus to the primary visual cortex (V1) and extrastriate areas (V2, V3, V4, and MT). From the visual cortex, information is further processed along the ventral "what" pathway that projects towards the inferior temporal cortex and the dorsal "where" pathway that projects towards the posterior parietal cortex

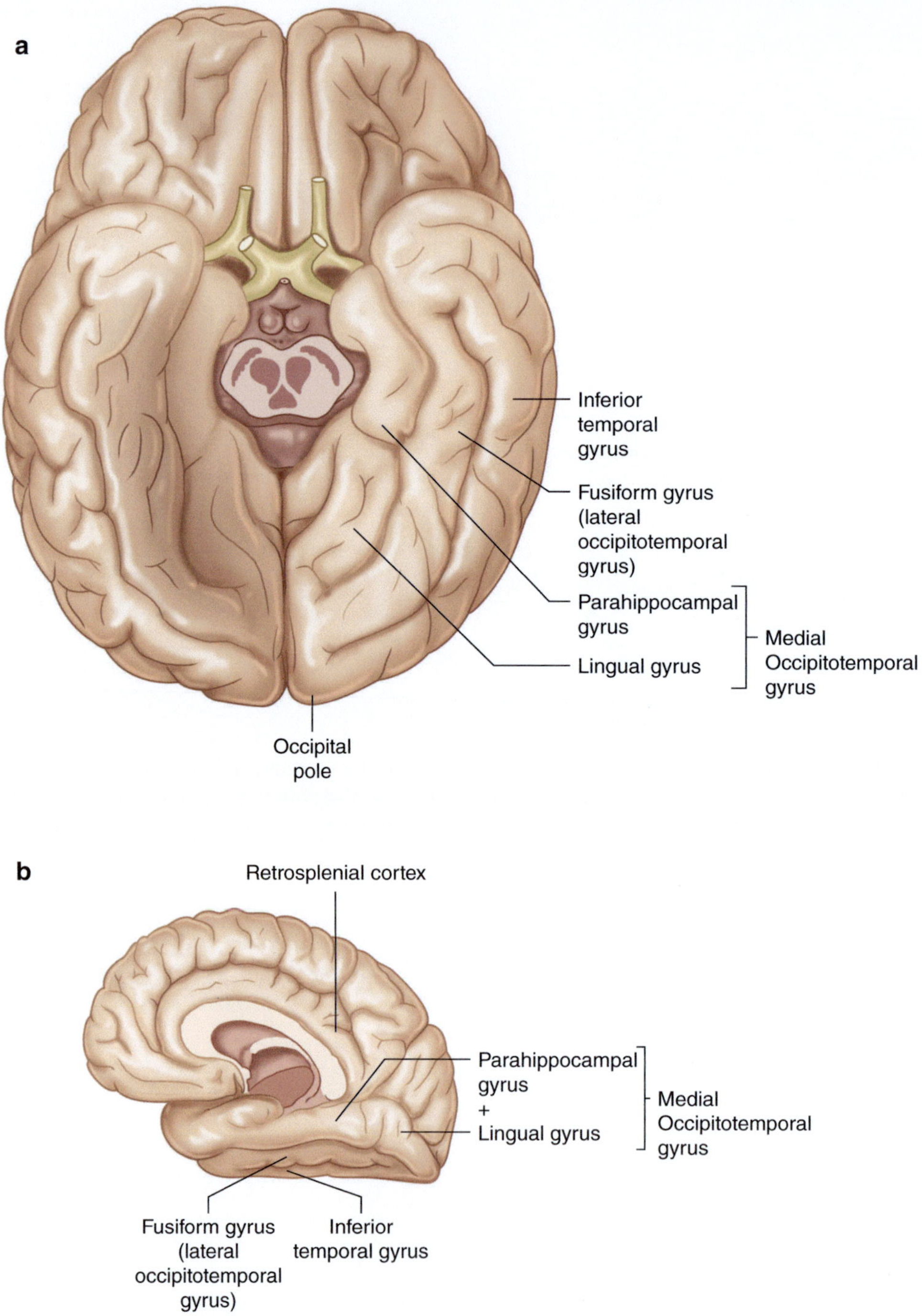

Fig. 4.2 Occipitotemporal regions involved in visual perception. (**a**) Ventral surface of the brain showing the occipital pole, inferior temporal gyrus, fusiform gyrus, parahippocampal gyrus, lingual gyrus, and medial occipitotemporal gyrus. (**b**) Medial surface of the brain showing the retrosplenial cortex, fusiform gyrus, inferior temporal gyrus, parahippocampal gyrus, lingual gyrus, and medial occipitotemporal gyrus

4.1 Sensory Vision: From the Eye to the Brain

4.1.1 Transforming Light into Neural Signals

The first stage of visual processing involves transforming light captured by the eyes into neural signals that can be sent to the brain for further processing. More specifically, light that has reflected off objects in our surroundings passes through the lens of the eye and is detected by cells that are in the retina lining the back of the eye (Fig. 4.3). These cells are called photoreceptors and transform light into neural signals, a process called visual phototransduction. The visual field refers to the total area of space that can be seen with the eye during steady fixation. Light coming from the left visual field is detected by photoreceptors in the right side of the retina whereas light coming from the right side is detected by cells in the left side of the retina.

There are two types of photoreceptors: rods and cones. Rods are most sensitive to low light levels and are therefore most active when it is dark. Cones on the other hand, are most sensitive to high levels of light and can code different colours and are therefore most active in daylight. In response to detecting light, photoreceptors release neurotransmitters that activate bipolar cells that in turn activate ganglion cells. Bipolar cells and ganglion cells are, just like photoreceptors, distributed across the retina. Their axons gather and exit the back of the eye forming the optic nerve that carries information to the brain.

4.1.2 Neural Signals Travel from the Eye to the Brain

Most of the axons forming the optic nerve (also known as cranial nerve II) of each eye terminate in the lateral geniculate nucleus (LGN) of the thalamus (see Box 4.2). What is important to know is that while some of the axons of each optic nerve project to the thalamus in the same hemisphere, others cross to the other hemisphere at an intersection called the optic chiasm (from Greek, meaning cross or crossing) (Fig. 4.4). The axons coming from the ganglion cells located in the retina towards the nose cross over and project to the thalamus in the opposite side of the brain. This means that posterior to the optic chiasm, the representation of the left visual field for both eyes is

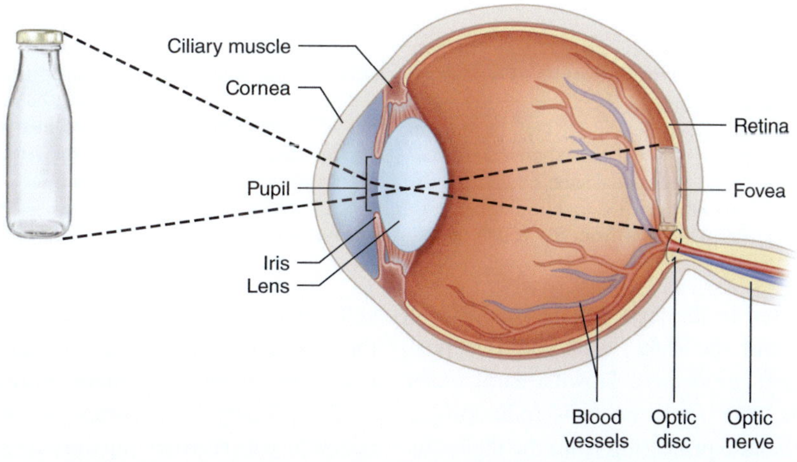

Fig. 4.3 Illustration of how light enters the eye and reaches the retina. Light passes through the cornea and the lens, through the centre of the eye, and is captured by cells in the retina. Note that light coming from the right is captured in the left of the retina (in the back of the eye) and light from the left is captured in the right of the retina (in the back of the eye)

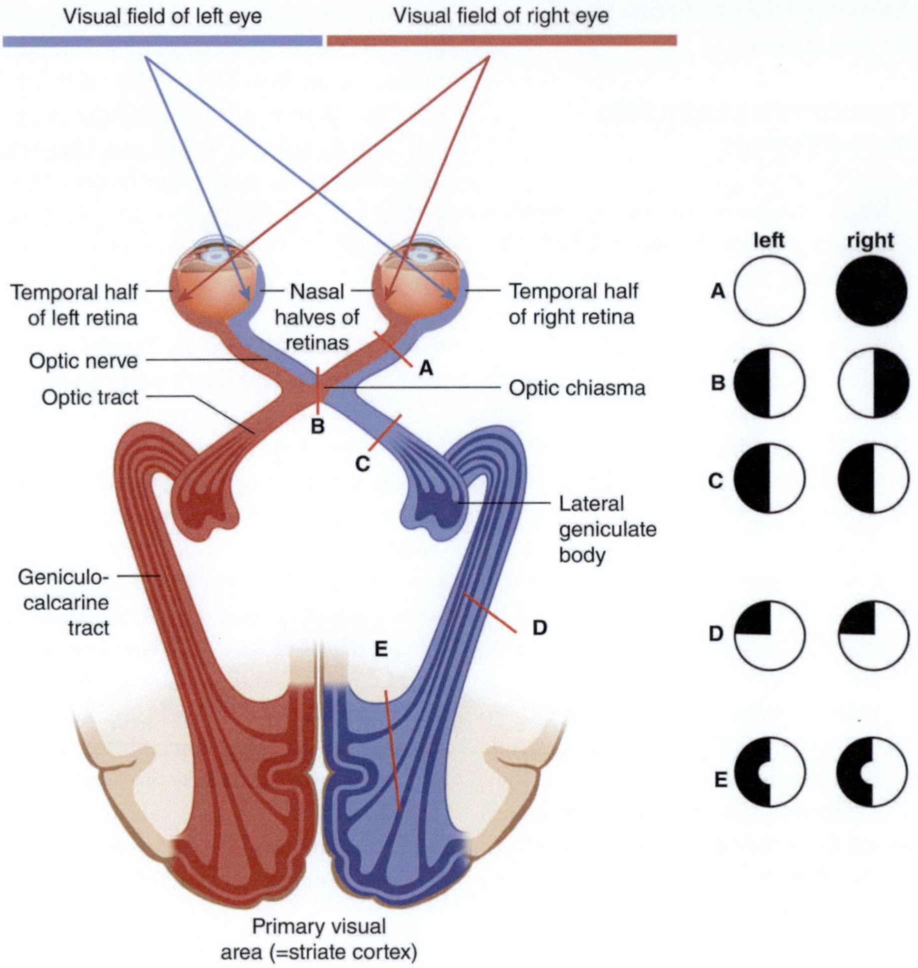

Fig. 4.4 On the left is a visual representation of how information from the left and right visual fields is detected in the retina and projected along the visual pathways to V1. Light from the left visual field i detected by cells in the right side of the retina in both eyes, whereas information from the right visual field is detected by cells in the left side of the retina in both eyes. Information is then projected along the visual pathways from the retina to V1. Note that a large proportion of axons forming the optic nerve behind each eye cross to the opposite hemisphere at the optic chiasm. This means that the left visual field of the left and right eye are represented in the right V1, whereas the right visual field of the left and right eye are represented in the left V1. On the right is a visual illustration of visual field loss for each eye corresponding to lesions different places along the visual pathways

further processed in the right hemisphere, while information from the right visual field is processed in the left hemisphere. Downstream, axons of cells in the LGN form the optic radiations, a white matter bundle projecting from the thalamus to the primary visual cortex (also called V1). Due to the crossover in the optic chiasm, the right primary visual cortex receives information from the left visual field and the left visual cortex processes information from the right visual field. It is worth mentioning that a small proportion of ganglion cells in the retina, rather than projecting to the thalamus and then V1, project to the midbrain that is involved in eye movement coordination.

The primary visual cortex (V1) is located in the occipital pole surrounding the calcarine sulcus. V1 has a retinotopic organisation, meaning that the visual field is represented in a similar topographic way in V1 as in the retina (Fig. 4.5). Central vision is represented in the occipital pole and peripheral vision represented more anteriorly. Central vision is overrepresented in V1. This means that when

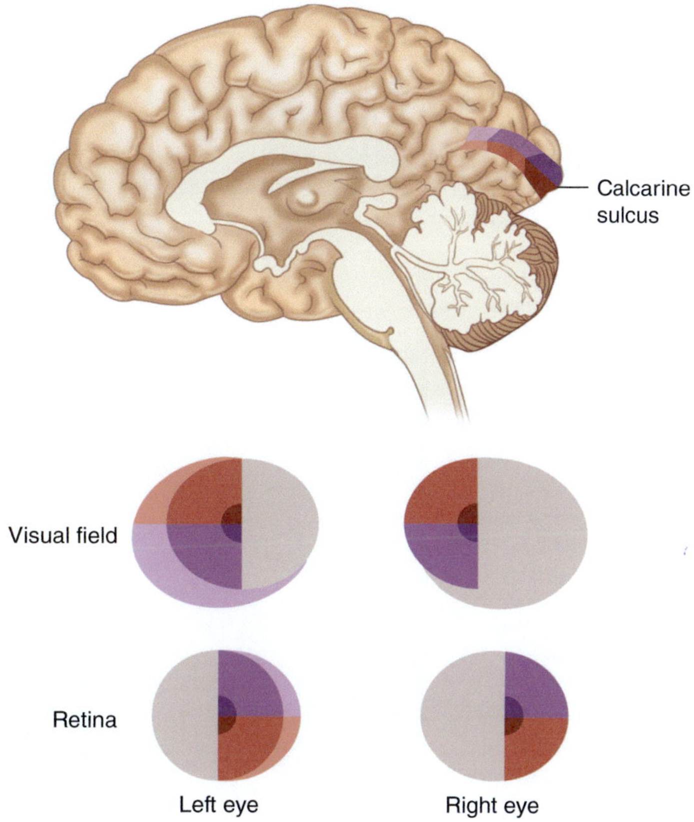

Fig. 4.5 Retinotopic representation of the left visual field in the retina and V1 in the right hemisphere. The central visual field is represented posteriorly in V1 (darker), whereas the peripheral visual field is represented more anteriorly (lighter). Note that the central visual field is disproportionally represented in V1 compared to the peripheral visual field. The upper visual quadrant is represented below the calcarine sulcus (illustrated in red) and the lower quadrant is represented above the calcarine sulcus (illustrated in purple)

compared to the retina, a larger proportion of V1 is dedicated to processing the central visual field than the peripheral visual field. This so-called "cortical magnification factor" is expressed as the number of millimetres of cortical surface that is dedicated to a degree of visual angle. In humans, cortical magnification declines rapidly when moving from central to peripheral vision.

Another concept that is important to understand in relation to visual perception is the concept of receptive fields. A neuron's *receptive field* refers to the region of visual space where changes in luminance influence the activity of the neuron. The size and properties of these receptive fields change through visual processing from the retina, through the LGN and primary visual cortex. The portion of space that a neuron is responsive to can differ according to their position on the retina (retinotopic) and may be very simple (responding to light/no light), or more complex, for instance responding to lines with certain angles or even combinations of lines or movement within a certain part of space.

As mentioned earlier, the left visual field from both eyes is represented in V1 in the right hemisphere, and vice-versa. Similarly, the upper visual quadrants are represented in the cortical areas below the calcarine sulcus, and the lower visual quadrants are represented in the cortical areas above the calcarine sulcus (Fig. 4.5). This is why some people say that "our brain sees the world upside down."

Understanding the visual pathways from the retina to the occipital lobe as well as the basic retinotopic organisation of V1 is crucial for understanding the types of visual field impairments that can be caused by a brain injury.

4.1.3 Impairments Caused by Lesions of the Optic Radiation and V1

4.1.3.1 Visual Field Impairments

There is a systematic relationship between a patient's lesion location and their visual field loss (Fig. 4.4). This means that it is possible to deter-

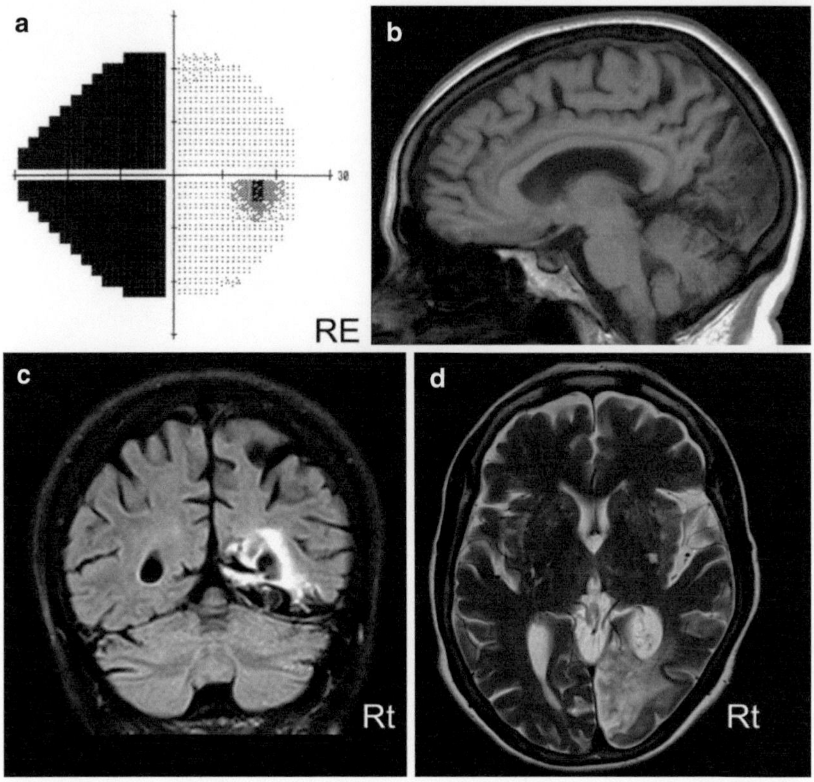

Fig. 4.6 Visual field of the right eye (**a**) and brain scan (**b**, **c**, and **d**) from a patient with a left homonymous hemianopia following right occipital stroke. (**a**) Result from an automated perimetry of the right eye with a darkened area indicating left hemianopia without macular sparing. (**b**) A sagittal view of the right hemisphere showing a lesion in the occipital lobe. (**c**) A coronal view showing a lesion in the right occipital lobe. (**d**) An axial view showing a lesion in the right occipital lobe. (Leff and Starrfelt (2014). Hemianopic Alexia. In: Alexia. Springer, London)

mine the approximate location of a brain injury based on a visual field assessment, and conversely it is also possible to predict a patient's visual field loss relatively precisely based on a patient's structural brain scan. Damage to either optic nerve in front of the optic chiasm will affect vision in only one eye (Fig. 4.4a), whereas damage to the visual pathways posterior to the optic chiasm will lead to affection of the same portion of the visual field in both eyes (Fig. 4.4 c–e). When a visual field deficit affects the same side in both eyes, it is called a homonymous visual field loss. More specifically, a lesion in the right occipital pole will lead to a full or partial loss of the left (opposite) visual field for both eyes, whereas a lesion in the left occipital pole will lead to a full or partial loss of the right (opposite) visual field for both eyes. Many patients who have a visual field deficit caused by unilateral posterior stroke assume that they have lost vision in one eye when in fact they have a partial visual field loss in both eyes. Importantly, many patients learn to compensate for their visual field deficits without having full comprehension of what part of vision is affected.

The most common visual field impairments that are seen following a stroke are a full loss of the contralateral field in both eyes (Fig. 4.4c or) or the loss of a quadrant in both eyes (Fig. 4.4d). Figure 4.6 shows the lesion and visual field measurement of a patient with a right hemisphere stroke causing left homonymous hemianopia. In some cases of homonymous hemianopia caused by an occipital lesion, the central portion of the visual field can be preserved. This is called macular sparing (Fig. 4.4e). A visual field loss can also be far more limited. The term scotoma is used to refer to the loss of an isolated area of visual field that is surrounded by preserved vision.

Visual field loss can have a wide range of consequences. One of the core problems for patients with homonymous hemianopia is that they struggle to get a full overview of their surroundings and often overlook stimuli. They typically experience bumping into things that are in their blind field. Traffic can be particularly dangerous as patients may overlook vehicles coming from one side (Fig 4.7). Patients with upper visual field loss risk banging their heads into, for example,

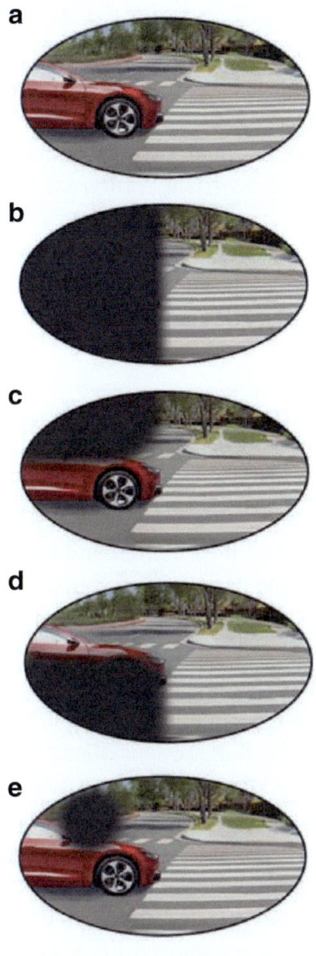

Fig. 4.7 Illustration of the consequences of different types of visual field deficits when crossing a road at a zebra crossing with a car approaching from the left. (**a**) Preserved visual field. The patient can see the car. (**b**) Left homonymous hemianopia. The patient cannot see the car. (**c**) Left upper homonymous quadrantanopia. The patient can see the lower part of the car. (**d**) Left lower homonymous quadrantanopia. The patient can see the upper part of the car. (**e**) Scotoma. A small area of the visual field is missing but the patient can still see the car approaching

kitchen cupboard doors, whereas patients with lower visual field loss risk bumping into furniture or stumbling when walking on uneven surfaces. Visual field loss can also have a large impact on reading. Patients with right homonymous hemianopia often make more mistakes, skipping whole words or the ending of words and sentences, whereas patients with left homonymous hemianopia typically struggle with line breaks as they can find it difficult to plan precise eye movements to the start of the next line. Whether a patient has macular sparing or not can have important clinical implications. For example, reading performance is more severely affected in patients without macular sparing than in patients with macular sparing. Scotomas, depending on their size and location, can be more or less compromising. Even the smallest scotomas, if located centrally, can have important consequences for patients.

Peter, the patient described at the start of the chapter, had partial visual field loss in both the left and right visual field because his lesion affected both hemispheres. His reading was slow and laborious. Thorough assessment revealed that his reading difficulties were caused by his visual field loss. For most patients with sensory vision impairments like reduced acuity, texts with larger font size are easier to read, but this was not the case for Peter. Peter found reading headlines of newspaper articles far more challenging than reading small print in the body text of articles. While this might seem counterintuitive, this is quite typical for patients with visual field impairments, as text that can fit into their preserved visual field can be read but larger letters tend to be affected by the visual field loss. Indeed, the larger the font size, the larger the proportion of text occluded and is thus invisible to the patient.

4.1.3.2 Visual Hallucinations Following Visual Field Loss

A large proportion (13–40%) of patients with homonymous visual field loss experience visual phenomena (hallucinations) in the blind visual field. These hallucinations may come in many variations and are most common after stroke and neurosurgery. They often do not appear immediately following damage, but rather following a period of latency and will usually subside with time. Some patients describe simple hallucinations such as flashes of light or geometric patterns and others experience seeing complex hallucinations including images of objects, people, or landscapes. The hallucinations can be static or moving and can last anything from seconds to hours. The disorder is likely a consequence of top-down processes playing a more dominant role in visual processing when bottom-up input is damaged. The hallucinations are typically more frequent in situations with low lighting, like in the evening if lights are not turned up. Charles Bonnet syndrome is used to refer to the condition when patients experience complex types of hallucinations. In contrast to hallucinations experienced by some psychiatric patients, visual hallucinations following visual field loss are restricted to the visual modality. This means that they are not accompanied by for example auditory or olfactory hallucinations. Most patients with Charles Bonnet syndrome are fully aware that what they are experiencing is a hallucination and they rarely experience the hallucinations as threatening. Despite this, patients can find the experience unsettling, as hallucinations are typically associated with psychiatric disorders. For this reason, patients frequently do not report hallucinations to health care professionals in fear of being diagnosed as mentally ill. This, and the lack of awareness about the condition amongst health care professionals, likely contribute to the syndrome being underdiagnosed. It is important to inform patients that hallucinations are a normal and common consequence of visual field loss, and it is crucial that the rehabilitation team refrain from interpreting the hallucinations as a sign of psychological instability. For further reading about visual hallucinations following brain injury see Fraser & Lueck (2021).

4.1.3.3 Blind-Sight

Studies have demonstrated that some patients with visual field loss caused by damage to the occipital cortex have some preserved visual processing abilities in their blind visual field. In experimental settings, patients have been asked to respond to stimuli that are presented in their blind field. The results indicate that patients may be able to move their eyes towards the location of targets in their blind visual field, determine the orientation of a target, the direction of motion of a target, and distinguish between simple shapes such as an X and an O. Typically, patients perform the tasks with surprising accuracy given their field loss, but none the less make multiple errors. As the patients have no conscious experience of vision in their blind field, they often find the tasks bizarre and need a fair amount of encouragement to participate. The most likely explanation for blindsight is that while most visual pathways leaving thalamus project to V1, some bypass V1 and project directly to other visual areas (extrastriate cortex, see below). This may mean that some basic aspects of visual processing can occur without contribution from V1. For more information about blindsight, read Danckert et al. (2021)

4.2 Visual Perception: Visual Cortex and Beyond

Primary visual cortex (V1) provides coarse processing of visual information and can be considered the starting point of perceptual vision. Basic information about edges of objects, their orientation, colours, and movements are represented in V1 in a non-specific manner. One must move beyond V1 to surrounding secondary visual cortex to find areas that are specialised in processing specific types of visual information. Areas V3 and V4 that are more ventrally located (towards the bottom of the brain) are specialised in basic form and colour processing, whereas area V5 that is more dorsally located (towards the upper part of the brain) is specialised in processing movement and location (see Fig 4.1). Following V1 processing, the next stage involves decoding which aspects of visual input go together (integration) and which do not (segmentation). For example, to identify and recognise a table, the tabletop and the legs of the table must be integrated as they are part of the same object. They must also be segmented from other stimuli such as chairs around the table. These mid-level computations are thought to begin in V1 and the lateral parts of secondary visual cortex.

Visual information from primary and secondary visual cortex is further processed along two main streams (Goodale & Milner, 1992). The ventral visual stream projects from the ventral parts of the visual cortex towards the ventral temporal lobes. It processes information necessary for identifying objects in the visual field and enables the recognition of *what* is being observed. The dorsal visual stream projects from the superior parts of the visual cortex primarily towards the parietal lobes. This stream processes visual spatial information that encodes *where* objects are placed in the surroundings and provides information needed to guide movements in relation to these objects. The two streams are intricately connected, and they rely strongly on one another to ensure accurate interaction with the environment. They are, however, separate to the extent that lesions along either stream can result in radically different impairments. Some patients, following lesions affecting the dorsal stream, can recognise a cup but are not able to reach for it. Other patients, following lesions to the ventral stream, are able to grab a cup quickly and smoothly, but are not able to recognise what they are reaching for. Note that the word "object" here is used in the most general sense: It can refer to a concrete object like a cup or a car that is within the reach and might be handled or interacted with. The ventral stream is also used to recognise written words on a page, and a mountain or a lake in the distance. The dorsal stream processes the information necessary for us to identify where these objects are, point towards them, track their shape, and conduct movements in relation to them. For example, catching a ball requires recognizing the ball (ventral stream), identifying its location, processing the speed and direction of its movement, and positioning the arm and hand appropriately (dorsal stream). To explain what happens along the ventral and dorsal stream, nearby, concrete objects will be used as an example.

4.2.1 The Ventral "What" Stream

Following the segmentation and integration processes, information is processed further to enable the perception and recognition of objects. First, to recognise an object, the perceived input must be matched to knowledge in the visual long-term memory about how objects look. This knowledge is commonly called structural representations. These representations are stored in the temporal lobe and include information about which parts an object consists of and how they are placed in relation to another (e.g. a table consists of a large rectangular shape with a certain amount of long thin rectangular shapes below). Once an object is recognised, knowledge about it needs to be retrieved. For example, a table can be used for placing items on, it is typically used during meals, and it is tightly associated with other objects such as chairs or plates. This knowledge is referred to as semantic representations or semantic memory that are thought to be stored in the temporal lobe.

Visual recognition processes are therefore dependent on input from V1 (so-called bottom-up processing) as well as stored perceptual knowledge and expectations (top-down processes). Note that even though memory and expectations come into play here, visual perception is considered an automatic and unconscious process, which means that it is difficult, if not impossible, to consciously modify the experienced percept. Most of the time this works fine, and objects are perceived accurately, but top-down processes can also lead to visual illusions, where the perceived image does not accurately reflect the visual input. Such illusions can affect the experience of light and darkness, colour, shape, size, and even object identity. See Fig. 4.8 for an example.

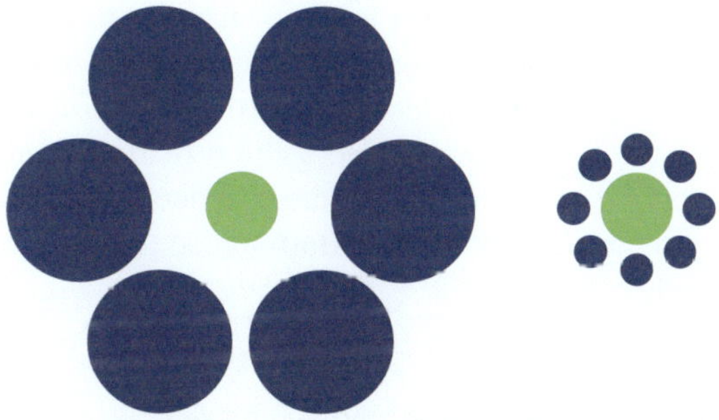

Fig. 4.8 Which of the two green circles is larger? Most likely, you perceive the green circle on the right as larger than the one on the left. In reality, they are both exactly the same size. This illusion illustrates how we do not always perceive the world as it is. Our perception of an object is influenced by context, often in an automatic (unconscious) manner. In this case, the difference in size perception is caused by the surrounding visual cues. The green circle that is surrounded by large blue circles appears smaller. Despite the green circles taking up the same space on the retina, you cannot force yourself to perceive them as the same size. This demonstrates the automatic nature of many perceptual processes. This illusion is commonly referred to as the "Ebbinghaus illusion" or the "Titchener circles"

When objects are processed through the ventral visual stream, the edges, contours, and simple shapes processed in low and mid-level vision come together to represent an object in a view- and viewer-invariant fashion. This means that even when moving towards, away from, or around an object, it will be perceived as the same object, even if it changes low level properties on the retina and in early visual cortex. A bicycle may come towards you and become bigger on your retina, it may go from being in the shade to being in direct sunlight and appear brighter, and it might even change direction so you suddenly see it from the side instead of the front, but you will recognise it as the same object none the less.

At lower levels of processing, all stimuli undergo the same operations or processing regardless of the type of object that are observed, but this changes in the anterior parts of the occipital lobes and the ventral parts of the temporal lobe. Some types of visual input seem to be processed in specific ventral occipital temporal areas. This is the case for faces and seems also to be the case for written words. Indeed, brain regions within the ventral stream have been named to reflect this specificity: the Fusiform Face Area (FFA) and the Visual Word Form Area (VWFA). These areas are both thought to be a link between the perception and recognition or visual memory of a face or a word and are crucial for fast and automatic recognition of faces and words. For other objects, more general-purpose systems are at work. See Bartolomeo (2022) for further reading.

4.2.2 The Dorsal "Where" Stream

While there is high agreement that the ventral stream is responsible for identifying stimuli, the role of the dorsal stream remains somewhat debated. Overall, however, this processing stream contributes to visuo-spatial coding important for locating and interacting with objects in the environment. On a general level, the main distinction between the ventral and dorsal stream is that the ventral stream enables the formation of allocentric representations, while the dorsal stream enables the formation of egocentric representations. Allocentric representations carry information about where objects are in relation to each other, and how the parts of an object are placed in relation to one another, regardless of the viewpoint. Egocentric spatial representations on the other hand, carry information about where objects are placed in relation to the viewer, information that is necessary to guide actions towards objects in the surroundings. While the specific role of the dorsal stream remains debated, there is broad agreement that the parietal lobes (that the dorsal stream projects towards) integrate somatosensory information about the position of our body parts (processed in the somatosensory cortex) with visual information about where stimuli are placed in relation to us, to coordinate precise movements when interacting with the environment. For further reading see Gallivan and Goodale (2018).

4.2.3 Disorders of the Ventral Stream

4.2.3.1 Cerebral Achromatopsia

Cerebral achromatopsia is a colour perception impairment caused by brain injury. While some patients have a complete loss of colour perception and describe seeing the world in shades of grey, others have a reduction in perception of some specific hues. The deficit is typically caused by lesions involving the medial occipitotemporal gyrus and the lingual gyrus (see Fig. 4.2). Colour perception plays an important role in human everyday life. It is vital for recognising objects in our surroundings and colours are often used as symbols, for example, in traffic. As illustrated with Peter, who is described in the introduction, a loss of colour perception can also have consequences for a patient's mental health. Read more about colour vison and colour vision deficits in Bartolomeo (2021).

4.2.3.2 Visual Object Agnosia

A lesion in the ventral stream can give rise to visual agnosia, a loss of ability to recognise familiar objects in patients who have preserved visual sensory function. Patients with visual agnosia can recognise objects through other sensory modalities such as touch or sound and can name objects based on a description of the object's function. So, while a patient with visual agnosia may not be able to recognise a key visually, they can recognise it when touching it, and are able to answer the question: "What do you use to unlock a door?" You can read more about visual agnosia in Gerlach and Robotham (2021).

4.2.3.3 Prosopagnosia

Prosopagnosia refers to a severe impairment in recognising people by their faces. Patients with prosopagnosia (popularly called face blindness) after brain injury struggle to recognise their friends and relatives, and in some cases are not even able to recognise themselves in the mirror. The deficit affects not only the recognition of familiar faces that the patient could recognise prior to their injury, it also affects the ability to learn new faces, e.g. of staff in a hospital ward. Most patients with prosopagnosia also have other visual impairments, but in some cases the impairment can be surprisingly selective. Prosopagnosia can have important consequences for patients' lives and quality of life. Many patients avoid social settings and become more socially isolated as they want to avoid the embarrassment of not recognising people that they know well. Some patients learn to use alternative strategies to recognise people using specific features such as the shape of someone's ears, nose, or eyes, or by using other characteristics such as a person's hairstyle or posture, but these strategies are no way near as efficient as normal face recognition. Prosopagnosia has commonly been associated with right hemisphere damage to the lateral and inferior occipitotemporal cortex, and the Fusiform Face Area (in the fusiform gyrus) mentioned above is thought to play an important role in face recognition (see Fig. 4.2). Prosopagnosia can also follow bilateral lesions and is then typically even more severe. Peter, the patient described in the introduction, had bilateral lesions, and described one episode that illustrated the extent of his face blindness particularly well: Peter had gone to the local department store to buy clothes. When making his way towards the exit of the store, he walked down a corridor and saw someone walking towards him. The two of them got closer until they finally were standing opposite each other. To avoid each other, they both took a step in one direction and then in the other. Finally, hoping the other person would move, Peter barged straight ahead and … smashed his head into a mirror! It turned out that the person he had been trying to avoid was not a stranger but his own reflection in a mirror, which he had not recognised. He had not been making his way down a corridor but rather had entered a fitting room. Prior to his stroke, Peter was head of a large firm, and prided himself in being good at recognizing his employees and large network of collaborators. You can read more about prosopagnosia in Starrfelt and Barton (2022).

4.2.3.4 Pure Alexia

Pure alexia refers to a selective impairment in reading, following injury to ventral occipitotemporal cortex in the left hemisphere. Patients with pure alexia lose the ability to read fast and fluently, and in the acute phase following their lesion they typically try to identify the individual letters of a word, and then put them together. Some patients can do this, some also struggle with recognizing letters. What is intriguing about pure alexia is that the patients have preserved general language: They can speak and comprehend speech, and they are even still able to write. But they cannot read even what they have written themselves. Sometimes pure alexia is accompanied by mild problems in recognising visually presented objects (visual agnosia), and it is almost always associated with a right sided visual field deficit. The field deficit alone cannot explain the reading problems. Patients with reading problems caused by hemianopia alone (with more posterior lesions) read much faster than patients with pure alexia and can recognise individual letters without problems. Patients with pure alexia commonly regain some reading ability with time and proceed from struggling with letters or spelling out loud to just reading very slowly. There is a clear effect of word length (the number of letters in a word) on the time it takes them to read a word. This is called the word length effect and might be in the range of 200 extra milliseconds per letter to more than one second per extra letter in a word. Typical readers do not show this effect on reading words up to 6 or 7 letters. So, while pure alexic patients' reading improves with time, they remain very slow readers even years after their injury. While some training methods have succeeded in improving reading speed somewhat in patients with pure alexia, they invariably remain poorer readers than before their injury unless their impairment remits within the first 3–6 months following injury. You can read more about pure alexia and other visually based reading deficits in Starrfelt and Woodhead (2021).

4.2.4 Disorders of the Dorsal Stream

4.2.4.1 Simultanagnosia

Patients with simultanagnosia can only perceive a limited number of objects at a time, and in extreme cases only one. Classical patients experience one object as "disappearing" as soon as another object is present in the visual field. This can be so extreme that the cup they are trying to reach might disappear from their sight when their hand enters their visual field. For this reason, patients have trouble recognizing scenes, complex pictures, or get an overall impression of their surroundings. Simultanagnosia is considered an attentional deficit: the visual attention of these patients is so limited that they only experience seeing one or two objects at a time. Patients with simultanagnosia often seem confused and visually disoriented, which is no surprise. Imagine if you experienced that objects you were looking at just disappeared. Simultanagnosia following lesions to the dorsal stream is typically due to bilateral lesions to the posterior parietal cortex, which is quite rare. It does however occur after oxygen deprivation, for example following cardiac arrest or carbon monoxide poisoning. Simultanagnosia also occurs in late stages of some degenerative diseases.

4.2.4.2 Optic Ataxia

Optic ataxia has traditionally been used to refer to an impairment in performing visually guided actions caused by bilateral parietal lesions. Patients with optic ataxia cannot reach out precisely to grasp an object that is in front of them. Today, it is acknowledged that the impairment can be the result of either mislocating the target or the hand in relation to oneself when reaching for something.

4.2.4.3 Ocular Apraxia

Ocular apraxia is a disorder affecting the ability to initiate voluntary eye movements. Patients struggle to control their eye movements to find a target and once they fixate on a stimulus, their gaze can become locked on a specific detail. For more information about simultanagnosia, optic ataxia, and ocular apraxia, see Pisella et al. (2021).

4.2.4.4 Topographical Disorientation

Brain injury can lead to impairments in the ability to orient and navigate in spatial surroundings, also known as topographical disorientation. Wayfinding problems can be caused by a variety of conditions that can be associated with specific lesion locations. Patients with egocentric disorientation have intact visual recognition abilities but they are unable to compute egocentric spatial relationships and are unable to localise landmarks relative to themselves. The deficit has been associated with lesions in the posterior parietal cortex. Patients with heading disorientation, on the other hand, who typically have lesions in the retrosplenial cortex (Fig. 4.2), are able to localise landmarks relative to themselves, but they are unable to figure out which direction to take to get from one place to another. Patients with landmark agnosia have an impairment in the recognition of landmarks meaning that they cannot use environmental features to guide orientation. Peter's wayfinding problems were likely due to landmark agnosia, as he described not being able to use landmarks to find his way from one place to another, as all corner shops look the same to him. The deficit is associated with ventral stream lesions to the fusiform and lingual gyri. The last condition that should be mentioned is anterograde disorientation in which patients are unable to orient themselves in novel environments only. The disorder has been described following lesions to the parahippocampal cortex (Fig. 4.2). For more about topographical disorientation read Iaria & Slone (2021).

4.2.4.5 Visuo-spatial Neglect

Visuo-spatial neglect is an attentional deficit, observed after parietal lesions. It is not considered a visuo-perceptual disorder, but rather a visuo-spatial one. Patients with visual neglect are unable to respond to or direct their attention to visual stimuli in one visual field, even when they do not have a visual field deficit (Vallar & Ronchi, 2022). For more information about neglect see Box 4.3.

Box 4.3 Understanding Visuo-spatial Neglect: An Impairment of Spatial Awareness and Attention

Visuo-spatial neglect (also known as hemineglect, neglect syndrome, visual neglect, and hemi-inattention) can be an important challenge for effective neurorehabilitation following brain injury. The term is used to refer to a range of disorders in which a person is unable to orient towards or respond to stimuli from one side of space or the body. Visuo-spatial neglect is not a perceptual disorder per se, but rather a deficit in attention and awareness that can affect what a person consciously perceives. Visuo-spatial neglect occurs most commonly following damage to the right hemisphere, affecting a patient's ability to attend to the left side of space. The clinical presentation of neglect can vary greatly and examples of behaviours include: only eating food from the right side of a plate; only putting make-up onto the right side of their face; bumping into furniture placed to their left; forgetting to put their left shoe on, or forgetting that they have a hemiparesis. Neglect after damage to the left hemisphere is less common (in which case it is the right side of space that is overlooked) and mostly occurs in the acute stage of recovery. Various sensory modalities can be affected by neglect (including visual, auditory, and tactile perception); however, visual neglect is the most common and prominent type. Neglect is mostly associated with damage to the right parietal lobe in relation to stroke, where it may be observed in 20–50% of survivors in the acute phase. It is less common in the chronic phase, but it is still reported to be observed in 5–30% of stroke survivors with right-hemisphere lesion depending on assessment methods and population. Various clinical tests and assessments are used to evaluate the presence and severity of neglect, including standardised neuropsychological tests and functional measures.

Neglect often co-occurs with other cognitive impairments, such as anosognosia (lack of awareness of deficits) and apraxia (difficulty performing purposeful movements). Neglect can significantly impair daily functioning, including activities of daily living, mobility, navigation, and safety awareness. Neglect is often challenging in neurorehabilitation, since the individual lacks awareness of their neglect and of their other deficits. For example, patients with co-occurring hemiparesis may lack awareness of the side of their body that requires functional training and therefore "forget" to perform the training. Patient with neglect and anosognosia often underestimate the consequences of their injury and have unrealistic goals in rehabilitation.

The core aim of rehabilitation is to improve awareness of and attention to the neglected side. Neglect interventions can be grossly classified into two categories: top-down and bottom-up interventions. Top-down interventions involve training

(continued)

Box 4.3 (continued)
conscious strategies that improve a patient's ability to direct their attention towards the unattended side. These include using visual cues, visual scanning training, using the light-house strategy, or mirror therapy. Bottom-up interventions require less patient awareness of the deficit and involve manipulating a patient's sensory environment to improve the automatic unconscious attentional processes. Bottom-up interventions include prism adaptation therapy, optokinetic stimulation, vestibular and galvanic stimulation, and mirror therapy.

It is also important to modify the environment to reduce the impact of neglect. This may involve arranging the environment to encourage scanning towards the neglected side, positioning objects within the attended side of a patient's visual field or using visual reminders.

Advances in technology, such as virtual reality and gaming platforms, are also being explored to facilitate neurorehabilitation of individuals with neglect (see Chap. 16). These platforms provide immersive and engaging experiences that seek to promote attention and spatial awareness.

4.3 The Oculomotor System

An important part of the visual system that has not been addressed in this chapter is the oculomotor system. As it is only the central part of the visual field that is processed at a high level of definition, eye movements are needed to ensure detailed processing of our surroundings. The oculomotor system is highly complex and controls various types of eye movements. Saccadic eye movements (fast "eye jumps") ensure that a stimulus is placed centrally in the visual field to allow high-definition processing. Smooth pursuit eye movements on the other hand ensure that fixation can be maintained on targets that move across the field of vision. The oculomotor system relies on the integrity of a wide range of functions that are localised throughout the brain. For example, the visual cortex, prefrontal cortex, frontal eye fields, supplementary eye fields, posterior parietal cortex, the cerebellum, and areas in the brainstem are all involved in the planning and execution of voluntary saccades. Oculomotor functions are often compromised after brain injury and deficits can have important consequences on how an individual perceives the world. To learn more about the oculomotor system read Horn & Leigh (2011).

4.4 Assessment of Brain-based Visual Impairments

When assessing vision, general principles of clinical assessment should be applied. The clinical assessment should be based on a combination of information from various sources including medical records, detailed history taking, observations of the patient's behaviour, as well as performance on tests. Medical records may include information about general neurologic and ophthalmologic history that can be particularly relevant for ensuring appropriate interpretation of the patient's visual deficits. Medical records may also provide insights as to when a patient's difficulties started and how they have progressed, which can be crucial for determining the aetiology of an impairment.

If visual impairments are suspected, history taking should include questions about some of the core aspects of vision including acuity, visual field, colour perception, visual overview of surroundings, vision in different lighting conditions, ability to recognise different types of stimuli such as objects and faces, as well as reading abilities. As patients often struggle to answer general questions about their abilities, concrete questions about specific situations should be preferred. For example, instead of asking a patient whether they have reading problems, the clinician can ask whether the patient has recently tried to read something, and if so, whether they in that specific situation could read at a similar pace as usual and with the same precision. It is also worth asking patients whether they have experienced falls or experienced bumping into things or people as this can be a sign of visual problems. It is important to be aware that insight (i.e. the patient's own knowledge, experience, or report of problems) can vary greatly in patients with visual impairments. Therefore, one cannot conclude that a patient has preserved vision solely because they do not report any symptoms. For instance, some patients with a complete homonymous hemianopia following stroke are totally unaware of their impairment and report no changes in their visual perception.

Observations of a patient's behaviour can give clues as to whether a patient has a visual impairment. Does the patient walk confidently from one location to another? Does the patient bump into things? Can the patient reach out to shake the clinician's hand or to grasp an object?

Behavioural tests are usually the main part of the clinical assessment for visual impairments. Before initiating assessment, it is worth asking the patient to describe their environment, to name some objects in the room and to read a simple bit of text. This can give a first impression of the extent of the impairments and help guide choice of tests.

Assessing sensory vision is a priority and includes the assessment of visual acuity and visual field. To ensure that results are not confounded by recognition problems, visual acuity tests that do not involve recognising letters or complex shapes should be the preferred choice. As visual field loss is common following posterior brain injury, a visual field assessment should be standard procedure for these patients. There are various types of visual field assessments available, ranging from confrontation testing to formal automated perimetry. Confrontation testing is the most common method for screening for visual field loss in neurological patients. It involves a clinician sitting opposite a patient and asking them to fix their gaze on the clinician's nose. The clinician then precedes to ask the patient to respond to stimuli presented in one of the four visual fields. This method is obviously highly accessible; however, it has limited precision and only provides information about the peripheral visual field. Automated perimetry tests are the Gold Standard and provide the most precise assessments. However, they can be challenging to perform with neurological patients with mobility problems or limited attentional capacity. In addition, access to such tests can be limited on neurological wards. As a compromise between the two methods, various computer-based visual field screening tests have been developed. Some of these tests, such as the computerised-Visual Field Test (Nordfang et al., 2019), can be administered on laptops at bedside making them more accessible for patients and staff. They are often shorter and easier to perform for patients with limited attentional capacity.

There are various test batteries available to assess visual impairments after brain injury. Some cover sensory and perceptual aspects of vision while others focus on visual perceptual and visual spatial impairments. Specific tests of intermediate visual perceptual processes such as perceptual integration and segmenting are also available. A wide range of tests to assess specific functions such as colour perception, face recognition, and reading also exist. As the manifestation of visual impairments can be highly individual, the use of a whole test battery is rarely relevant. More often, selecting a subset of tests is more appropriate (Gerlach & Robotham, 2021).

Assessing visual abilities in patients with other impairments such as aphasia or visuo-spatial neglect can be challenging. In patients with aphasia, tests involving matching tasks or multiple-choice response may be preferred. When assessing visual perception in patients with visuo-spatial neglect / visual attentional disorders, tasks in which stimuli that are presented vertically rather than horizontally or one at a time in the non-neglected side are preferred.

4.5 Rehabilitation of Brain-based Visual Impairments

Spontaneous improvement of visual perceptual functions is common after brain injury. However, patients rarely regain their full visual abilities.

This means that the majority of patients have some persistent visual perceptual impairments. Research into interventions to restore visual perceptual functions is limited. Many clinicians have designed their own rehabilitation strategies based on clinical experience, but there is little research evaluating the effectiveness of such interventions. Consequently, there are no evidence-based professional guidelines for rehabilitation of brain-based visual perceptual impairments. This chapter covers the somewhat limited interventions described in the scientific literature. When the evidence-base is lacking, suggestions are provided for rehabilitation strategies based on the understanding of the visual system and the specific visual perceptual condition.

4.5.1 Hemianopia

Some spontaneous recovery of hemianopia can occur in the first months after a brain injury. However, patients rarely make a full recovery, and most are left with visual field deficit. Peli prisms are small prisms that are attached to a patient's glasses as a form of substitutive treatment. The prisms move the missing portion of the visual field towards the centre of a patient's vision. Patients need time to get used to these glasses before they can benefit from them, and only some patients find them useful. Producing prisms is costly, making them difficult to get hold of. The most promising compensatory rehabilitation option for hemianopia is visual scanning training. In visual scanning training, patients learn to make eye movements to their blind visual field to bring it into view. Traditionally this has been administered as paper and pen training in which a patient must search for specific words on a page or find post-it notes on the walls of a long corridor. More recently, however, various computerised scanning training programs that patients can complete at home have become available. These programs either focus on improving reading or improving spotting items on the screen (visual search). Regardless of the format used, it seems like intense repetition is the key to success. To benefit from the training, patients are expected to practice several times per week for several months. Although promising, the evidence supporting these programs is still limited, and the extent to which the training effects generalise to everyday tasks such as reading a book or finding the salt on the table remains unclear. There is some evidence that vision therapy including saccadic training can improve some aspects of visual awareness in real life (Smaakjær et al., 2018). For a detailed review of rehabilitation of visual field impairments see Leff and Barton (2021).

4.5.2 Hallucinations

There are a few reports available of individual patients being successfully treated with medication for their visual hallucinations after visual field loss. Although the patients described improved over a few days or weeks, it is unclear whether they improved due to the medication or spontaneously as hallucinations commonly disappear in the first few weeks after a brain injury. In other words, there is no strong evidence that medication helps patients with hallucinations. As mentioned earlier, there is a lack of awareness related to hallucinations following visual field impairments. It is therefore important to explain to all patients with visual field loss that hallucinations are common after a brain injury, as this knowledge can in itself be reassuring for patients. Similarly, informing patients that the hallucinations typically reduce over time and might eventually disappear is usually sufficient to reduce distress and worry. Hallucinations rarely interfere with daily activities, so most patients do not require further interventions (Hazelton et al., 2022).

4.5.3 Ventral and Dorsal Stream Disorders

It is not always possible to diagnose specific ventral and dorsal visual stream disorders in an individual patient because the conditions often overlap and interact. Rehabilitation is therefore rarely focused on one specific disorder, instead covers a range of visual perceptual issues that are addressed collectively. The few intervention case studies available describe individually tailored rehabilitation programmes. Interventions aimed at restoring the visual functions include therapist led table-top tasks like drawing complex geometrical figures, matching colours, sorting sticks, or building mosaics. Other interventions are more physical like balance training in a virtual environment. Neurofeedback has recently been gaining research interest too. There are indications that neurofeedback training in visual attention and physical interventions might improve visual perception skills, but the evidence is of very low quality. In addition, evidence that the trained skills lead to improvements in daily life is lacking. For reviews of rehabilitation of visual impairments after brain injury read Hazelton et al. (2022) and Leff and Barton (2021).

For agnosia, compensation strategies are currently the recommended approach. Patients are advised to use other senses like touch to recognise objects. Contextual information, such as the location, time of day, and surrounding sounds, can all support the patient in recognising objects in daily life. For instance, it might be easier for a patient to recognise a cup when they are in a café at 10 am than recognising that same cup on a shelf in a large department store. Using memory actively can also be an important strategy. Patients are usually more independent in their own environment compared to unfamiliar surroundings. Useful advice can be to keep objects in fixed places in the house, like keys on a hook near the door. Some patients will have some preserved visual functions that enable them to compensate for their difficulties in recognising objects. For instance, in a patient with intact colour vision, colour coding sharp objects in the kitchen with some red tape might prevent them from cutting themselves on a knife. Read more about rehabilitation of visual agnosia in Heutink et al. (2019).

Interventions aiming to improve face recognition abilities in cases with prosopagnosia have generally not been particularly successful. For example, intense training with a set of faces has been demonstrated to lead to limited improvements in recognising the trained faces in a test setting. However, it had no impact on face recognition in daily life. Compensatory strategies are commonly used spontaneously by patients with prosopagnosia that do not have more general visual recognition impairments, and these may include recognizing people by their voice or gait, distinctive features like scars or moles, or more changeable aspects like hairdos or clothing style. For instance, Peter, the patient presented in the introduction of the chapter, described that his wife wore very distinctive glasses to make herself more easily recognisable. Wearing brightly coloured clothing or agreeing on a very specific meeting place will also help a patient with prosopagnosia. For this condition, psychoeducation of the patient and people in the patient's environment (e.g. family, friends, and colleagues) can make a big difference. For example, encouraging people to introduce themselves to the patient on every occasion may help avoid socially awkward situations. For more about rehabilitation of prosopagnosia see Leff and Barton (2021) or Heutink et al. (2019).

Patients with pure alexia commonly show some degree of spontaneous recovery, but rarely regain fluent reading even following compensatory of restorative training. Some find compensatory strategies like apps that read text out loud helpful. Others can benefit to some degree from restorative techniques tailored to the severity of their reading impairment. This also holds for patients with hemianopic alexia, where a visual field deficit impairs fluent reading. For more on rehabilitation of alexia, see Leff and Starrfelt (2014).

Rehabilitation for simultanagnosia should also be multi-faceted with aspects of psychoeducation, building on strengths in other domains (e.g. memory, touch), and training in everyday life. Compensation strategies are currently the recommended approach. Especially decluttering can make it easier for patients with simultanagnosia to perceive their environment. This means avoiding patterned curtains, wallpaper, or clothes and removing objects like paintings, pictures, or ornaments from the living space. This is especially important in a work setting where, e.g.

open space offices can make it very challenging for an individual with simultanagnosia to focus on their work. Similarly, reducing competition from other senses such as noise and smells can help so the patient does not waste resources on processing background noise. Keeping regularly used objects in fixed places will also highly benefit a patient with simultanagnosia. Furthermore, verbal cueing can support a patient in directing their attention to a particular object. For instance, a patient with simultanagnosia was trained to take the lift down to the garden in her care home by letting her talk through the different steps while finding her way. Saying "now I need to find the lift button. It is round, shiny, and at the same height as my hip" helped her to detect the button amongst many other visual stimuli. Read more about rehabilitation of dorsal steam disorders in Heutink et al. (2019).

Taken together, there is currently limited evidence for restorative interventions for visual perception conditions after a brain injury. This means that the current advice is to use compensatory strategies that can substitute the lost visual capacities. The two key strategies are making adaptations to the environment and relying on other senses. It is important to note that a patient rarely has one condition only and impairments can interact. Rehabilitation therefore needs to be tailored specifically to the patient. To maximise coping and confidence of the patient, rehabilitation should build upon their strengths.

Review Questions

- If a patient has a right homonymous hemianopia after a stroke, where is their lesion in the brain?
- What kind of impairments can be caused by damage to the ventral pathway?
- If a patient with posterior stroke has normal visual acuity and no visual field deficit, can it be assumed that their visual functions are fully preserved?

References

Bartolomeo, P. (2021). Color vision deficits. *Current Neurology and Neuroscience Reports, 21*(10), 58. https://doi.org/10.1007/s11910-021-01137-8

Bartolomeo, P. (2022). Chapter 10—Visual objects and their colors. In G. Miceli, P. Bartolomeo, & V. Navarro (Eds.), *Handbook of clinical neurology* (Vol. 187, pp. 179–189). Elsevier. https://doi.org/10.1016/B978-0-12-823493-8.00022-5

Danckert, J., Striemer, C., & Rossetti, Y. (2021). Chapter 16—Blindsight. In J. J. S. Barton & A. Leff (Eds.), *Handbook of clinical neurology* (Vol. 178, pp. 297–310). Elsevier. https://doi.org/10.1016/B978-0-12-821377-3.00016-7

Fraser, C. L., & Lueck, C. J. (2021). Chapter 17—Illusions, hallucinations, and visual snow. In J. J. S. Barton & A. Leff (Eds.), *Handbook of clinical neurology* (Vol. 178, pp. 311–335). Elsevier. https://doi.org/10.1016/B978-0-12-821377-3.00014-3

Gallivan, J. P., & Goodale, M. A. (2018). Chapter 23—The dorsal "action" pathway. In G. Vallar & H. B. Coslett (Eds.), *Handbook of clinical neurology* (Vol. 151, pp. 449–466). Elsevier. https://doi.org/10.1016/B978-0-444-63622-5.00023-1

Gerlach, C., & Robotham, R. J. (2021). Chapter 9—Object recognition and visual object agnosia. In J. J. S. Barton & A. B. T. H. O. C. N. Leff (Eds.), *Handbook of clinical neurology* (Vol. 178, pp. 155–173). Elsevier. https://doi.org/10.1016/B978-0-12-821377-3.00008-8

Goodale, M. A., & Milner, A. D. (1992). Separate visual pathways for perception and action [Review] [61 refs]. *Trends in Neurosciences, 15*(I), 20–25. https://doi.org/10.1016/0166-2236(92)90344-8

Hazelton, C., Thomson, K., Todhunter-Brown, A., Campbell, P., Chung, C. S., Dorris, L., Gillespie, D. C., Hunter, S. M., McGill, K., Nicolson, D. J., Williams, L. J., & Brady, M. C. (2022). Interventions for perceptual disorders following stroke. *Cochrane Database of Systematic Reviews, 11*(11), CD007039. https://doi.org/10.1002/14651858.CD007039.pub3

Heutink, J., Indorf, D. L., & Cordes, C. (2019). The neuropsychological rehabilitation of visual agnosia and Balint's syndrome. *Neuropsychological Rehabilitation, 29*(10), 1489–1508. https://doi.org/10.1080/09602011.2017.1422272

Horn, A. K. E., & Leigh, R. J. (2011). Chapter 2—The anatomy and physiology of the ocular motor system. In C. Kennard & R. J. Leigh (Eds.), *Handbook of clinical neurology* (Vol. 102, pp. 21–69). Elsevier. https://doi.org/10.1016/B978-0-444-52903-9.00008-X

Iaria, G., & Slone, E. (2021). Chapter 11—The relationship between mental and physical space and its impact on topographical disorientation. In J. J. S. Barton & A. Leff (Eds.), *Handbook of clinical neurology* (Vol.

178, pp. 195–211). Elsevier. https://doi.org/10.1016/B978-0-12-821377-3.00009-X

Leff, A., & Barton, J. J. S. (2021). Chapter 19—Rehabilitation of visual disorders. In J. J. S. Barton & A. Leff (Eds.), *Handbook of clinical neurology* (Vol. 178, pp. 361–386). Elsevier. https://doi.org/10.1016/B978-0-12-821377-3.00015-5

Leff, A., & Starrfelt, R. (2014). *Alexia: Diagnosis, treatment and theory*. Springer London. https://doi.org/10.1007/978-1-4471-5529-4

Nordfang, M., Uhre, V., Robotham, R. J., Kerry, S. J., Frederiksen, J. L., & Starrfelt, R. (2019). A free and simple computerized screening test for visual field defects. *Scandinavian Journal of Psychology, 60*(4), 289–294. https://doi.org/10.1111/sjop.12546

Pisella, L., Vialatte, A., Khan, A. Z., & Rossetti, Y. (2021). Chapter 13—Bálint syndrome. In J. J. S. Barton & A. Leff (Eds.), *Handbook of clinical neurology* (Vol. 178, pp. 233–255). Elsevier. https://doi.org/10.1016/B978-0-12-821377-3.00011-8

Smaakjær, P., Tødten, S. T., & Rasmussen, R. S. (2018). Therapist-assisted vision therapy improves outcome for stroke patients with homonymous hemianopia alone or combined with oculomotor dysfunction. *Neurological Research, 40*(9), 752–757. https://doi.org/10.1080/01616412.2018.1475321

Starrfelt, R., & Barton, J. J. S. (2022). Prosopagnosia. In S. Della Sala (Ed.), *Encyclopedia of behavioral neuroscience* (2nd ed., pp. 597–604). Elsevier. https://doi.org/10.1016/B978-0-12-819641-0.00047-5

Starrfelt, R. & Woodhead, Z. (2021). Reading and alexia. In: Barton, J.J.S. & Leff, A.P. (Eds). *Handbook of Clinical Neurology*, (Vol. 178, pp 213-232). Elsevier. https://doi.org/10.1016/B978-0-12-821377-3.00010-6

Vallar, G., & Ronchi, R. (2022). Unilateral spatial neglect. In S. Della Sala (Ed.), *Encyclopedia of behavioral neuroscience* (2nd ed., pp. 605–618). Elsevier. https://doi.org/10.1016/B978-0-12-819641-0.00144-4

Sensorimotor Control

5

Jens Bo Nielsen and Carmelo Bellardita

Abstract

This chapter offers an overview of the neurobiology of human movement. The functions of specific areas and sites within the nervous system and how their integrative action ensures various aspects of movement will be described. A sequential approach will be adopted, commencing with the muscle and spinal cord, progressing through the brain stem and descending motor tracts, the motor cortex, and finally the basal ganglia and the cerebellum. While this may suggest serial processing, it is essential to recognize that the processing underlying human movements relies on parallel and integrated activities within and between the networks. The chapter concludes with a synthesis of the different elements and a description of how three critical movement behaviors are generated: reaching and grasping, balance and posture, and locomotion. Throughout the text, the implications of basic neurobiology in the context of neurorehabilitation will be emphasized.

Keywords

Movement neuroscience · Reflexes · Voluntary movements · Muscles · Spinal cord and brain stem function · Locomotion · Balance and postural control · Basal ganglia · Cerebellum

J. B. Nielsen (✉) · C. Bellardita
Department of Neuroscience, University of Copenhagen, Copenhagen, Denmark
e-mail: jbnielsen@sund.ku.dk; cbellardita@sund.ku.dk

Box 5.1 Case Story

Jenny suffered a stroke the day after her 70th year birthday, which left her with severe paresis on the left side of her body. MR showed an infarct corresponding to the right internal capsule. Jenny was initially unable to stand up and maintain balance so remained in bed for the next 2 days. Encouraged by the physical therapists at the neurorehabilitation unit and with their initial help, she gradually found a way to maintain balance and walk slowly back and forth to the bathroom. Over the next weeks, although she remained weak and unable to feel and sense most of the left side of her body, she regained many of her abilities and managed to walk further and for a longer time. At the same time, she experienced that she would feel stiff in the early morning and in cold weather and that her muscles would often feel as if they tensed up without her intent. When she complained about this to her medical doctor, she was prescribed antispastic medication on the assumption that her symptoms were caused by spasticity. This made her feel more relaxed, but at the same time she also felt drowsy during most of the day, and she found that she quickly became tired when physically active and therefore ended up spending most of the day sitting down. Her functional recovery proceeded slowly, but 2 years later she was still unable to walk for longer distances and she was

(continued)

J. B. Nielsen et al. (eds.), *Neuroplasticity-based Neurorehabilitation*,
https://doi.org/10.1007/978-3-031-81120-3_5

Box 5.1 (continued)
unable to use her left hand except for support in tasks done primarily by the right hand. She therefore mostly stayed confined in her home except when her daughter visited and took her out in a wheelchair.

5.1 Introduction

When the early morning craving for a cup of coffee strikes, it takes little conscious effort for most people before they find themselves gradually waking up with the cup in their hand. Regardless of the preferred coffee-making method, the brain is an experienced guide through the necessary steps, just as it has done on countless mornings before. Once the idea of "coffee" has come to mind, the brain handles all the complex neural processes involved in planning which muscles to activate for each movement and ensuring that they are active at the right time and with the right intensity. Rarely do things go wrong, leading to accidental scalding with the warm coffee.

This is the hallmark of a well-functioning brain in an adult. After years of learning from mistakes during childhood and youth (remember all those spilled glasses of soda?), adults can fully appreciate the luxury of having a nervous system that responds precisely and efficiently to every command. This liberates cognitive resources that allow thinking of other things (or nothing at all) while brewing and drinking the coffee. This automatization of subprocesses in overlearned actions and thoughts is referred to as schemas in a cognitive neuropsychological framework (see Chap. 9).

The ease with which movements are made should not be taken for granted. The ability to make movements with little effort relies on the integrated coordination of neural networks spanning the entire nervous system, from the cortex to the muscles and back. This system of interrelated networks is remarkably adaptable and resilient, capable of finding efficient solutions to disruptions by reorganizing activities within the networks. However, there are also numerous points where things can go awry, evident from the wide array of injuries that necessitate neurorehabilitation. Whether a central, peripheral, motor, or sensory injury is involved, one of the primary consequences remains consistent: movements are no longer effortless but require conscious control and effort. The subjective experience of patients undergoing neurorehabilitation is more than anything that movement is difficult—if not impossible—and that it requires tremendous conscious resources and attention. That cup of coffee in the morning may become a high mountain to climb.

This chapter will describe the various neural pathways involved in movement and how their disruption results in movement disorders that necessitate neurorehabilitation. Although the networks are highly integrated and the motor areas are tightly coupled to sensory areas, a serial approach will be retained starting with the muscles and spinal reflex mechanisms, proceed with the control of movements by the primary motor cortex and end up with the initiation, planning, and optimization of movement by cortical and subcortical networks including the premotor areas, basal ganglia, and cerebellum. At the end of the chapter, these different parts will be brought together in an integrative description of three different movement abilities: (1) Posture and balance, (2) locomotion, and (3) reaching and grasping.

Box 5.2 Anatomy
The primary motor cortex (M1) is depicted in Fig. 5.1, responsible for initiating and executing voluntary movements. Adjacent areas such as the supplementary motor area (SMA) and premotor cortex (PMC) contributing to motor planning and coordination are also shown in Fig. 5.1. The connections between these cortical regions and the spinal cord, represented by the descending corticospinal tract (CST), facilitate the transmission of motor commands to the muscles, depicted in 5.6B. Additionally, subcortical structures including the basal ganglia (Fig. 5.7) and cerebellum, form loops with the cortex to modulate and refine motor output. These subcortical loops play crucial roles in motor learning, coordination, and

(continued)

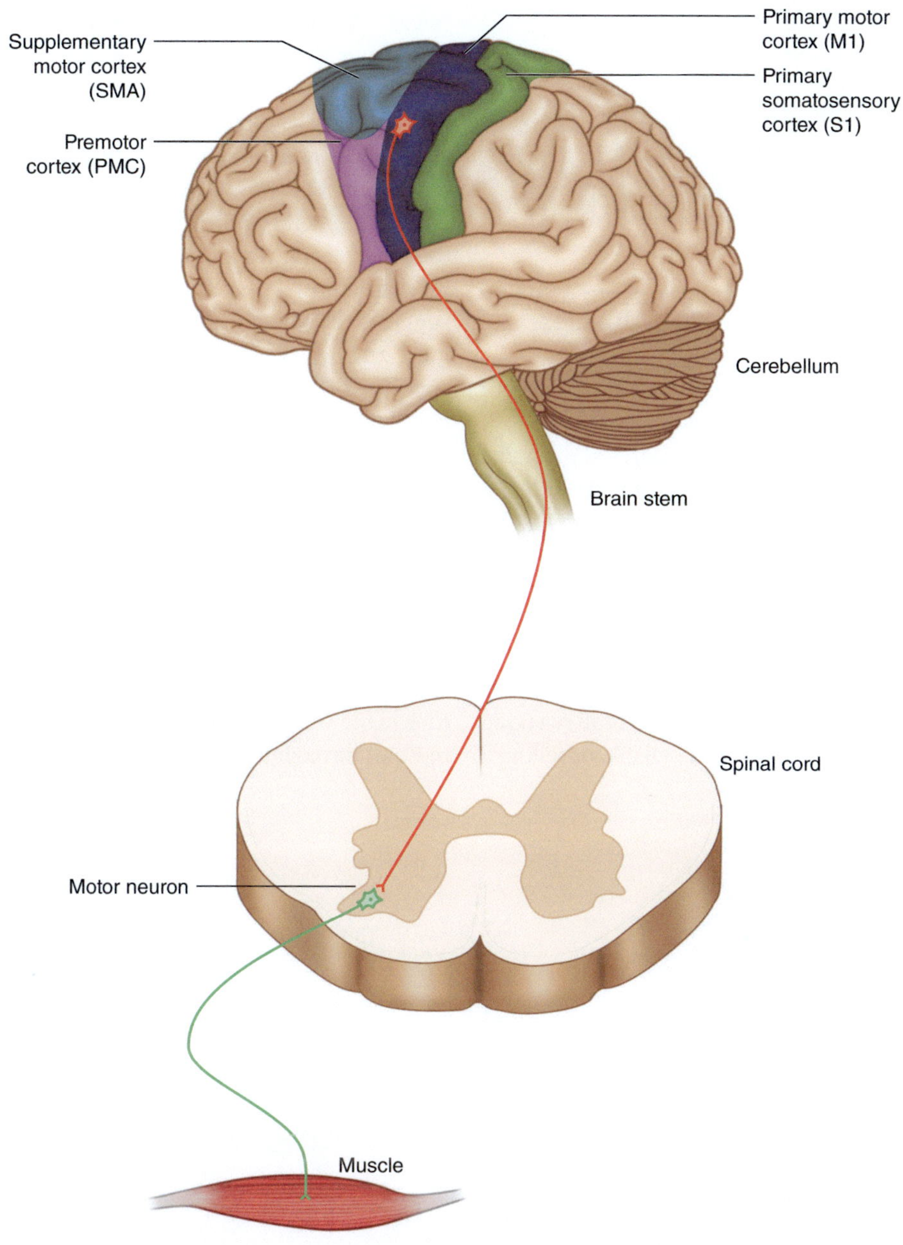

Fig. 5.1 Cortical areas involved in sensorimotor control. The somatosensory cortex (SI) in the postcentral gyrus is marked in green, the primary motor cortex (M1) in the precentral gyrus is marked in blue, the premotor cortex (PMC) in purple and the supplementary motor cortex (SMA) in turquoise. The connection from M1 to the spinal motor neuron is shown schematically in red and the motor neuron in green

Box 5.2 (continued)
the regulation of movement parameters. The brainstem serves as a relay center, integrating motor signals from higher brain regions and coordinating basic motor functions such as posture and balance.

5.2 The Prime Mover—Muscles

Skeletal muscles are specialized to convert the neural command from the nervous system into movement that can exert a mechanical force on the skeleton and allow interaction with the external world. Skeletal muscles allow walking and running, to reach out and grasp objects, manipulate objects with hands and fingers, to eat and drink, and to express the deepest feelings and thoughts through language—spoken or written. Charles Sherrington (1857–1952) expressed the importance of muscles in his famous quote, "to move things is all mankind can do—whether whispering a syllable or felling a forest". Without muscles we would be isolated within our brain—a fate that strikes people with locked-in syndrome following complete spinal cord injuries or amyotrophic lateral sclerosis.

Muscles use molecular mechanisms to create movement that are remarkably similar to those used by unicellular organisms that move through the water using undulating movements of a tail-like structure, a flagellum (Brunet, 2023). This suggests that the ability to move has ancient origins, tracing back to before the last common ancestor of all animals. Muscles are formed by bundles of single muscle fibers (muscle cells), which contain filaments (called actin and myosin) that are able to slide actively by each other and thereby pull at each end of the muscle fiber and make it shorter (Fig. 5.2).

Muscle contraction requires that many muscle fibers within the muscle shorten at the same time. This is ensured by the neural activation of the muscle fibers. The axons of individual motor neurons in the ventral horn of the spinal cord reach the muscles through the peripheral nerves and split up

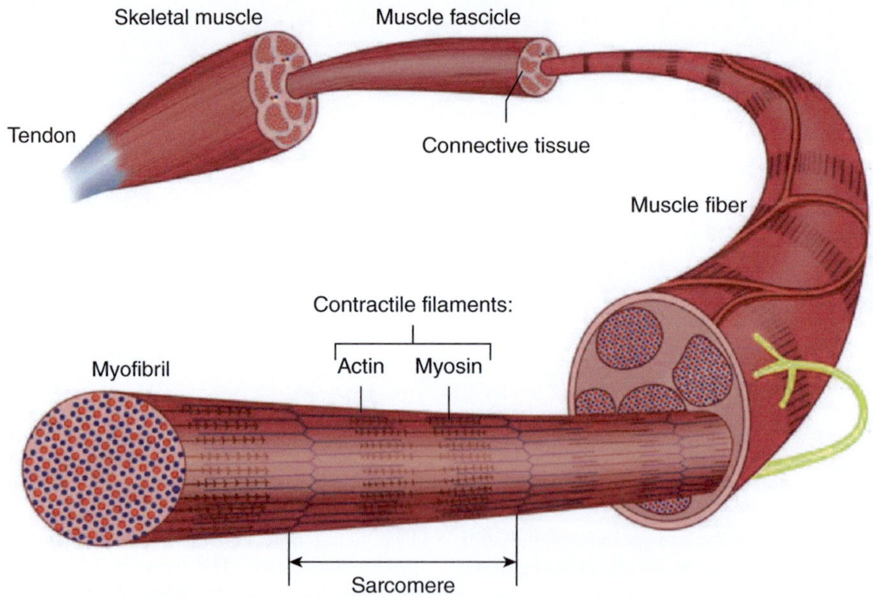

Fig. 5.2 The structure of a skeletal muscle
This figure depicts a muscle bundle with muscle fibers and myofibrils. Muscle fibers, represented by elongated structures, are organized into bundles, each containing multiple individual muscle cells. Within each muscle fiber, myofibrils are visible as densely packed, thread-like structures running parallel to the length of the fiber. Myofibrils consist of repeating units called sarcomeres, which contain contractile proteins responsible for muscle contraction. The alternating dark and light bands within sarcomeres represent the arrangement of thick (myosin) and thin (actin) filaments, respectively, giving rise to the striated appearance of skeletal muscle. Together, the organization of muscle fibers and myofibrils enables the efficient transmission of force generated during muscle contraction, facilitating movement and locomotion

in collaterals that innervate a multitude of muscle fibers (from 10 in small muscles to more than 1000 in large muscles). The motor neuron and the muscle fibers that it innervates form the functional unit of a muscle: the motor unit (Fig. 5.3). Each muscle fiber receives only a single collateral from the motor neuron. In this way, an action potential in the motor neuron reaches all the muscle fibers that the motor neuron innervates and ensures that all the muscle fibers of the motor unit shorten at the same time. Muscle contraction and movement require the coordinated activation of a number of motor units. In contrast, the shortening of an individual motor unit is insufficient to produce any real contraction and movement, and it is referred to as fasciculation or a small twitch of a part of a muscle. Sporadic activation of motor units is usually quite harmless, but it may also be indicative of an early sign of amyotrophic lateral sclerosis, where dying motor neurons discharge and cause muscle twitches without coordinated central neural control.

The size of a muscle contraction in relation to a voluntary movement is scaled both by how much the muscle fibers in individual motor units shorten when they are activated and by the number of motor units that are active. The shortening of the muscle fibers in individual motor units depends on the rate of the action potentials in the motor neuron. The higher the rate, the more the filaments in the muscle fiber pull on each other and the more the muscle fiber is shortened.

Motor units can be functionally categorized into slow motor units, fast-resistant motor units, and fast-fatigable motor units. The recruitment of these different motor unit types during a movement follows a strict order that relates to the type of motor unit—the so-called Henneman size principle (Gordon et al., 2004). Slow motor units, corresponding to type I motor units, are activated first during muscle contraction. They have motor neurons that are small and discharge at relatively low rates (Fig. 5.3). The corresponding muscle fibers (often called red muscle fibers) are also small and contain relatively few contractile filaments. They are therefore not able to produce force very much, which ensures that we can control and grade muscle force appropriately. They also contract slowly (the contractile filaments in the muscle fibers are slow in making contact with each other and especially releasing them again) and have high endurance due to a high capacity of using oxygen to generate energy from glucose. These features render type I motor units perfectly suited for maintaining low-intensity contractions over extended periods. This is also the likely reason why the ankle plantar flexor muscle, the soleus muscle, almost only contains type I motor units. When we stand the soleus muscle is almost constantly active to help us maintain an upright position. In contrast, the fast-resistant (type IIa) and fast-fatigable (type IIx) motor units, often associated with white muscle fibers, include larger motor neurons that fire at higher frequencies and muscle fibers with a greater number of contractile filaments. This configuration allows them to produce significantly more force and contract more rapidly, making them ideal for generating high forces swiftly. Type IIa fibers demonstrate some level of endurance, able to sustain activity by partially relying on aerobic energy production. However, type IIx fibers fatigue quickly due to their limited capacity for generating energy aerobically, relying instead on anaerobic processes that quickly deplete energy reserves. Consequently, type IIx motor units are typically engaged only for short durations during intense and rapid movements, reflecting their specialization for quick, powerful actions.

The corresponding characteristics of motor neurons and muscle fibers within a motor unit are essential for the functionality of the muscle and its ability to translate the neural signals from the nervous system into purposeful movements. This correspondence is partly achieved through chemical signals exchanged between the motor neuron and the muscle fiber. However, the activity level of the motor neuron plays a key role. The low rate of activity in the type I motor neurons triggers the development of type I muscle fiber. This results in the activation of specific genes that lead to the production of the contractile filaments and other proteins that characterize the type I muscle fibers. Conversely, the high rate of activity in type II motor neurons induces the characteristic properties of type II muscle fibers by activating a "type II genetic program" in the muscle fibers (Lomo et al., 1974).

The neural activity combined with mechanical (resistance), and metabolic (nutrients, hormones)

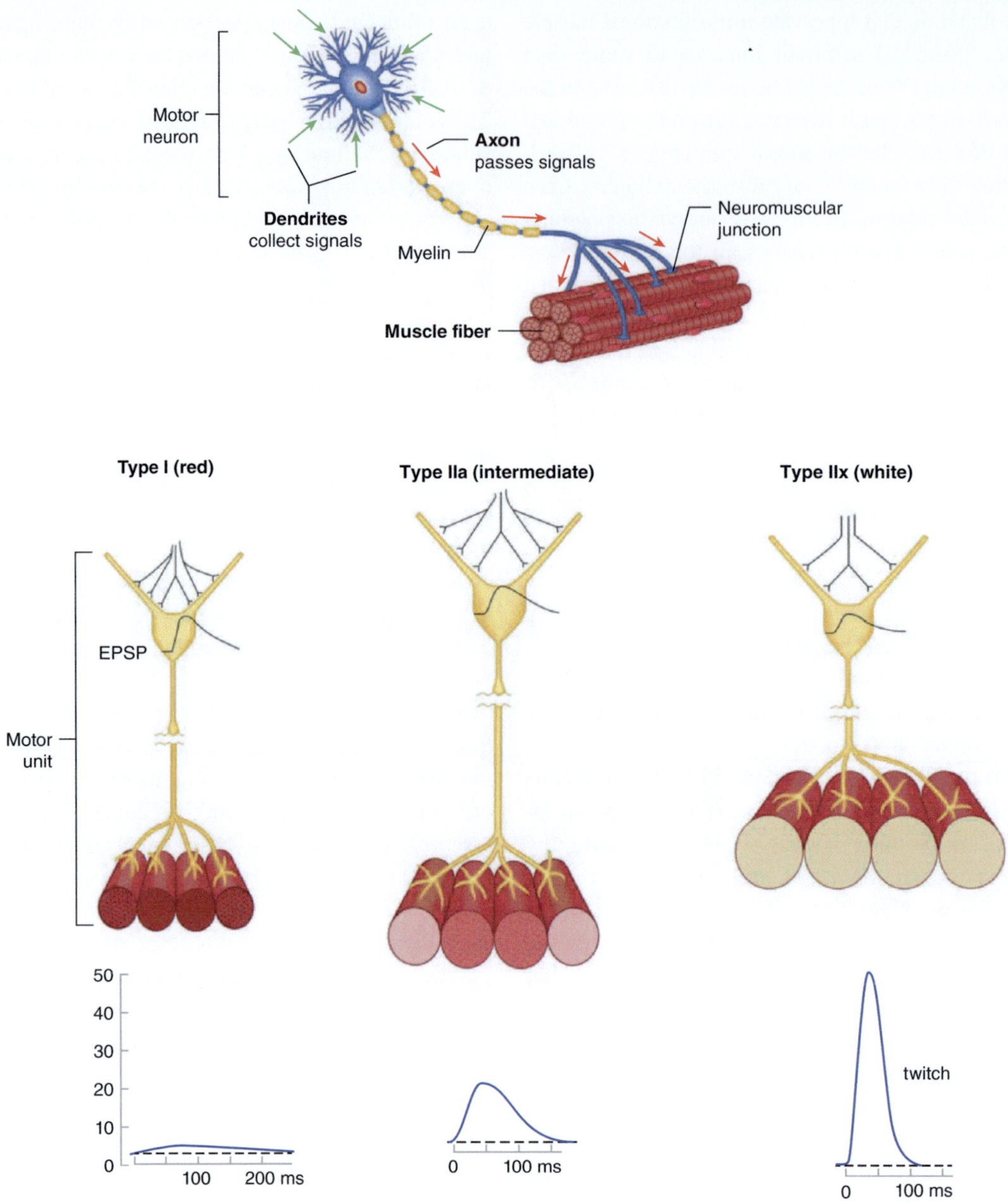

Fig. 5.3 Motor unit and properties
This figure illustrates the organization of a motor unit and provides a graphical representation of different motor unit types in humans. Each motor unit consists of a motor neuron and the muscle fibers it innervates. Motor neurons are depicted as neuron-shaped structures with dendrites extending toward the muscle fibers and axons connecting to them. The size of the motor neuron and the number of muscle fibers it innervates are represented proportionally, with larger motor neurons innervating a greater number of muscle fibers (large motor units) and smaller motor neurons innervating fewer muscle fibers (small motor units). Additionally, different motor unit types are depicted, including slow-twitch (type I) and fast-twitch (type II) motor units. Type I motor neurons, characterized by smaller cell bodies, receive stronger synaptic input compared to type II motor neurons, as depicted in the figure. They are recruited first in voluntary movements due to their lower activation threshold. Slow-twitch motor units, represented by type I motor units, are characterized by a slow contraction speed and high resistance to fatigue, making them well-suited for sustained contractions and endurance activities. In contrast, fast-twitch motor units, represented by type II motor units, exhibit rapid contraction and fatigue more quickly, making them suitable for generating rapid bursts of force. The combination of motor unit size, type, synaptic input strength, and cell body size contributes to the fine control and coordination of muscle activity required for various motor tasks

signals also induce the growth of the muscle fibers. With the use of muscles—and especially with strength training—the production of contractile filaments increases, empowering muscle fibers to significantly improve their the force generation capabilities. An increase in the number of contractile filaments lying in parallel within the fiber and pulling together at each end of the muscle fiber leads to a larger diameter of the muscle fibers. When muscles become larger and stronger in relation to training, this is therefore not because there are more muscle fibers, but because the individual muscle fibers become larger and contain more contractile filaments.

Conversely, the production of contractile filaments decreases when muscles are not used. The muscle fiber becomes thinner and weaker and eventually, muscle atrophy is observed. This is evident in spending days, weeks, or even months in bed due to disease, or when the muscles are not used to their full extent due to casting or other means of immobilization following bone fractures and other injuries. However, muscle atrophy and weakness are particularly pronounced and have the most significant functional impact on individuals with brain and spinal cord injuries. The muscles quickly react to the lack of neural activation following lesions that affect the motor system at either spinal or supraspinal level. Changes in gene expression of the muscles in response to the lack of neural activation have been determined already a few hours following spinal cord injury and structural and functional changes in the muscle fibers are measurable already one day later. This highlights the importance of initiating early mobilization in people with brain and spinal cord injury as soon as it is practically feasible after injury.

Muscle atrophy and muscle weakness are, however, not the only consequences of the reduced neural activation and use of muscles following brain and spinal cord injury. In complete spinal cord injured subjects almost all muscle fibers have been shown to be type II fibers (Biering-Sorensen et al., 2009). This is because the "default" genetic program that is activated in the absence of neural activation is the "type II program." This change in fiber type results from a functional adaptation to help muscles maintain force as the type II fibers are stronger than the type I fibers. However, at the same time, they are also fatigable and therefore contribute to increased muscle fatigue following brain and spinal cord injuries.

The muscle and its surroundings also respond in other ways to lack of neural activation and lack of use. The muscle fibers are surrounded by connective tissue, which ensures the structural stability of the muscle, and facilitate the transfer of the contraction of the muscle fibers into pulling of the tendon that the muscle is attached to. Reduced or absent neural activation of the muscles—combined with changes in mechanical and metabolic stimuli—following brain and spinal cord injury, quickly leads to increased production of connective tissue around the muscle fibers. This is especially the case if the muscle fibers are under constant tension due to immobilization in a position different from the neutral position of the joint. Unfortunately, this extra connective tissue is less elastic than what is found in healthy, active muscles and quickly leads to a reduced muscle's range of motion and flexibility. During a neurological examination, this condition appears as an increased resistance to joint movement, eventually leading to a reduced range of motion in the affected joint; that is, muscle contracture. Normally, the contractile filaments in the muscle fiber are only activated and contribute significantly to the resistance of the muscle when the motor neuron transmits an action potential. Yet, muscle contractures occur without any neural activation and they are accompanied by increased resistance to stretch of a muscle and reduced range of movement of the joint. This is primarily due to the accumulation of stiff connective tissue around the muscle fibers and a reduction in muscle fiber length which together results in the increased stiffness and reduced mobility. Therefore, the treatment should be directed against the accumulation of connective tissue by mobilizing the patient and facilitating normal use of the muscle. This treatment strengthens the muscle and improves motor control at the same time.

5.3 Spinal Control Mechanisms

The spinal motor neurons are located in the ventral horn of the spinal cord and send their axons through the peripheral nerves to innervate the muscles. Their activity and thereby the muscle contractions are determined by the integration of the neural activity in descending motor tracts from the cortex and brain stem, and sensory feedback from the muscles, tendons, joints, and skin, conveyed to the motor neurons either directly or through groups of spinal interneurons. The different segments of the spinal cord may be seen as evolutionarily ancient control units of the different parts of our body and especially our extremities. The neural populations and neural networks in these segments—and the communication between them—provides automatic control mechanisms that help to ensure that movements may be performed easily, precisely, and with little conscious effort.

5.3.1 The Stretch Reflex

The simplest of these networks is the monosynaptic stretch reflex (Fig. 5.4). Clinically the stretch reflex is used as part of the neurological examination to test spinal reflex excitability. Tapping a tendon with a hammer (for instance the patella tendon) elicits a reflex contraction of a muscle, for instance, the quadriceps muscle; that is, a knee jerk. The mechanism of this reflex or jerk is that stretch-sensitive receptors in the muscle (the muscle spindles illustrated in Fig. 2.2), are activated and transmit a barrage of action potentials in large-diameter sensory afferents (the Ia afferents) to the spinal cord where they synapse onto spinal motor neurons. If the barrage of action potentials is sufficiently large the spinal motor neurons will discharge and the muscle will contract. An absent or greatly reduced stretch reflex is seen following peripheral nerve lesions that interrupt the reflex circuitry or spinal cord

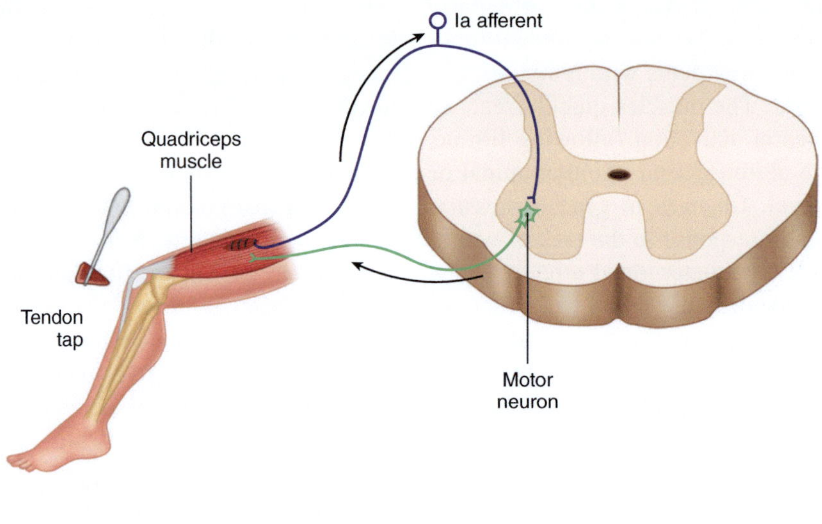

Fig. 5.4 The stretch reflex
This figure illustrates the knee jerk reflex, a monosynaptic Ia stretch reflex elicited by a tendon tap to the patella. The diagram depicts the key components involved in the reflex arc. When the patellar tendon is tapped, sensory neurons (Ia afferents) within the muscle spindle are stimulated, sending action potentials to the spinal cord via the dorsal root ganglion. In the spinal cord, these sensory neurons synapse directly onto alpha motor neurons in the ventral horn of the spinal cord. The alpha motor neurons then send efferent signals back to the muscle, causing contraction of the quadriceps muscle group

lesions that involve the spinal motor neurons tested by the reflex. Conversely, increased stretch reflexes (reflex hyperexcitability) are seen following lesions that involve the descending motor pathways, and this is usually taken as the characteristic sign of spasticity (see Box 5.3). The reflex hyperexcitability develops over weeks to months following the lesion and involves plastic changes in both the motor neurons themselves (upregulation of different receptors and membrane channels) and altered activity of inhibitory and excitatory spinal neurons that influence the motor neurons and their activation from the sensory afferents. Whereas the reflex hyperexcitability may be useful as a diagnostic tool in the neurological examination, it is doubtful whether it has any functional significance and can be used to guide treatment (Nielsen et al., 2020). There are three reasons for this. First, the reflex is hyperexcitable at rest but not during movement in patients with lesion of descending motor tracts (i.e., stroke, spinal cord injury, multiple sclerosis). Hyperexcitable reflexes are therefore not likely to be a functional problem for the patients. *Secondly,* the method used by doctors to test these reflexes, typically with a hammer, does not mimic how muscles are naturally activated during movements. During normal movements, the muscle spindles measure the stretch (or tension) in a muscle and are modulated by a specialized set of spinal motor neurons, the gamma motor neurons (see Chap. 2). The gamma motor neurons innervate the muscle spindles in parallel to the innervation of the muscle fibers by the alpha motor neurons. During movement alpha and gamma motor neurons are usually activated in parallel (Alpha-gamma co-activation). This ensures that the muscle spindles may provide feedback about muscle length (proprioception) throughout the movement and thereby through the reflex loop provide reinforcement of the activation of the muscle. This is referred to as automatic gain compensation and it consists of a positive feedback contribution similar to the servo mechanism that helps us steering the wheels in all modern cars. Because of this mechanism, less descending activation from the brain and hence less mental effort is necessary in order to move. If anything, the increased excitability of the stretch reflex following lesion of descending motor tracts may therefore be seen as a compensatory mechanism to facilitate the activation of the muscles further. It follows that diminishing the reflex through medication will make it even more difficult for a person with central motor lesion to activate the muscle than is the case due to the lesion. *Thirdly,* it is not only the monosynaptic stretch reflex that is activated by a tendon tap as part of the neurological examination. Muscle spindles have other sensory afferents than Ia afferents (called group II afferents—see Table 2.1) and these afferents are connected to specific groups of interneurons in the spinal cord which also influence the spinal motor neurons and contribute to the reflex contraction that is observed clinically. This is also the case of the Ia afferents, and the size of the muscle response thus also depends on the setting of these different neurons and neuronal networks in the spinal cord. Both Ia and II afferents also ascend in the dorsal columns (Fig. 2.3) and have connections to supraspinal neurons that may also be activated and contribute to the muscle response (transcortical reflexes). The knee jerk and the other reflexes elicited by a tendon tap are thus complex responses that are not easily interpreted.

5.3.2 Integrating Load- and Force Feedback to Control Movement

Hyperexcitable stretch reflexes may be perceived as a sudden resistance to movement of a joint during the neurological examination—a "catch." Often this catch is followed by a pronounced and sudden decrease in resistance- called a clasp-knife phenomenon. The clasp-knife phenomenon is also observed in case of lesion to the descending motor pathways and has historically been related to the activation of force-sensitive receptors in the tendons, the Golgi tendon organs (illustrated in Fig. 2.2). The sensory afferents from tendons trigger a reflex that acts in contrast to the stretch reflex, the inverse stretch reflex or autogenetic inhibition. This leads to the inhibition of the motor neurons supplying the muscle, suggesting that this reflex may support the clasp-knife phenomenon. However, it is now known that the clasp-knife phenomenon is more simply explained by the inactivation of the spinal motor neurons when a large part of them have been activated synchronously in the stretch reflex. It has been further discovered that the influence of force feedback from muscle tendon on the spinal cord is much more complex and that autogenetic inhibition plays a minimal or negligible role in both normal and abnormal movements. During normal gait, the Golgi tendon organ activation does not generate the autogenic inhibition, but instead, it provides excitation to the motor pool (Pearson et al., 1998). This means the feedback from tendon sensors helps to increase muscle activity, especially during critical phases of walking, such as when pushing the body forward. This is of fundamental functional importance in the control of gait. Tendon organs in the Achilles tendon sense the greatest amount of force, leading to the most significant activation when the Triceps surae muscles are active. Consequently, this causes a pull at the tendon while the foot is on the ground, supporting the weight of the body in the late stance phase of walking. The positive feedback from the tendon organs through the excitatory spinal pathways at this time in the gait cycle helps in pushing the body forward so that the center of gravity moves in front of the supporting leg. If not for the opposite leg, which has been swinging forward at the same time, this would result in falling. However, as soon as the opposite foot hits the ground and supports the body weight, activity of the force-sensitive tendon organs in the Achilles tendon rapidly declines, which helps to diminish activity in the Triceps surae muscles and initiate swing. When this positive feedback mechanism is not functioning optimally, which is the case in patients with lesions of the descending motor pathways, forward propulsion and transition between extension and flexion during gait become impaired. These same spinal circuits also integrate information from other types of sensors in muscles and joints, as well as from the skin, to automatically adjust leg muscle force to match the ground conditions during walking. This automatic adjustment is crucial for walking effortlessly across different surfaces without consciously thinking about each step. This is taken care of automatically by the sensorimotor reflex mechanisms built into the spinal cord neural circuitry. However, when these are not working appropriately following lesion of the descending motor pathways, significant conscious attention may be necessary, which will be experienced by the patient as having to devote much more effort to the simple task of walking than what is normally required. This may quickly lead to a much higher cognitive load and development of fatigue. Antispastic medication may be of little help in this relation.

5.3.3 Reciprocal Inhibition

More than one muscle is involved in the control of all our joints in order to allow us to make movements in different directions. Some of these muscles will inevitably pull in opposite directions and when one of the muscles contracts (the agonist), the opposite (antagonist) muscle will be stretched. Since all the muscles are equipped with muscle spindles, the stretch of the antagonist would result in a stretch reflex if not for one important mechanism: Reciprocal inhibition (Fig. 5.5). When we make a movement in one direction, spinal inhibitory neurons are activated to suppress both the sensory feedback signals from muscle spindles in the antagonist and the spinal motor neurons supplying the antagonist muscle themselves. This is possible because the descending motor fibers that activate agonist motor neurons have collaterals to the spinal neurons that inhibit the antagonist motor neurons.

Studies have repeatedly demonstrated that reciprocal inhibition is diminished in patients with lesions of the central motor pathways, and

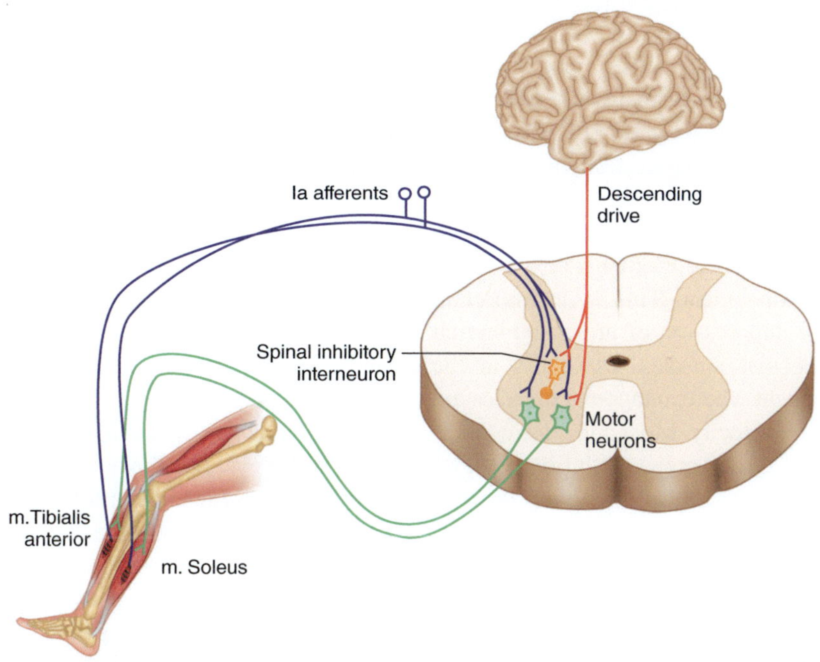

Fig. 5.5 Reciprocal inhibition
This figure illustrates reciprocal inhibition from ankle plantar flexors (m. soleus) to ankle dorsi flexors (m. tibialis anterior) via inhibitory interneurons in the spinal cord. Sensory afferents are represented in blue (or purple?) while motor neurons are depicted in green. Inhibitory interneurons responsible for mediating reciprocal inhibition are shown in orange. Additionally, descending control of interneurons and motor neurons through the corticospinal tract from the brain is depicted in red. This diagram demonstrates the neural circuitry underlying reciprocal inhibition, a mechanism by which the activation of one muscle group leads to the inhibition of antagonist muscle activity, contributing to coordinated movement and postural control

this may contribute to impaired coordination of muscles and increased co-activation of antagonists during standing and walking. However, a reduced reciprocal inhibition with a greater co-contraction of antagonist muscles may also be the result of a functional adaptation that results in stabilization of joints in patient with weak muscles. Studies have indeed demonstrated that reciprocal inhibition is reduced during co-contraction and that subjects who frequently use co-contraction of antagonists to maintain specific body positions, such as ballet dancers, show very little reciprocal inhibition (Nielsen, 1998). Interventions to diminish co-contraction should therefore be carefully considered in the individual patient.

5.3.4 Gating of Sensory Feedback and Reflex Activation

Reciprocal inhibition is not the only mechanism that prevents stretch reflexes in antagonist muscles at the onset of an agonist contraction. A distinct population of GABAergic neurons in the spinal cord specifically project to the terminals of the sensory afferents to modulate the release of neurotransmitters from the sensory terminals onto motor neurons. This form of regulation is called presynaptic inhibition to distinguish it from the postsynaptic inhibition exerted directly on the soma or dendrites of motor neurons. Presynaptic inhibition is an effective way of gating the effect of sensory feedback on the spinal motor neurons. During voluntary movements, presynaptic inhibition of sensory afferents from the muscle spindles of the active muscles is thus diminished, allowing the positive feedback to optimally facilitate the activation of the muscle. At the same time presynaptic inhibition of sensory afferents in antagonistic muscles is increased, preventing involuntary activation in response to stretch reflex or other reflexive activity during the movement. This is an important mechanism for suppression of unwanted stretch reflex in antagonist muscles, especially at the onset of movement where antagonist muscles are stretched at high velocity. Most antispastic medication increases GABAergic inhibition, leading to a general depression of reflex activity through presynaptic inhibition, among other processes. Unfortunately, this equally affects muscles that require suppression of stretch reflex activity (antagonists) and those that do not (agonists) during voluntary movement.

5.3.5 Withdrawal Reactions and Spinal Circuitries Mediating First-Order Pain Reactions

The retraction of a hand, which is accidentally put on a hot stove, usually happens so quickly that the pain is only realized later. The retraction of the hand is a complex reaction, but the initial part of the reaction is a well-defined spinal reflex also called the flexor reflex because it involves flexion of all joints in the limb to which a painful stimulus is applied. The reflex is seen in all animals with limbs and is well preserved through evolution. This highlights its functional importance in removing the limb away from harm. The reflex pathway involves a series of spinal neurons some of which excite flexor motor neurons and others inhibit extensor motor neurons controlling the limb. The axons of some of the neurons also cross the midline of the spinal cord and cause the opposite effects in that limb: Excitation of extensors and inhibition of flexors. This makes functional sense since it is necessary that at least one leg remains on the ground when one is withdrawn/lifted from a painful stimulus. It should be noted that in humans' withdrawal of one arm is never accompanied by extension of the other when we stand up—only when we crawl on all four. This illustrates that the withdrawal reaction is more complex than a simple hard-wired and stereotyped reflex. It is also highly context dependent and may be completely suppressed by will. This is possible because the spinal circuitry is tightly controlled by descending pathways from the brain stem and cortex and because supraspinal centers contribute to the functional withdrawal reaction.

In patients with lesions of the descending motor pathways, the flexor reflexes may consequently also become uncontrollable and hyperexcitable. This is especially the case in patients with complete spinal cord lesion, where even light touch of the skin may cause powerful flexor reflexes that develop into spasms. These may be painful and cause significant discomfort for the patient. At the same time, the flexor reflex and crossed extensor reflex circuitries are a fundamental part of the spinal circuitry, which generates the basic locomotor rhythm for walking and running. Treatment directed at suppressing unwanted flexor reflexes and spasms therefore needs to be balanced against a wish to recover gait function following brain and spinal cord injuries.

5.3.6 Spinal Locomotor Network

In animals with complete spinal cord lesion, stimulation of skin afferents easily elicits flexor reflexes similar to what is seen in patients with spinal cord injury. In the animals, the flexor reflexes are often followed by repeated bursts of alternating extension and flexion, which may involve all four limbs and develop into rhythmic alternating activity similar to that seen during locomotion. The spinal network of neurons responsible for this basic locomotor rhythm is often called the spinal central pattern generator (CPG) (Kiehn, 2006). In animals, it may be activated easily by stimulation in the brain stem (see next section), pharmacologically, or by providing sensory input from the moving belt of a treadmill. Animals with complete spinal cord transection thus produce functional locomotion when placed on a treadmill with a moving belt and even adapt the rhythmicity according to the speed or tilt of the treadmill. Although there is a similar CPG network in the human spinal cord, it is not as easily activated as in animals and requires supraspinal input in order to produce functional locomotor activity. Intensive gait training may promote considerable recovery of gait ability only if there is some minimal preservation of functional connection to the spinal cord from supraspinal centers. There is proof-of-concept that the effect of gait training may be enhanced pharmacologically by medication that increase the excitability of the spinal network such as a range of monoaminergic drugs as well as glutamate or by electrical stimulation of the spinal cord, either through the skin or through implanted electrodes (see Chap. 18). Despite promising reports of improvements in gait function following implantation of electrodes (Lorach et al., 2023), gait training on a treadmill or over ground with or without the help of robotic assistive devices is still the main approach to obtain functional recovery of gait in clinical practice. Future clinical studies will determine whether pharmacological interventions, spinal stimulation, or other forms of stimulation of the nervous system have sufficient beneficial effects to play a role also.

5.4 Brain Stem Motor Control Circuitries

The brain stem is a large brain area at the interface between supraspinal center involved in action planning, selection, and initiation and the spinal cord where the spinal neurons transform neural activity into body movements. The brainstem mediates the integration of sensory feedback from different modalities into descending motor commands to instruct spinal circuits in the generation of complex behavior. A large number of nuclei with excitatory neurons (glutamatergic), inhibitory neurons (GABA and Glycinergic), and modulatory neurons (monoamines) allow the brainstem to mediate and orchestrate the neural activity underlying a range of actions, from more stereotyped movements such as breathing and walking to more complex movements such as reaching, grasping and facial expression.

5.4.1 Breathing

The alternating inspiration and expiration of air through our airways, which ensures that oxygen reaches our bloodstream in exchange for CO_2, depends on the rhythmic activity of a network of neurons located in the brain stem. Three different centers have been identified with distinct functional roles and activity patterns in relation to respiration. It is the interaction of the neurons in these centers, which generates the respiratory rhythm. Their rhythmicity is driven by inputs from both mechanoreceptors in the lungs and chemoreceptors that respond to changes in blood CO_2. In humans as well as in many other animals it is essential that the activity of the respiratory centers is controlled and integrated with other movements and that brain areas involved in producing sounds/spoken language have the capability to utilize the air within the airways to generate sounds. During galloping horses breathe in and out in synchrony with the movement of the legs and humans as well as other animals need to stop breathing when the head is temporarily underwater or when eating or drinking. In such instances as well as in the production of sounds, control of respiration from the motor cortex and integration of sensory information from the mouth and throat is necessary. Cortical control is exerted in humans both by direct connections to the motor neurons controlling the respiratory muscles (and the throat, tongue, and lip muscles) and the respiratory centers in the brain stem.

Clinically, high cervical spinal injuries are critical since they may compromise the basic locomotor rhythm and require permanent artificial respiration if the person survives the initial injury. For patients with lesions above the brain stem, compromised speech, swallowing, and coughing are the main clinical problems that are related to the respiratory system. Speech depends crucially on the ability to use the respiratory system to push air through the airways and make the vocal cords vibrate. This requires precise coordination with the respiratory system and breathing exercises may therefore be helpful in promoting functional recovery of speech. Swallowing is generated by a brain stem reflex circuitry which is activated when a bolus of food activates sensory receptors in the back of the mouth. It is essential that the airways are simultaneously closed, and respiration is paused to prevent that food or drink from entering the airways. In patients with brain injury corresponding to the brain stem or above the swallowing reflex is often either not fully coordinated or is not activated sufficiently quickly to avoid food or drink from entering the airways causing discomfort, distress, and potentially serious harm. Training in swallowing and modification of food and drink to ease swallowing are therefore important as part of neurorehabilitation in many patients.

Coughing is the next line of defense in the respiratory system. Coughing is also a reflex, which is integrated with the respiratory centers in the brain stem, and it is also often deficient in patients with brain injuries. Various strength training exercises that ensure that the expiratory muscles are strengthened are of importance in this relation. Voluntary coughing exercises may play a role also.

5.4.2 Postural Control and Balance

Several nuclei that are located as part of the reticular system in the brain stem project to the spinal cord (reticulospinal tract) and are involved in controlling the axial muscles and coordinating their activity with activation of the extremities (Fig 5.6a). The vestibular nucleus also projects to the spinal cord (vestibulospinal tract) and is responsible for integrating proprioceptive, visual, and vestibular information to control balance. Together these nuclei and descending tracts are involved in controlling the position of the body when we move in the field of gravity. It is their integrated activity, which is responsible for the basic (anti-gravity) muscle activity which is often referred to as "muscle tone" in the clinic and often misinterpreted as spasticity or confused with altered muscle and connective tissue properties (see Box 5.3).

5.4.3 Brain Stem Control of Locomotion

It was found originally by a Russian research group in the 1960s that stimulation of a specific site in the midbrain (which they named the mesencephalic locomotion region (MLR)) may elicit locomotion in animals (Leiras et al., 2022). Subsequent work has identified specific neuronal populations, which when activated optogenetically (the neurons are genetically modified to respond to light of certain wavelengths), may initiate locomotion and induce intact animals to walk, trot, or gallop depending on stimulation frequency (Leiras et al., 2022). Other neuronal populations have been shown to stop locomotion when activated, probably through inhibition of the neurons, which initiate and control speed of locomotion.

The neurons from MLR have short- and long-range projections in the reticulospinal tracts to the spinal CPG neural circuitry. Many of these release monoaminergic neurotransmitters, but the details of the interaction of the MLR and the spinal CPG have not been worked out.

The MLR is controlled directly from the motor cortex as well as more indirectly through the basal ganglia (see Sect. 5.5). There is evidence that the basal ganglia exerts a static inhibitory effect on the MLR at rest and that locomotion is initiated when this inhibition is removed. Locomotion stops when the inhibition from the basal ganglia is increased. It is likely that the problems in initiating gait and the slowing of gait observed in patients with Parkinsons disease are related to malfunctioning of the basal ganglia control of the MLR.

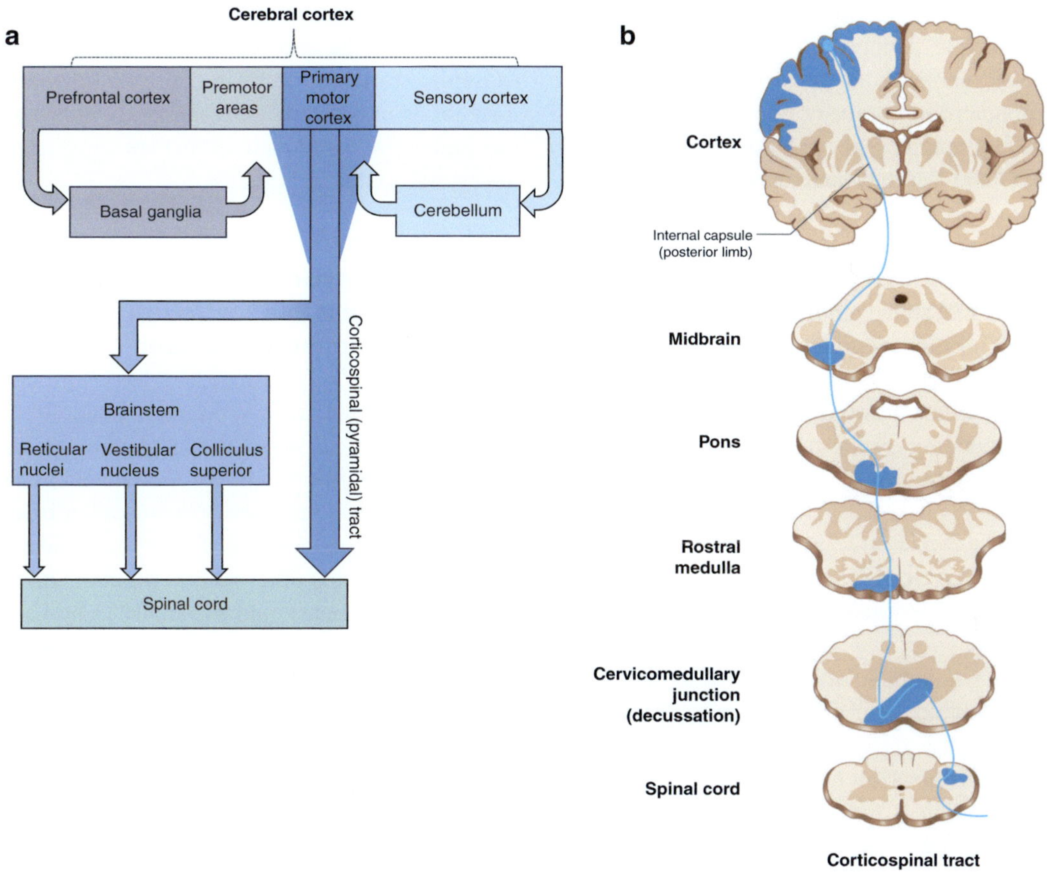

Fig. 5.6 Overview of descending control of movement (**a**) A diagram illustrating the connections involved in motor control is depicted. Connections from the motor cortex to the spinal cord and brainstem are represented by white arrows. Connections from the frontal cortex to the basal ganglia, and back via the thalamus to the premotor cortex, are shown by gray arrows. Additionally, connections from the sensory cortex to the cerebellum, and back via the thalamus to the primary motor cortex, are depicted by blue arrows. (**b**) On the right side of the figure: Anatomical slices at different levels of the nervous system illustrate the path of the corticospinal tract. The corticospinal tract, responsible for transmitting motor signals from the motor cortex to the spinal cord, is highlighted in each anatomical slice

5.4.4 Fight or Flight Reactions

Several brain stem nuclei are closely coupled to the amygdala and surrounding structures involved in emotional processing and control (see Chap. 11). This is the basis of various stereotyped reactions or behaviors generally called Fight or Flight reactions. One of the simplest reactions is the startle reaction or startle reflex. This reaction is elicited by unexpected sounds, which cause activation of cervical spinal motor neurons through a brain stem pathway from the inner ear. Through association of the sound with painful stimuli, the startle reflex may become exaggerated through the regulatory control of the gain of the reflex by the amygdala. In relation to locomotion, a scared animal may have to select whether to take flight or to freeze in order not to be discovered. This selection of behavior involves connections from the amygdala to the brain stem neurons involved in initiating or stopping locomotion as described in the previous section. The emotional modulation of brain stem nuclei and circuits is also the basis for the unconscious variations in "muscle tone" that may be experienced during daily life, and which may be especially evident in unconscious patients following brain injuries. All people may experience "tensing up" now and again or that it may be difficult to relax when stressed, unhappy, anxious, or angry. In a safe environment in company with good friends and family, people may on the other hand be able to "relax" and "let the shoulders down." Such experiences may be related to the influence of the amygdala on the reticular nuclei and networks in the brain stem. Through their descending projections to the spinal cord, these monoaminergic neurons in turn modulate the excitability of the spinal networks and especially the spinal motor neurons, which become either more or less excitable depending on the modulatory control from the brain stem.

5.5 Cortical Control of Movement

Although automatic mechanisms in the spinal cord and brain stem play important roles in the neural control of movements as described in the previous sections, all human movements are ultimately initiated and controlled by the cortex. Whereas injury of the motor cortex or the descending motor tracts to the spinal cord (the corticospinal tract, Fig 5.6b) and brain stem (corticobulbar) leaves humans paralyzed or with severe paresis, most other animals recover considerable ability to move even following complete ablation of the motor cortex. As already mentioned, this is not because the automatic mechanisms in the spinal cord and brain stem have become obsolete in humans. It is because human movement relies to a much larger extent on cortical control of the spinal cord and brain stem circuitries than in other animals as part of a general "encephalization" of the primate and especially human brain through evolution. This is what has enabled humans to let their imagination—their conscious ideas and plans—use their bodies as a tool to manipulate objects, change the world around them, and create art. The downside is that it has also made humans exceptionally vulnerable to brain injuries involving the motor cortex and the corticospinal tract. Interruption of the blood supply in some of the tiny blood vessels that supply the motor cortex or the capsula interna where the corticospinal tract descends close to the basal ganglia and the lateral ventricles; for example, stroke is the main cause of functional disabilities in humans. Only stroke in other apes has functional consequences that are comparable in severity to that in humans.

5.5.1 The Corticospinal Tract Is Responsible for Voluntary Movement in Humans

The corticospinal tract in humans contains far more descending axons than in any other species (close to one million) and the individuals axons split up and make far more collaterals that innervate a much larger number of neurons in the spinal cord than in any other species (Lemon, 2021). It is only in primates, and especially in humans, that some of these collaterals innervate the spinal motor neurons directly, making it possible for the cortex to control the activity of the muscles directly (Lemon, 2021). In all other species, the corticospinal tract controls the muscle activity indirectly through spinal interneurons which are part of the spinal reflex circuitry. This probably more than anything is what has enabled humans to walk on two legs in a challenging environment, use their hands for tool making, and control their throat, tongue, and facial muscles to communicate with each other.

5.5.2 The Primary Motor Cortex Is Organized Somatotopically

Eighty to ninety percentage of the axons in the corticospinal tract cross the midline at the level of the brain stem (at the anatomical landmark, the pyramids; thereby the alternative name for the corticospinal tract: The pyramidal tract, Fig 5.6b) (Lemon, 2021). The left side of the body is therefore represented in the motor cortex of the right hemisphere and vice versa. Different parts of the body are represented in different parts of the cortex (so-called somatotopic representation similar to the primary somatosensory cortex, Fig. 2.4) with muscles of the lower limb represented medially whereas muscles of the upper limb are represented more laterally. This is possible to demonstrate directly in awake volunteers using transcranial magnetic stimulation (see Box 3.4). When the coil of the magnetic stimulator is placed over the right hemisphere of the brain close to the midline, stimulation elicits movement of leg muscles on the right side, whereas stimulation more laterally causes movement of fingers and hands. Even more laterally stimulation elicits movement of the muscles of the face. Characteristic of this somatotopic organization is that muscles are not represented based on their anatomical size but on their functional role. Thus, muscles that control fine, precise movements—like those in the face, hands, and those governing speech such as the tongue and throat—have a disproportionately larger representation in the human cortex. In contrast, axial muscles that control posture and larger limb movements have a much smaller representation. This brain architecture emphasizes functionality over size, prioritizing sophisticated control of movements that are vital for human interaction and the manipulation of our environment.

5.5.3 Activity in Related Populations of Corticospinal Cells Is Used for Activation of Synergistic Muscle Groups During Coordinated Movements

A more detailed analysis of the organization of the cortex shows a very complex organization within the cortical representation areas. Corticospinal neurons projecting to specific muscles are located interspersed with neurons that project to other muscles. Each muscle in the hand is thus controlled from several different corticospinal neurons located in different parts of the hand representation area of the cortex and interspersed with cortical neurons controlling other muscles in the hand (Lemon, 2021). Additionally, the axon of each individual corticospinal neuron divides when it reaches the spinal cord and excites an average of 5–6 different motor neurons in the spinal cord. In addition, other motor neurons (often motor neurons of antagonist muscles) are inhibited via local spinal inhibitory interneurons. This means that there is both pronounced divergence (single cortical cells supply several spinal motor neurons) and convergence (several cortical cells activate a single spinal motor neuron). The functional significance of this is that the motor cortex is not a simple piano where activation of a certain area (a keypress) leads to activation of a specific muscle (a tone). The connection between the cortex and the spinal cord (and the brain stem) is a network with complex possibilities of modulation of its activity. Therefore, when we wish to move our index finger, corticospinal neurons, which project to the motor neurons controlling the muscles of the index finger become active, but they do not only excite motor neurons of muscles controlling the index finger. They also excite motor neurons of muscles controlling the other fingers and the hand—and motor neurons of antagonist muscles are inhibited. The advantage of this organization is that it is not necessary to depolarize the spinal motor neurons from a resting state far from their firing threshold each time we want to use that muscle in a movement. The excitability of the spinal motor neurons is maintained close to their firing threshold by ongoing corticospinal activity even at rest (and during sleep) and they may thereby be easily recruited in a movement by small changes in the activity of the corticospinal neurons. Changing the direction of a movement also only requires small changes in the activity profile across the population of corticospinal neurons.

5.5.4 The Direction of Movement Is Coded in the Weighted Activity of Corticospinal Neurons

This was demonstrated originally in monkeys who were trained to move a handle in different directions (Georgopoulos & Carpenter, 2015). When moving the right arm to the left (toward the body), corticospinal neurons projecting to motor neurons of the anterior part of the deltoid muscle will increase their activity. Conversely, corticospinal neurons projecting to motor neurons of the posterior part of the deltoid will become active when the movement is to the right. Other nerve cells connected to other muscles will correspondingly have increased or decreased (or perhaps unchanged) activity depending on the direction of movement. This means that the direction of any movement is coded in the activity of the entire population of motor neurons and that the direction of movement can be determined if the activity of the population of neurons is known. This is the background for the development of brain-computer interphases (BCI) as described further in Chap. 16. Recording the activity of a defined population of cortical neurons may be translated by a computer algorithm into commands for the movement of a robotic device.

5.5.5 The Representation of Muscles in the Motor Cortex (Motor Maps) Is Plastic

Learning-related plastic changes in the representation of muscles in the motor cortex are well-documented in relation to acquisition of new skills and optimization of movements. Experiments using transcranial magnetic stimulation have documented that the representation of muscles, that are used in a new motor task, expands following training of the task (Perez et al., 2004). This expansion only lasts for some minutes, but it is followed by long-lasting changes in the representation when the training is repeated over days and weeks. The initial short-lasting change in representation likely reflects a change in the communication within the existing neural network such as down-regulation of inhibitory connections to the corticospinal neurons involved in the task. The long-lasting changes on the other hand appear to reflect structural changes within the network such as outgrowth of neurites and establishment of new synaptic connections. Importantly, the long-lasting changes are only seen when training remains challenging and continued improvement of performance takes place. This has important implications for the design of neurorehabilitation efforts as discussed further in Chap. 15.

Plastic changes in muscle representation also take place in response to any change in the environment, the body, or the nervous system itself. Rapid changes in the representation of muscles are thus observed following immobilization of a limb or following the restriction of sensory information from an extremity (Werhahn et al., 2002). This illustrates clearly how the organization of the cortical network is adapted according to the sensory information from the body and the environment and is also consistent with the basic principle of the establishment of an internal model that is updated by sensory information (Chap. 8). Amputation of a body segment has also been shown to cause rapid changes in the cortical representation of muscles (Karl et al., 2001). The corticospinal neurons, which used to control the muscles of the amputated body segment, relatively quickly participate in the control of muscles belonging to body segments that are represented in adjacent areas of the cortex (but not necessarily adjacent body segments). The representation of the face thus greatly expands following amputation of the hand. Similar changes in the representation are also seen following lesions in the CNS. One example is that spinal cord lesion at C6 leads to expansion of the representation of the deltoid muscle, which has motor neurons located in the spinal cord above C6. These (spontaneous) plastic changes are not necessarily beneficial and may prevent re-establishment of a normal representation in M1 following lesions. In neurorehabilitation, a main goal may therefore be to start functional training as quickly as possible and direct the plastic changes toward establishment of an as normal representation as possible. Here it is important also to consider the interaction between the two hemispheres. While it has been shown that ipsilateral connections from the non-injured hemisphere may be upregulated and compensate for the loss of contralateral connections from the injured side, there is also evidence that this may diminish plastic changes within the injured hemisphere due to an inhibitory/suppressive influence from the functioning hemisphere. This may be a further argument in favor of constraint-induced movement therapy in which patients with injury on one side are prevented from using their non-injured side as compensation (Box 15.2).

5.5.6 Cortical Control of Brain Stem Nuclei Is Responsible for Predictive (Anticipatory) Postural Reactions

All movements of our extremities require that the rest of the body maintains a stable position. In order to lift the right leg to the side while standing, we need first to shift our body toward the left and ensure that the center of gravity is positioned safely above the left foot, otherwise, we will fall to the right when we lift the right leg. This is an integrated part of the motor plan for all our movements regardless of the initial position of the body. Some milliseconds before the motor cortex transmits a motor command through the corticospinal tract to activate the muscles that lift the right leg, a command has been transmitted to the reticular and vestibular nuclei in the brainstem, where it is integrated with vestibular, visual, and proprioceptive information in order to activate the appropriate muscles in the body that will ensure the body position. These control mechanisms are automatically adjusted according to the initial position of the body and the demands imposed by the desired movement. Following years of practice, the cortex and brainstem nuclei are able to predict the sensory consequences of most of our movements and adjust the muscle activity throughout our body appropriately (see also Chaps. 7 and 8). Many muscles involved in this predictive postural control are in the core of the body and the motor neurons involved in controlling trunk muscles are innervated by the reticulospinal and vestibulospinal pathways.

5.6 Initiation of Voluntary Movement

When movements are made as part of daily life, it is difficult to determine whether any given movement is initiated completely voluntarily in the absence of any external stimulus, or whether it is a reaction in response to a sound or a visual stimulus. Although the question of whether movements are voluntary or reflexive in nature is Millennia old, the answer is simple and probably not surprising: movements are to a varying extent a mixture of the two. This is the very nature of the (conscious) presence of a human being in an external world and the human ability to sense that world and interact with it. Movements in daily life are made in continuum between the most voluntary and the least voluntary.

An athlete who is waiting for the starting signal before initiating a 100 m sprint is at one end of this continuum, whereas the President of the USA, who is about to decide whether to press a red button or not is at the other. In the first case, it is essential to react as quickly as possible and conscious considerations would only slow down the reaction. The decision on when and how to move must be predetermined and prepared to respond to the sound of the starting gun. In the second case, however, there is (hopefully) ample time for conscious considerations that lead up to the decision to move.

The electrical activity recorded from the brain (EEG) is very different in these two situations. In the first case, no clear movement-related activity will be observed from the brain until after the sound of the starting gun (unless the subject makes a false start). However, in the second situation increased EEG activity will be observed over the frontal areas of the brain up to 1 s prior to the start of the movement. This so-called readiness potential probably reflects the communication in networks involved in deciding and planning the movement (Neafsey, 2021).

When these areas are stimulated in patients undergoing brain surgery in local anesthesia, the patients often report an urge to move and may sometimes initiate movements. Patients with lesions in these areas often experience deficits in the initiation or suppression of movements. This can have the form of akinesia or mutism when language areas are involved. When prompted, patients may be able to generate movements, but they lack the urge to perform self-initiated movements. Other patients may experience an uncontrollable urge to grasp objects in their vicinity, which can have an almost compulsive character (alien hand syndrome; anarchic hand syndrome).

The prefrontal motor areas involved in initiation of movement form a subcortical loop with the basal ganglia (Fig. 5.6a). At rest, the basal ganglia exert a continuous inhibitory effect on brain stem circuitries and the premotor cortex through the thalamus. Excitation of the basal ganglia from the prefrontal cortex results in removal of this inhibitory effect so that initiation of movement can proceed. This depends crucially on dopaminergic innervation from the substantia nigra. In Parkinsons disease (Chap. 21), dopaminergic innervation is deficient and patients with Parkinsons disease therefore characteristically have difficulty initiating movements, their movements are slowed down, and they often halt their movements and "freeze" unable to continue moving. In contrast, patients with damage of the basal ganglia, which is the case in genetic disorders such as Huntington's disease and following injury (stroke, etc.), suffer from involuntary irregular movements (dyskinesias) that can have a dancing character (chorea). The basal ganglia are also thought to be involved in dystonias where involuntary continuous muscle activity is observed at rest or provoked by voluntary movement. Dystonias are also seen secondary to other disorders (stroke and cerebral palsy) as well as in a primary genetic form.

5.7 Planning of Movement

Once the decision to make a movement has been made, the plan of the movement has to be worked out. As already mentioned, automatic mechanisms are built into the spinal cord and brain stem neural circuitries, which simplifies the task of the cortex in ensuring that muscles throughout the body are activated at the right time and to the right extent. In order to do this, the (posterior) parietal cortex integrates proprioceptive information from the body with visual information about the surroundings and transmits this to the premotor cortex where it is used to form specific movement commands taking the organization and connectivity of the corticospinal neurons and the automatic brain stem and spinal cord neural circuitries into account. The communication between the premotor cortex and the posterior parietal cortex is bidirectional and facilitates that sensory information is used to guide movement, that the sensory areas are informed about the intention of movement (efference copy see Chap. 8) and that the two may be compared to each other to optimize movement. In addition to this, the cortex makes use of two important subcortical motor loops, the frontal cortex-basal ganglia-thalamus-premotor cortex and the parietal cortex-cerebellum-thalamus-primary motor cortex loops, to plan, control and optimize movement (Fig. 5.6a).

5.7.1 Premotor Cortex and Supplementary Motor Area

The SMA receives input from the basal ganglia and parietal association areas processing sensory information from muscles, joints, and skin. In contrast, the PMC primarily receives input from parietal association areas involved in visual information processing. This anatomical distinction aligns with their functions. PMC neurons are active in tasks requiring visual information, like object location. In contrast, SMA is active in tasks relying on internally stored knowledge, with little emphasis on visual input. PMC is thought to code movements in extrapersonal space using visual coordinates, while SMA utilizes information about the individual, such as muscle and joint positions, for movements based on internally stored coordinates. Because of this PMC appears to be more involved in "new" movements that have not been practiced and therefore require significant visual guidance, whereas SMA appears to be more involved in "old" well-practiced movements that can be "done with closed eyes." This is illustrated by a shift in activity from PMC to SMA in relation to learning of new sequences of movement. In the initial learning phase, where visual information about the sequence is required, neurons in PMC tend to be more active than neurons in SMA, whereas the opposite is the case when the sequence has been stored in memory and can be performed without visual information.

The premotor cortex is especially engaged in tasks involving the manipulation of objects, contributing to the planning and coordination of hand movements required for dexterous and skilled actions. It integrates sensory information about the properties of objects, such as size, shape, and texture, to guide appropriate hand movements.

The premotor cortex also contains mirror neurons, which are neurons that are activated both when an individual performs a specific action and when they observe someone else performing the same action (Rizzolatti & Sinigaglia, 2016). According to some theories mirror neurons in the premotor cortex may contribute to understanding and imitating hand movements, fostering social learning and communication. However, the role of mirror neurons in direct imitation is debated. The process of imitation might involve additional cognitive mechanisms, and mirror neurons might serve more as a part of a broader network for action understanding rather than direct imitation. Mirror neurons are also often implied in social cognition and empathy, but their role in generating complex social behaviors like empathy is likely to be more nuanced. Other brain regions and processes are likely involved in the intricate nature of social interactions and emotional understanding.

5.8 The Basal Ganglia

The basal ganglia is a complex network of sub cortical nuclei that play a multifaceted role in motor control, reward processing, and cognitive functions. It comprises the caudate nucleus, putamen, subthalamic nucleus, and substantia nigra (Fig. 5.7).

The primary function of the basal ganglia in motor control function lies in its ability to select and initiate appropriate actions while inhibiting competing ones. The primary input nucleus, the putamen, receives glutamatergic signals from the cortex with information about the current state of the body, the external environment as well as the intended movement. The output from the basal ganglia is predominantly inhibitory, mediated by gamma-aminobutyric acid (GABA), and is directed toward the thalamus and brainstem nuclei. Two principal pathways within the basal ganglia regulate inhibition, yet they do so in complementary ways: the direct pathway facilitates a form of excitation by reducing inhibition on the thalamus, thereby promoting movement, while the indirect pathway enhances inhibition on the thalamus, thus suppressing movement.

Dopamine serves as a key neurotransmitter to fine-tune the activity of the direct and indirect pathways. Dopamine from the substantia nigra modulates movement by exciting the direct pathway to enable desired actions and inhibiting the indirect pathway to lessen suppression of unnecessary movements. In Parkinson's disease, the substantia nigra is damaged, leading to a significant decrease in dopamine production. This reduction disrupts the balance between the direct and indirect pathways, leading to the symptoms that characterize the disease, such as bradykinesia (slowness of movement), rigidity, tremors at rest, and postural instability. The lack of dopamine tilts the balance toward more inhibition of movement through the indirect pathway and less facilitation via the direct pathway, making voluntary movements more difficult and less coordinated for people with Parkinson's.

The basal ganglia are also implicated in reinforcement learning, where the brain adapts its motor strategies based on the outcomes of previous actions. Dopamine release, particularly in response to rewarding experiences, reinforces neural circuits associated with successful motor behavior, contributing to the learning and optimization of motor skills. As motor skills progress from the initial learning phase to automatic execution, the basal ganglia play a role in the gradual transfer of control from conscious, effortful processing to more automatic, less consciously monitored movements.

The basal ganglia's role extends beyond motor control, encompassing cognitive and affective functions. Aberrations in basal ganglia function are associated with a spectrum of neurological and neuropsychiatric conditions. A comprehensive understanding of the pathophysiology of these conditions is essential for developing targeted therapeutic interventions and this is therefore a very active research field.

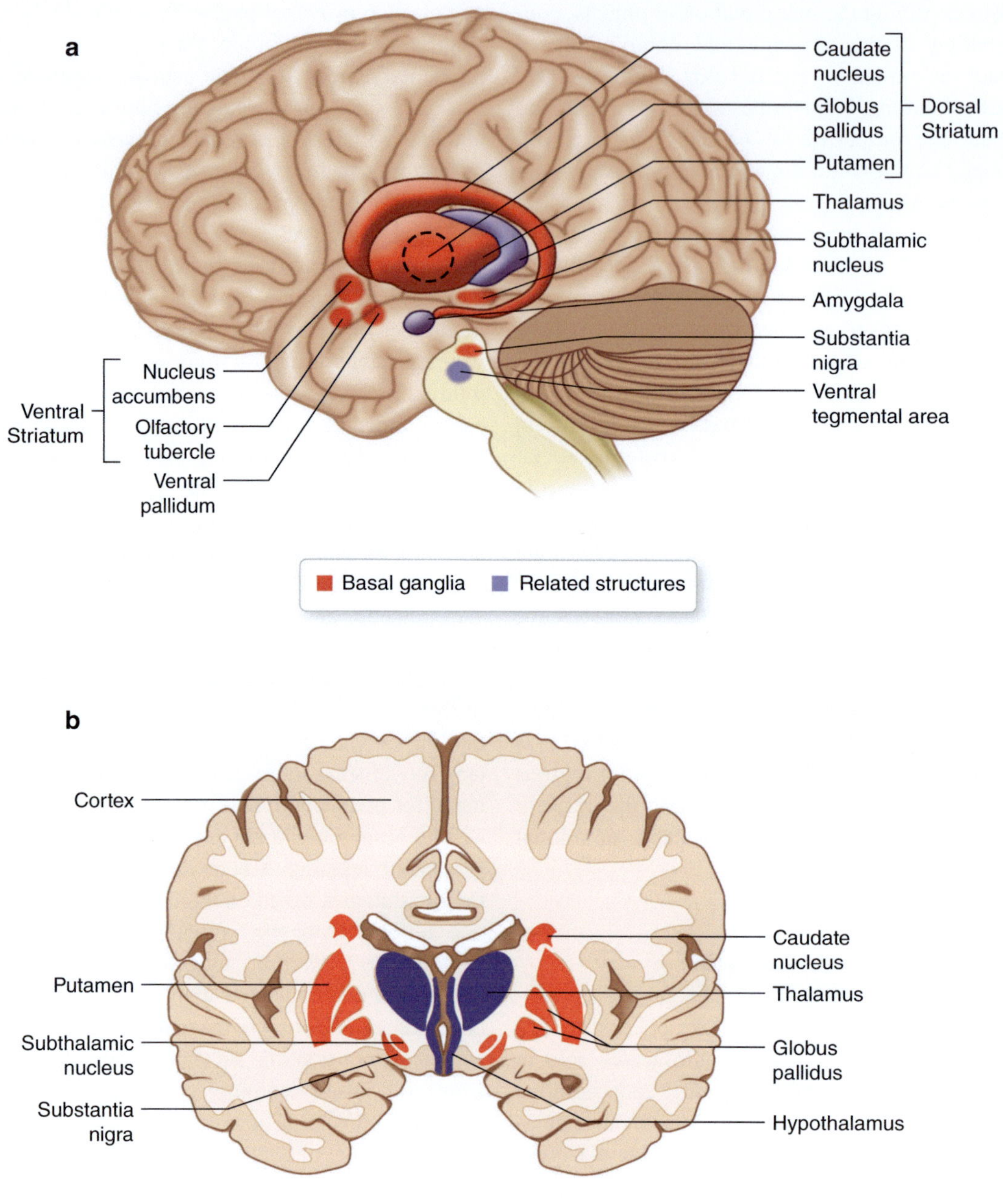

Fig. 5.7 Basal ganglia
(**a**) A three-dimensional depiction of the basal ganglia and their internal connections is shown, emphasizing their interconnectedness. The basal ganglia include the caudate nucleus, putamen, globus pallidus, subthalamic nucleus, and substantia nigra. These structures are intricately interconnected through various pathways and play a role in motor control and cognition. Positioned adjacent to the thalamus, the basal ganglia communicate with this relay center for sensory and motor signals. (**b**) A frontal slice through the brain at the level of the basal ganglia is displayed, highlighting their anatomical relation to the thalamus and the ventricles

5.9 The Cerebellum

The functional organization of the cerebellum and its connections with the cerebral cortex are described in Fig. 5.8.

5.9.1 The Cerebellar Hemispheres Are Involved in Initiation of Movement

The cerebellar hemispheres are integral components of a neural circuit involving the cerebral cortex (Fig. 5.8). They receive input from association areas in the frontal and parietal lobes and, through the thalamus, project back to the primary motor cortex. Learned subroutines for executing the movement, programmed within the cerebellar hemispheres, and updated through climbing fibers (further elaborated below), are activated through this neural circuitry.

5.9.2 The Cerebellum Is Involved in Motor Adaptation

The cerebellum processes information from two types of nerve fibers: moss fibers and climbing fibers. Moss fibers offer general input from various sources, including the cortex, balance sense, brainstem, spinal cord, and proprioception. On the other hand, climbing fibers, originating from the nucleus olivaris inferior in the medulla oblongata, establish a direct connection with cerebellum output cells known as Purkinje cells. The activation of climbing fibers induces a long-lasting change in the synaptic effect of moss fibers on Purkinje cells, playing a crucial role in

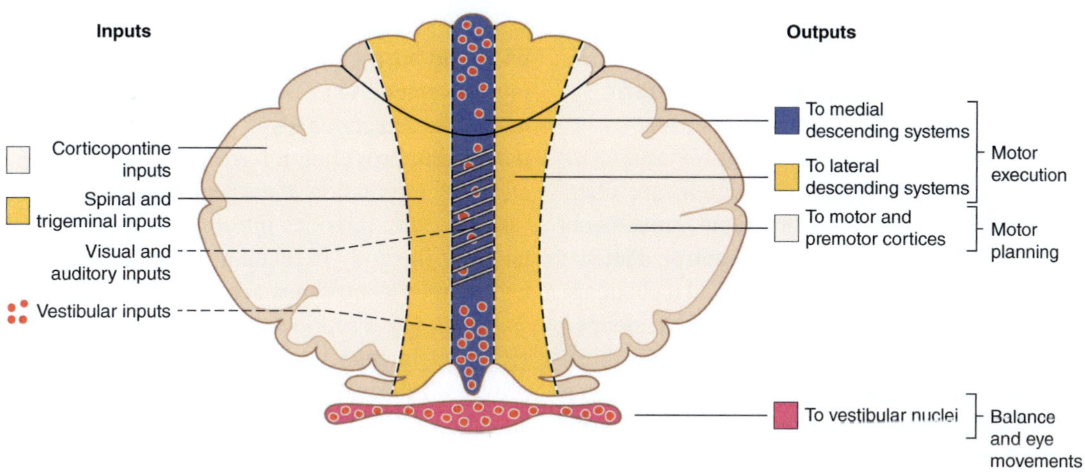

Fig. 5.8 Input and output of the cerebellum
The cerebellum is divided into distinct regions, each with specific functions in motor coordination, balance, and eye movements.

Inputs to the cerebellum are primarily received from various brain regions, including the spinal cord, brainstem nuclei (such as the pontine nuclei), and cerebral cortex. These inputs synapse onto granule cells in the cerebellar cortex.

Outputs from the cerebellum are primarily directed toward two regions: Deep cerebellar nuclei: The cerebellar cortex projects excitatory signals to the deep cerebellar nuclei, including the fastigial, interposed, and dentate nuclei. These nuclei send efferent signals to various brain regions, including the thalamus and brainstem, to modulate motor function. Vestibular nuclei: In addition to motor outputs, the cerebellum also influences vestibular function through connections with the vestibular nuclei in the brainstem. Specific regions of the cerebellum are involved in different aspects of motor control: Motor planning and execution: These functions are primarily associated with the lateral cerebellum, including the lateral hemispheres and the dentate nucleus. Balance and coordination: The vermis and intermediate cerebellum, along with the fastigial nucleus, play crucial roles in maintaining balance and coordinating movements. Eye movements: The flocculonodular lobe and its associated fastigial nucleus are involved in controlling eye movements, particularly vestibulo-ocular reflexes.

updating motor programs and facilitating motor learning.

In monkeys, climbing fibers become active during the recalibration of movement direction or force, signaling a discrepancy between planned motor programs and the actual movement. They contribute to altering Purkinje cell activation, thereby updating the motor program. Climbing fibers are also involved in the vestibulo-ocular reflex, ensuring precise activation of eye muscles to maintain gaze during head movements. The same vestibular afferents that activate the vestibular nuclei in the brainstem and contribute to the reflex also connect to moss fibers in the cerebellum. Through Purkinje cells, they inhibit these vestibular nuclei, determining the reflex strength. If the reflex is too strong or weak, climbing fibers signal the error to the cerebellum, adjusting Purkinje cell activation until the reflex reaches an optimal state.

5.9.3 Lesion of the Cerebellum Causes Ataxia and Movement Tremor

Clinically, lesions in the cerebellum are characterized by severe uncoordinated movements (ataxia) and impaired postural control. Patients with extensive cerebellar damage find it challenging to maintain balance, exhibit a wide-stepped walking pattern, and struggle with precise object reaching. Hand and arm movements become jerky, often resulting in overshooting (dysmetria) and subsequent overcompensation. These movements exhibit significant fluctuations in agonist and antagonist activity at around 10 Hz, leading to intention tremor.

Movements lack the usual smooth trajectory, displaying distinct subcomponents (dyssynergy). Speech is notably affected, showing a fragmented, syllable-separated pattern. In lesions affecting specific functional areas of the cerebellum, symptoms align with the compromised functions. For example, vestibulocerebellar lesions result in isolated balance issues and nystagmus.

5.10 Generation of Movement Behaviors

5.10.1 Postural Control and Balance

Humans and other animals live on planet Earth, and the nervous system of all animals is inherently aware of this reality. As Newton was the first to realize (or at least the first to put into mathematical formulas), the mass of the Earth exerts a gravitational pull on all objects in its vicinity. From the time humans are born and begin to move, the nervous system undergoes a learning process, integrating the influence of gravity into the movements and adjusting them based on variations in Earth's gravitational pull. This adaptation allows humans, with some practice, to move purposefully both in weightlessness within a spaceship and in 1/sixth of Earth's gravity when walking on the moon.

The nervous system employs three different sensory systems to control the position of the body and ensure that balance is maintained during movement. (1) The vestibular system in the inner ear detects changes in head position and movement, providing information about acceleration and orientation of the head in space. (2) The visual system provides information of the orientation of the body in relation to the surroundings and thereby contributes significantly to postural stability. (3) Proprioceptive information from receptors in muscles, tendons, joints, and skin provides information about body position, pressure, and touch. This input is essential for the nervous system to create a representation of the body's spatial orientation.

Information from these three sensory systems is integrated in specialized areas responsible for processing spatial orientation and balance in the brainstem (vestibular nuclei, inferior olive, and reticular formation) and cerebellum (vestibulocerebellum). Under normal circumstances, the three systems, thus, work together toward the same goal: To ensure that the body maintains its position in the gravitational field and that movements may be performed without jeopardizing balance. Although each system has distinct responsibilities related to posture and balance, there is significant overlap and each of the three systems can substitute for the others. The adaptive (plastic) capacity of the nervous system also ensures that movements may still proceed when one, and to some extent, two of the three systems are impaired. People do not fall when they close their eyes and blind people are naturally able to move around and perform purposeful movements using other senses. People with lesions of the inner ear also learn with time to compensate for the loss of information from the vestibular system and can manage most situations with information from the visual and proprioceptive systems only. Deafferented people (Chap. 2) who have lost all proprioception may also learn to use visual information to maintain posture and balance (Yousif et al., 2015). However, with closed eyes or in the dark, they lose balance and fall.

The integration of the vestibular and proprioceptive systems is also evident from the automatic regulation of body posture that can be demonstrated in experimentally decerebrated animals who rely only on control of muscle activity from the brainstem and cerebellum. Vestibular input provides information about the head's position in gravity and proprioceptive input from the neck about the body's orientation relative to the head. Combination of these two inputs may therefore provide the necessary information to automatically regulate the position of the different body segments in the most purposeful way. For example, when an animal leans its head backward and extends its neck against gravity, it indicates that the animal is about to move upward. Accordingly, the forelimbs are flexed and the hindlimbs are extended. Conversely, the forward tilt of the head in gravity and flexion of the neck corresponds to an animal about to move downwards and accordingly the forelimbs are extended and the hindlimbs flexed. Similar automatic adjustment of the position of the arms and legs may be seen when newborn human babies are positioned differently in the gravitational field. It is also these automatic adjustments of static postural muscle activity that explain the pattern of "increased muscle tone" or "hypertonia" seen in some children with cerebral palsy (Chap. 19), and which is often misinterpreted as spasticity.

In contrast to other animals, human babies do not cope with the realities of gravity at birth but require around 1 year of practice before they take their first wobbly steps. Part of the reason for this delayed development is the generally late development of the human nervous system, but human bipedal gait also plays a significant role. Walking on four legs poses less of a risk of losing balance than the bipedal gait that humans have been equipped with through evolution. Letting a tall erect body balance on top of a narrow and relatively short platform of a foot is a challenge to balance in itself, but on top of that humans throw their body forward with each step so that the center of gravity is moved in front of the supporting leg and the only way to avoid falling is to quickly move the other leg forward. In four-legged locomotion the center of gravity is always securely placed between hindlimbs and forelimbs and the risk of falling is close to zero (but not quite zero which is the subject of several funny cat videos on YouTube).

The priority of maintaining posture and balance when performing movements within the gravitational field means that automatic adjustment of postural muscle activity is an integrated part of all movements. When reaching for that cup of coffee in the morning, it may seem that the brain is only concerned with which muscles to activate in order to bring the hand close to the cup, but in fact, the motor cortex ensures that appropriate muscles are activated throughout the body to ensure that body position and balance is maintained when the arm is lifted. An arm is quite heavy and may easily disturb balance if sufficient counterweight is not ensured by increasing muscle activity in the core muscles. The reticulospinal and vestibulospinal pathways are responsible for sending this command to the spinal cord before the muscles in the arm are activated through corticospinal activity. Another example is when opening a door. Well before the muscles in the arm are used to pull the door open, ankle plantar flexor muscles are activated to prevent the body from being pulled toward the door. These automatic adjustments are called anticipatory postural reactions and are part of predictive motor commands established through prior experience. Sensory error signals that are picked up by the cerebellum and relayed to the parietal and frontal sensorimotor areas to update the motor programs are essential for this adaptation and for establishing an optimal predictive model that may ensure that the correct adjustments of posture and "muscle tone" are made under all circumstances.

In the case of sudden external perturbations, visual, vestibular, and proprioceptive information is also integrated in the brainstem and cerebellum to maintain balance if possible. These stumbling corrective responses are elicited from the brain stem and cerebellar circuitries and involve coordinated activation of muscles throughout the body.

Higher cognitive functions, including attention, spatial awareness, and executive functions, contribute to maintaining balance. The prefrontal cortex and other brain regions play a role in integrating cognitive processes with sensory and motor functions for effective postural control.

5.10.2 Reaching and Grasping

When reaching for that cup of coffee in the morning, a series of computations takes place in a range of areas and networks in the brain. Visual information about the position of the cup is processed in the visual areas of the occipital lobe (dorsal stream—"Where" pathway—see Chap. 4) and proprioceptive information about the position of the body and body segments is processed in the somatosensory areas of the parietal cortex (see Chap. 4). These two separate modalities are combined in the posterior parietal cortex and used to determine the most optimal path for reaching toward the cup. The plan for this is laid out in the premotor cortex based on the visual and proprioceptive information. It is not a plan that is worked out de novo for each movement, but rather a decision of which pre-learned and well-rehearsed movement plan should be set in motion. Already before reaching for the cup, parallel visual processing informs the brain about the shape of the cup (ventral stream—"What" pathway—see Chap. 4), and the relevant neurons in the premotor cortex are activated to ensure that the hand is opened, and the fingers are ready to grasp the cup in the most optimal way. The movement toward the cup is generated when the appropriate populations of corticospinal neurons are called into action, and they activate the relevant populations of spinal motor neurons. The movement direction is determined by the weighted activity of the population of corticospinal neurons (the population vector), where individual corticospinal neurons increase or decrease their activity depending on their connectivity to the spinal motor neurons and thereby their "preferred" direction of activity. When the hand touches the cup and/or the visual system determines that the hand is sufficiently close to the cup, the nervous system will make the fingers squeeze the handle, lift the cup, and bring it to the mouth. The activation of the appropriate populations of corticospinal neurons and further processing in the intricate neural networks of the spinal cord ensures that the muscles controlling the fingers, which squeeze, the handle are activated at the exact same time as the muscles in the elbow, which lift the hand. Because this movement has been trained in different situations daily, adults generally become very good at it. When the movement has been optimized through experience, the sensory (visual and proprioceptive) feedback elicited by the movement corresponds to the predicted sensory feedback and the internal model for the movement is confirmed. This is experienced by the individual as being the "agent" of the movement. In those rare cases when the fingers slip and the cup is not lifted appropriately, the sensory feedback from the movement will differ from the predicted sensory feedback and an error signal will be used to update the internal model. The cerebellar loop connecting the lateral cerebellar hemispheres with the parietal lobe plays an important role in this ongoing adaptation and optimization of movement (Fig. 5.6a).

5.10.3 Locomotion

The ability to move from one place to another is vital for all animals. This behavior, perhaps the most fundamental of all, has been a driving force behind the evolution of the nervous system in animals. The ability of the nervous system to coordinate body segments and ensure propulsion of the body through water, over ground or in the air in pursuit of prey or for escape from predators has always—and is still—essential for survival.

Human bipedal walking is different from walking in other animals, yet it is built upon billions of years of nervous system evolution. This evolution initially facilitated swimming and later adapted to support quadrupedal movement on land. Although human ancestors adopted habitual two-legged walking only 3–5 million years ago, it is not surprising that the human nervous system shares a fundamental design with other animals. The key distinction lies in a few essential differences that are critical for the specialized human walking pattern.

The spinal cord originated from interconnected local populations of neural cells (ganglia) responsible for controlling specific body segments during movement. It is not surprising, therefore, that the neural network in the spinal cords of four-legged animals can generate and coordinate basic muscle activity in all four limbs for efficient locomotion. Animals with a complete transection of the spinal cord can still generate locomotor activity, with different limbs fully coordinated and sensory feedback, if intact, adjusting limb movements based on ground properties.

The human spinal cord has retained this network of locomotor-generating neurons, crucial for coordinating muscle activity at various joints in the two legs during walking and running. However, individuals with a complete spinal cord lesion are incapable of producing locomotor activity, even with intensive training, and even relatively minor lesions of the corticospinal tract and other supraspinal motor pathways have major effects on the ability to walk. This is not because the network does not exist in humans or is not used for walking; rather, it is much more reliant on supraspinal control compared to animals. The likely reason is that human bipedal gait is more unstable, requiring greater supraspinal coordination to prevent falls compared to animals.

The biomechanics of human bipedal gait are fundamentally distinct from other types of walking. In a four-legged gait, the center of mass is consistently positioned between the hind- and forelimbs, and forward propulsion is achieved by pushing the body forward with the hindlimbs, primarily involving the large muscles around the hip. In contrast, in humans, the center of mass is in front of the single supporting leg, and with each step, the body essentially falls forward but is prevented from hitting the ground by the swinging motion of the opposite leg.

Significantly, only the ankle plantar flexors contribute substantially to forward propulsion in humans. During the stance phase, these muscles produce a brief burst of activity, sufficient to push the body forward, allowing gravity to complete the motion. This unique mechanism makes human bipedal gait highly energy-efficient, a key factor in its evolutionary success along with the freeing of the hands.

However, this gait pattern is inherently unstable, resulting in falling as an adverse side effect. To counter this, humans have evolved extensive supraspinal control networks, surpassing those seen in other animals. This includes direct monosynaptic connections from the motor cortex to spinal motor neurons, facilitating quick and efficient corrections and gait modifications when needed. Despite these adaptations, falling remains a significant challenge for many neurological patients and elderly individuals, underscoring the ongoing complexity of maintaining stability in human bipedal locomotion. Visual steering of gait is of fundamental importance for gait in all species but especially in humans for the same reason. Visual surveillance of the terrain is necessary to avoid obstacles and ensure accurate foot placement. This is less of a concern for a four-legged animal. The visual control of gait relies largely on cortical processing and corticospinal control, but quick corrections of steps may also be controlled through visual connections to brain stem nuclei. A large part of the balance control necessary for walking is also exerted automatically by the integration of vestibular, proprioceptive, and visual information in the vestibular nucleus and conveyed from there to the spinal cord circuitry.

The cortex is ultimately responsible for starting and stopping gait, but the basal ganglia and the locomotor centers in the brain stem play important roles. Freezing of gait in Parkinson's disease is a clear indication of this role.

Functional gait also requires that it is adapted to changes in the environment or in the physical properties of the body. Gait needs to be adapted to different properties of the ground whether on a concrete pavement, on a sandy beach, or on the moon. With age body segments change their dimensions and physical properties, and the muscle neural control must adapt accordingly. The ability of humans to walk forwards with one leg and backward with the other leg on a split-belt treadmill is a testimony to the extent of this adaptability. The cerebellum and its ability to modify the central motor programs in the cortex, the brain stem, and the spinal cord play an essential role in this adaptation.

Box 5.3 Involuntary Muscle Activity

Lesions to the brain and spinal cord do not only cause reduced ability to voluntarily activate and coordinate muscles, but also different types and forms of involuntary muscle activity, such as spasms, cramps, dystonia, and tremors. These may be a nuisance and even cause pain to the patient. They may also interfere with the ability to recover and maintain function. Clinically, a distinction has been made between spasticity-related signs and symptoms, which are related to lesion of the corticospinal tract and/or motor cortex, dystonia, and dyskinesia, which are related to basal ganglia disorders and intention tremors which are related to cerebellar disorders. In clinical practice these different types of involuntary muscle activity may be difficult to distinguish and may also be observed in one and the same patient.

Spasticity is often defined as an exaggerated neural reaction to stretch of a muscle (i.e., exaggerated stretch reflex), but the signs and symptoms that are attributed to spasticity clinically are not universally related to muscle stretch, and an exaggerated stretch reflex is in itself not the cause of the patients complaints (Nielsen et al., 2020). Although exaggerated stretch reflex activity in the form of exaggerated tendon jerks or the sensation of a catch during the neurological examination when stretching a muscle rapidly, is useful for diagnostic purposes, it is important to consider that the reflex in itself does not require treatment and that it is only a surrogate measure of the underlying pathology. The different signs and symptoms that are merged under the heading "spasticity" have different underlying pathophysiological mechanisms and require different treatment depending on the functional status of the patients. It therefore makes more sense to put focus on the individual signs and symptoms and objectively evaluate if and how they contribute to the functional challenges of the patients.

Spasms are frequent in patients with spinal cord injury and are characterized by being elicited by sensory stimuli such as skin brushing, muscle stretching, or relatively imprecise stimuli such as a filled bladder or similar. In all likelihood, spasms are generated by activation of the spinal flexor reflex circuitry, which is involved in withdrawal reactions to painful stimuli. There is likely also considerable overlap with occurrences of muscle cramps generated by aberrant activation of nerve terminals in the muscles. This should be considered when deciding on possible treatment.

The term "increased muscle tone" is often used almost synonymous with spas-

(continued)

Box 5.3 (continued)
ticity and has the underlying assumption that it is caused by ongoing "involuntary" muscle activity when the patient attempts to be at rest. When this is not verified by measurement of Electromyography (EMG) from the muscle, there is a risk of confounding ongoing muscle activity with altered elastic properties of the muscle, connective tissue and joint secondary to immobilization and disuse. In their ultimate form these changes in stiffness and resistance to movement of the joint cause reduced range of movement and manifest contractures. The word "contracture" is in its own right one of those unfortunate misleading words, which have caused considerable confusion. There is no contraction involved in a contracture—either in the sense of active myosin-actin interaction or constriction of the tissue in other ways. Because of this, treatment directed at neural mechanisms are unlikely to be of any benefit for the patient.

Increased "muscle tone" should also be considered carefully in the context of gravity and the conscious and emotional state of the patient. It is exceedingly difficult to evaluate whether muscle activity is "involuntary" and "unwanted" in patients with reduced consciousness and awareness. Such patients may not be able to communicate and may not be able to "relax" when asked to do so during a neurological examination. The same concern applies to any patient with reduced skills of communication, including children. There is no need of using antispastic treatment to reduce muscle activity that is neither involuntary nor unwanted. The clinical challenge is to determine when this is the case or not. Objective biomechanical and electrophysiological (EMG) techniques are often required for this. With the development of small portable measuring devices such techniques may now be applied bedside as part of routine diagnostics.

Increased "muscle tone" is also difficult to differentiate from dystonia, which is usually associated to lesions of the basal ganglia (secondary dystonia) or specific genetic disorders (primary dystonia). Many patients with stroke or cerebral palsy show involuntary muscle contractions either at "rest" or provoked by voluntary movements, which resemble dystonia, but are often referred to as spasticity. This has led to the introduction of the term "spastic dystonia" to denote ongoing involuntary muscle activity in patients who have paresis and muscle weakness and other signs of lesion of the corticospinal tract or the motor cortex. However, this conflation of symptoms that are traditionally associated to lesion of either the basal ganglia (dystonia) or the corticospinal motor system (spasticity, paresis), is not generally accepted as it may confuse treatment.

Dyskinesias in the form of dancing (chorea), writhing, wriggling, waving, or swaying movements are the hallmark of basal ganglia disorders and are generally referred to as hyperkinetic disorders (in contrast to Parkinson's disease as a hypokinetic disorder). The simplified understanding of dyskinesia is that it is caused by malfunctioning basal ganglia that are unable to exert the normal inhibitory control of the premotor cortex and brain stem. Often dyskinesia is triggered by voluntary movements and in cases where only one side is affected (as in hemiballism caused by stroke affecting the subthalamic nucleus), perfectly normal voluntary movements may be seen on one side, while involuntary dyskinesias are triggered on the other.

Tremor is involuntary rhythmic muscle activity, which is classically described in relation to Parkinsons disease (resting tremor especially in hands and jaw with characteristic 3–5 Hz frequency) and cerebellar disorders (intention tremor which is

(continued)

Box 5.3 (continued)
only seen during movement and with frequency of around 10 Hz). However, neurologically intact individuals also display so-called physiological tremor at 10 Hz to a varying extent. It is especially evident in the fingers where it may often be noticed with the naked eye, but otherwise may be detected using accelerometers. It is likely generated by the cortical-cerebellar-thalamic circuitry, which has been shown to be active at frequencies around 10 Hz and which is also a significant component of the alpha rhythm measured in EEG recordings. Physiological tremor may be attenuated with fatigue or from drinking coffee or taking other stimulants. Some suffer from abnormally pronounced 10 Hz tremor which may have a genetic background (familial tremor), but more often is seen for unknown reasons (essential tremor).

Review Questions
- Which neural mechanisms enable a human to walk on a high-wire between two skyscrapers?
- Why do people with brain injuries often experience cognitive load and development of fatigue when performing simple motor tasks?

References

Biering-Sorensen, B., Kristensen, I. B., Kjaer, M., & Biering-Sorensen, F. (2009). Muscle after spinal cord injury. *Muscle & Nerve, 40*(4), 499–519. https://doi.org/10.1002/mus.21391

Brunet, T. (2023). Cell contractility in early animal evolution. *Current Biology, 33*(18), R966–R985. https://doi.org/10.1016/j.cub.2023.07.054

Georgopoulos, A. P., & Carpenter, A. F. (2015). Coding of movements in the motor cortex. *Current Opinion in Neurobiology, 33*, 34–39. https://doi.org/10.1016/j.conb.2015.01.012

Gordon, T., Thomas, C. K., Munson, J. B., & Stein, R. B. (2004). The resilience of the size principle in the organization of motor unit properties in normal and reinnervated adult skeletal muscles. *Canadian Journal of Physiology and Pharmacology, 82*(8–9), 645–661. https://doi.org/10.1139/y04-081

Karl, A., Birbaumer, N., Lutzenberger, W., Cohen, L. G., & Flor, H. (2001). Reorganization of motor and somatosensory cortex in upper extremity amputees with phantom limb pain. *The Journal of Neuroscience, 21*(10), 3609–3618. https://doi.org/10.1523/JNEUROSCI.21-10-03609.2001

Kiehn, O. (2006). Locomotor circuits in the mammalian spinal cord. *Annual Review of Neuroscience, 29*, 279–306. https://doi.org/10.1146/annurev.neuro.29.051605.112910

Leiras, R., Cregg, J. M., & Kiehn, O. (2022). Brainstem Circuits for Locomotion. *Annual Review of Neuroscience, 45*, 63–85. https://doi.org/10.1146/annurev-neuro-082321-025137

Lemon, R. N. (2021). The Cortical "Upper Motoneuron" in Health and Disease. *Brain Sciences, 11*(5). https://doi.org/10.3390/brainsci11050619

Lomo, T., Westgaard, R. H., & Dahl, H. A. (1974). Contractile properties of muscle: Control by pattern of muscle activity in the rat. *Proceedings of the Royal Society of London - Series B: Biological Sciences, 187*(1086), 99–103. https://doi.org/10.1098/rspb.1974.0064

Lorach, H., Galvez, A., Spagnolo, V., Martel, F., Karakas, S., Intering, N., et al. (2023). Walking naturally after spinal cord injury using a brain-spine interface. *Nature, 618*(7963), 126–133. https://doi.org/10.1038/s41586-023-06094-5

Neafsey, E. J. (2021). Conscious intention and human action: Review of the rise and fall of the readiness potential and Libet's clock. *Consciousness and Cognition, 94*, 103171. https://doi.org/10.1016/j.concog.2021.103171

Nielsen, J. B. (1998). Co-contraction of antagonistic muscles in man. *Danish Medical Bulletin, 45*(4), 423–435.

Nielsen, J. B., Christensen, M. S., Farmer, S. F., & Lorentzen, J. (2020). Spastic movement disorder: Should we forget hyperexcitable stretch reflexes and start talking about inappropriate prediction of sensory consequences of movement? *Experimental Brain Research, 238*(7–8), 1627–1636. https://doi.org/10.1007/s00221-020-05792-0

Pearson, K. G., Misiaszek, J. E., & Fouad, K. (1998). Enhancement and resetting of locomotor activity by muscle afferents. *Annals of the New York Academy of Sciences, 860*, 203–215. https://doi.org/10.1111/j.1749-6632.1998.tb09050.x

Perez, M. A., Lungholt, B. K., Nyborg, K., & Nielsen, J. B. (2004). Motor skill training induces changes in the excitability of the leg cortical area in healthy humans. *Experimental Brain Research, 159*(2), 197–205. https://doi.org/10.1007/s00221-004-1947-5

Rizzolatti, G., & Sinigaglia, C. (2016). The mirror mechanism: A basic principle of brain function. *Nature Reviews Neuroscience, 17*(12), 757–765. https://doi.org/10.1038/nrn.2016.135

Werhahn, K. J., Mortensen, J., Kaelin-Lang, A., Boroojerdi, B., & Cohen, L. G. (2002). Cortical excitability changes induced by deafferentation of the contralateral hemisphere. *Brain, 125*(Pt 6), 1402–1413. https://doi.org/10.1093/brain/awf140

Yousif, N., Cole, J., Rothwell, J., & Diedrichsen, J. (2015). Proprioception in motor learning: Lessons from a deafferented subject. *Experimental Brain Research, 233*(8), 2449–2459. https://doi.org/10.1007/s00221-015-4315-8

Basic Principles of Learning and Memory

6

Lasse Christiansen and Jesper Lundbye-Jensen

Abstract

Every day humans learn something new: the name of the artist behind a catchy tune, the route to the mall, or how to transfer from bed to wheelchair. Regardless of the topic or task at hand, learning depends on the formation of memories that in term depends on the malleability of the nervous system. The iterative process of memory formation can be organized based on the time course of storage or based on the type of information. Selected sensory experiences are temporarily withheld and manipulated in the working memory before being 'consolidated' into long-term memory. From here, it can be 'recalled' and changed before being 'reconsolidated'. Based on the neural systems underpinning it, memory is typically viewed in a dichotomous manner distinguishing 'explicit' or 'declarative' memory from 'implicit' or 'non-declarative' memory. Returning to the examples above, it is easy to declare who composed a song, whereas the timing and intensity of muscle contractions necessary to transfer to the wheelchair is a procedure that cannot be readily declared. In this chapter, models of memory formation along with the organization of learning grounded in well-described clinical cases of amnesia are introduced. Motivated by the instrumental role of neuroplasticity in neurorehabilitation, the principal basis of memory and learning, namely network, and cellular neuroplasticity is discussed. Finally, hot topics in learning and memory research are introduced.

Keywords

Declarative memory · Non-declarative memory · Synaptic plasticity · Consolidation · Working memory · Medial temporal lobe · Prefrontal cortex

Box 6.1 The Story of Henry Molaison (HM): A Dichotomized Memory

HM (1926–2008) suffered from severe epilepsy, which was treated in 1953 by removing parts of his temporal lobes in both hemispheres. Following the resections, HM could no longer recall recent events, and he was incapable of forming new memories. More specifically, HM experienced that he could no longer turn an experience into a lasting memory. Every time he

(continued)

L. Christiansen (✉)
Danish Research Centre for Magnetic Resonance (DRCMR), Copenhagen University Hospital, Amager and Hvidovre, Hvidovre, Denmark

Department of Neuroscience, Faculty of Health and Medical Sciences, University of Copenhagen, Copenhagen, Denmark
e-mail: lassec@drcmr.dk

J. Lundbye-Jensen
Movement & Neuroscience, Department of Nutrition, Exercise & Sports, University of Copenhagen, Copenhagen, Denmark
e-mail: jlundbye@nexs.ku.dk

J. B. Nielsen et al. (eds.), *Neuroplasticity-based Neurorehabilitation*,
https://doi.org/10.1007/978-3-031-81120-3_6

Box 6.1 (continued)
saw his wife, he would greet her as if he saw her for the first time after the operation. Even if she just left the room for a minute. At the same time, HM displayed preserved general intelligence, could maintain, and manipulate items in mind through active rehearsal, and could remember childhood episodes. As such, he could have an informed conversation and relate the topic to childhood events, but minutes later he would not be able to remember ever having had that conservation. When HM during a visit from a neuropsychologist tried to trace a star-shaped line while looking in mirror, he was surprised how easy he found this task. What HM was not aware of, because he could not remember, was that he tried this task on several occasions before during visits from the same neuropsychologist. What can be learned from HM's symptomatology? Why did HM forget recent but not distant experiences and episodes? Does the neural underpinnings of memory formation differ from those that support short-term memory or learning how to master mirror drawing?

Box 6.2 Anatomical Structures Involved in Learning and Memory
The medial temporal lobe (MTL) is heavily involved in learning and memory and compromises key structures such as the hippocampus essential for forming new memories and spatial navigation, and the amygdala crucial for emotional memories (see Fig 11.4). Also, the neocortex is involved in long-term memory storage, which includes the instrumental role of the prefrontal cortex in working memory and consolidation of declarative memories (see Fig. 9.3). The basal ganglia are important for procedural learning and habits (see Fig. 5.7). The thalamus serves as a relay station, directing sensory information to appropriate areas of the cortex. Within the midbrain, integral structures such as substantia nigra pars compacta (SNc) and the ventral tegmental area (VTA) also contribute to learning and memory by influencing synaptic plasticity and reward signals.

6.1 The Organization of Learning and Memory

Everyone has an idea of what *memory* and *learning* mean. They are interweaved phenomena that can be studied from numerous perspectives spanning many disciplines incl. psychology, cognitive, computer, and neural sciences. The internal and dynamic process of *learning* relies on effective *memory* formation and storage. Directly assessing learning is challenging, so it is indirectly estimated by measuring memory formation through observable changes in specific behaviors or in the underlying neural alterations. If someone rehearses a poem but cannot remember it the following day, to what extent have they truly learned it? A memory, be that of a phone number or a movement, can be short or longer lasting. The latter depends on successful long-term storage and retrieval, and it can be argued that learning is the sum of the encoded and consolidated memory and the ability to retrieve the consolidated memory.

Most people associate memory with *episodic memory*, i.e., an event or episode that occurred at a point in someone's life. Or maybe *semantic memory*, which is more in line with general knowledge encompassing the 'memory' or understanding of concepts, language, and facts. Both semantic and episodic memory are *explicit* or *declarative* memories but differ in the perspective in that episodic memories are egocentric and unique, whereas semantic memories are not (see Fig. 6.1).

The same collision between two cars may be stored as vastly different episodic memories in the brains of the two drivers, whereas they share the semantic memory that a *full stop* means stop.

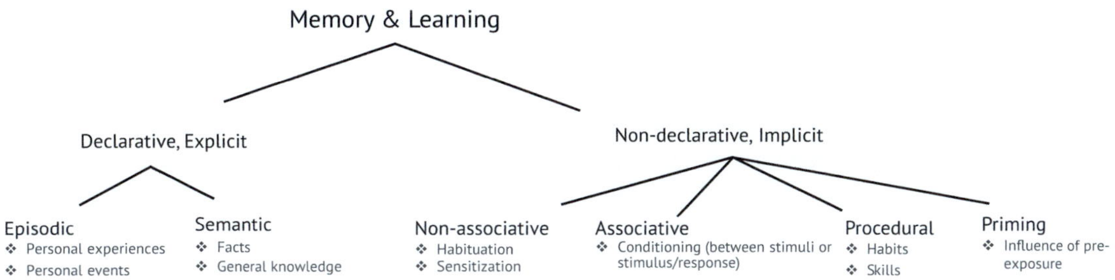

Fig. 6.1 Organization of long-term memories

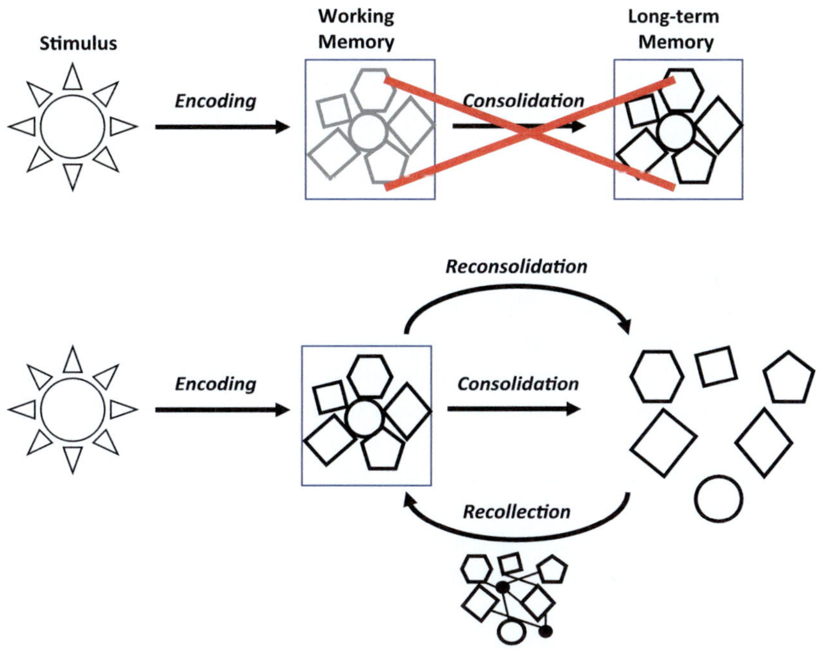

Fig. 6.2 Iterative memory formation. Memory is not a serial, unidirectional process but involves numerous iterations where the memory is recollected into the working memory before being reconsolidated into long-term storage

However, not all memories can be declared. Some aspects of memory are *implicit, procedural,* and *non-declarative.* This includes the ability to ride a bike but also the fear response to a venomous viper. Based on the symptomatology of patients like H.M., long-term memories are generally separated into two categories with a series of subcategories.

The segregation between explicit and implicit memory is based on the formation of long-term memories. The role of working memory in forming lasting representations from transient stimuli as well as the role in recollecting stored memories is introduced in Sect. 6.2.3. Regardless of memory type, memory formation is not a single process, nor a linear process comprised of a string of *memory stages* as depicted in Fig. 6.2 (top row). A memory is *encoded, consolidated,* and then recalled, *retrieved,* or rather *recollected* (as argued below) before being subjected to *reconsolidation* again and again (Fig. 6.2 top row). Based on this, memory formation, and thereby learning, should be seen as an iterative process that can be augmented or interrupted on multiple time points.

6.2 Explicit, Declarative Memory

Common for both the episodic and semantic division of explicit memory is the need for attention. Neither experiences nor facts are transformed into neural representations and incorporated into existing schemes of knowledge without attention. This simple fact is the cornerstone in many modern views of education, where time-consuming activities that engage pupils or students are favored.

6.2.1 Explicit Memories are Complex and Difficult to Measure

Most people (but not HM) can store explicit information and experiences as lasting representations that can be *recollected* later on. The term *recollect* is in many ways preferable to *recall* especially when it is episodic rather than semantic memory. The reason for this is, that the representation of an episodic memory is not a fixed or continues entity. Rather it is bits and pieces stored in widely distributed circuits in the cortex in modality relevant areas. These bits and pieces need to be recollected when an experience is remembered. Episodic memories are often multimodal. A childhood memory of a vacation on a Greek island may include the sound of cicadas, the smell of thyme, the heat from the sun, and the sunlight being reflecting in the water at the sandy beach. The modalities are interconnected in that the smell of thyme can facilitate the recall of how cicadas sound, and thereby the recollection of the full multimodal childhood experience. Practically, this can enhance the recollection of explicit memories as evident from the studies showing how students who study under exposure to, e.g., a specific olfactory stimulus recall more during a closed book exam if the same olfactory stimulus is presented. Due to the complexity of multimodal memories, these are hard to study in controlled settings and explicit memories are often operationalized as the ability to recall words or navigate a maze. The latter furthermore has the advantage of being applicable across species, which enables scientists to study memory at the cellular and synaptic level. One thing is studying the mechanisms of *how* memory is stored but *where* does the memory of, e.g., an episode reside? As illustratively depicted in Harry Potter, where prof. Dumbledore uses his wand to extract a memory trace in the shape of a silver string from his brain, the memory must be 'inside the skull' somewhere. The idea that an experience leaves behind a lasting memory trace—an 'engram'—has fascinated scientists for centuries. But what is an 'engram'? and where in the brain does it reside?

6.2.2 From Chasing the Engram to a Network Perspective

Over the course of the first three decades of the twentieth century, Karl Lashley searched for the *memory engram* by systematically removing small bits of the cerebral cortex in rodents. He could not identify a single bit that specifically impaired spatial memory functions. Rather, cognitive deficits increased with the proportion of brain resected. This led him to propose the concepts of *equipotentiality*, i.e., that the whole brain is important and of *mass action*, i.e., it is not the location but the extent of the lesion that matters. Subsequent work has demonstrated that the extent of a brain lesion in no way is the sole determinant of the resultant impairments. Even with large chunks of brain missing, one can uphold relatively normal cognitive functions incl. memory. When Lashley's fruitless search for the memory engram was coming to an end, Donald Hebb proposed that assemblies of cells work together to represent memories, which would mean that memories would be stored not in cells per se, but in the connectivity between cells, i.e., neural networks (see Chap. 13). Even though changes within a cell also take part in the multiscale process of forming memories, Hebb's postulate still holds true to this day. This is underlined by recent findings using lesion network mapping, where brain connectivity from, e.g., the 'Human Connectome Project' (a large-scaled project sponsored by the National Institutes of Health mapping structural and functional connectivity of the human brain) is overlaid with individual lesion locations associated with a specific symptomatology. Ferguson et al. (2019) used lesion network mapping to explore the relationship between brain lesions and anterograde amnesia.

Whereas both lesions located within and outside the hippocampal formations could cause severe anterograde amnesia, 95% of all lesions that resulted in anterograde amnesia were found in sites functionally coupled to the subiculum, which connects hippocampus to the entorhinal cortex. In relation to HM's symptoms, it is interesting that both subicula were resected during his surgery. In conclusion, a lesion (or a resection) of hippocampus impairs explicit memory formation but so does a lesion in the 'memory network'.

It should now be clear to the reader that a memory engram (be that MTL-dependent or not) is not a fixed or spatially confined entity. By the end of this chapter, the reader should be left with the take-home message that an explicit memory is a set of tuned cellular connections distributed in a dynamic network consisting of modality relevant cortices and subcortical loci connected to organizing nodes in the prefrontal and medial temporal lobes. In contrast, some forms of implicit learning occur only in the engaged circuit.

6.2.3 A Short-term, Working Memory Enables Us to Act in Real-time

H.M.'s clinical symptoms suggest that the process of forming long-term memory differs considerably from the ability to withhold new (or old) information present in mind. This dissociation does not imply that long-term memory is decoupled from short-term memory. These are coupled in time in a bidirectional manner as illustrated in Figs. 6.2 and 6.3. In this following paragraph, the term working memory (WM) is used to encompass both the short-lasting representation that fade if not rehearsed as well as the executive ability to manipulate the representation (Baddeley & Hitch, 1994). The description below is based on a representation of declarable information, which should be more intuitive to the reader. This does not imply that non-declarable information cannot be maintained 'present in mind'. As an example, following a motor action, a copy of the motor output is accessible for reinforcement for tens of second, which can be argued to constitute a short-term or working motor memory. However, as implicit memories can be formed independent of attention, the core roles of a working memory (incl. allocation of attentional resources) are easier to grasp in the declarative domain. Every day animals—including humans—encounter situations where the need for a system that enables us to filter, contextualize, and deal with the information at hand is tangible. In Fig. 6.3, a model of how the WM governs the processes of transforming a transient stimulus into a lasting memory is depicted. Far from all stimuli reach conscious representations

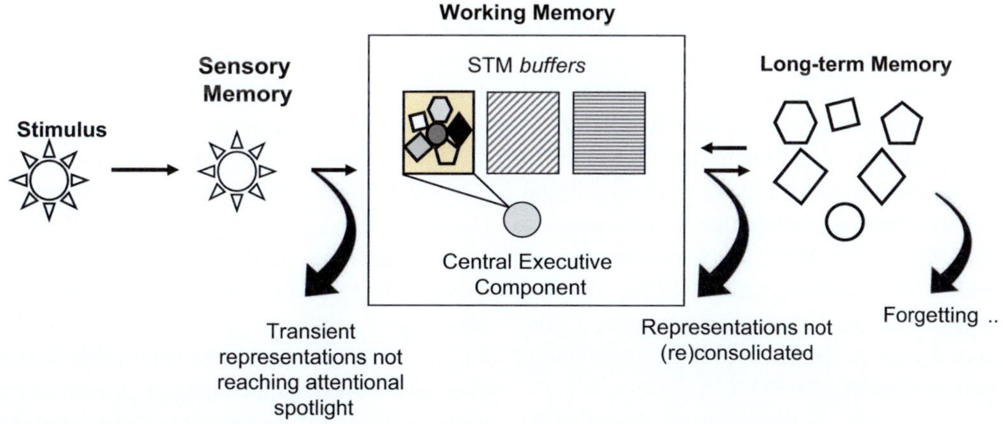

Fig. 6.3 A model of how the working memory (WM) governs the process of transforming a transient stimulus into a lasting memory. *STM* short-term memory

or perception and therefore fade quickly from the 'sensory memory'. A central executive component (see Chap. 9) directs attentional resources to the short-term memory 'buffer' that fits the sensory modality of the information. The executive buffers also mediate and filter the recollection of relevant memories needed for contextualization by interfacing with long-term memory (see, e.g., Baddeley, 2010). In Fig. 6.3, it can be seen how some, but far from all, of the temporary representation in the WM are further consolidated into long-term memory. It is that final, MTL-dependent process, that HM fell short off.

6.2.4 Persistent Prefrontal Activity Enables the Working Memory

To concretize and discuss the neural underpinnings of WM, it is worthwhile to consider the core objectives of the WM; to maintain and manipulate information. The ability to maintain information calls for sustained neural activity, which has been demonstrated in neurons in the prefrontal cortex of monkeys tasked with pairing matching stimuli, displayed seconds to minutes apart (Fuster & Alexander, 1971). However, it is unlikely that single neuron activity can represent the complex features of an image in the span between a stimulus and the response. Recent evidence shows that activity of hundreds (and likely thousands) of prefrontal neurons contains a low-dimensional, stable representation of object features (Murray et al., 2017). Reverberating activity in neural networks that occurs both between and within regions of the brain supplement sustained activity in prefrontal neurons. Results from neuroimaging studies have shown that different prefrontal regions support the tasks of manipulating versus maintaining information (D'Esposito et al., 1999). The WM functions needed to manipulate information can be further divided into a *what* and *where* that are contingent on ventral and dorsal prefrontal activity, respectively (Chap. 4; Nee et al., 2013).

In summary, the working memory withholds and manipulates information with the goal of transforming sensory information into neural representations and ensure appropriate actions based on both novel and stored information. These capabilities are ensured through sustained activity in single neurons and neural populations of the prefrontal cortex, as well as through reverberating activity throughout local and brain-wide networks.

6.2.5 Network Mechanism of Explicit Memory Consolidation

After a sensory stimulus has called upon attentional resources and has been through contextualization and filtering in the working memory, it can be transformed into a long-lasting (explicit) memory through the process of consolidation. As evident from HM's symptomatology, this process must somehow involve the MTL. A notion that is supported by neuroimaging studies in neurological uncompromised individuals as well. When humans are exposed to memory testing paradigms inside, e.g., an MR scanner, it is possible to pinpoint the site(s) with neural activity that relates to memory formation. Not surprisingly, converging evidence find MTL activity to predict successful encoding, i.e., items or navigations that are later successfully recollected. But also, prefrontal and posterior parietal cortical regions often display increased activity during functional magnetic resonance imaging. In relation to the formation of long-term explicit memory, a standard theory of consolidation has been proposed in which hippocampus is involved in the consolidation by linking cortical components together (see Fig. 6.4 for conceptual visualization).

Upon recollection of the memory during both sleep and awake hours and through extensive *replay* (see next section), hippocampus gradually strengthens the cortical representation and becomes less and less involved in storing and recollecting the memory. This model fits with the data from amnesic patients (like HM) who display severe anterograde amnesia as well as retrograde amnesia for recent but not distant episodic memories. In addition, in HM episodic but not

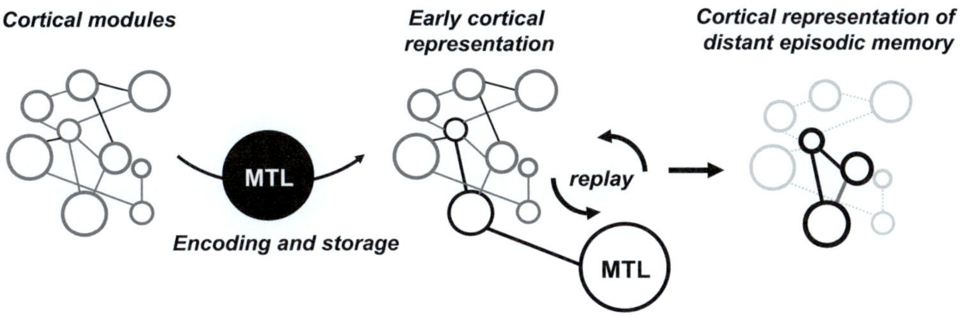

Fig. 6.4 Conceptual visualization of memory consolidation. The medial temporal lobe (MTL) is involved in the transformation into a neural lasting representation through repeated replay of neural activity until the neural representation exists in a robust MTL-independent form

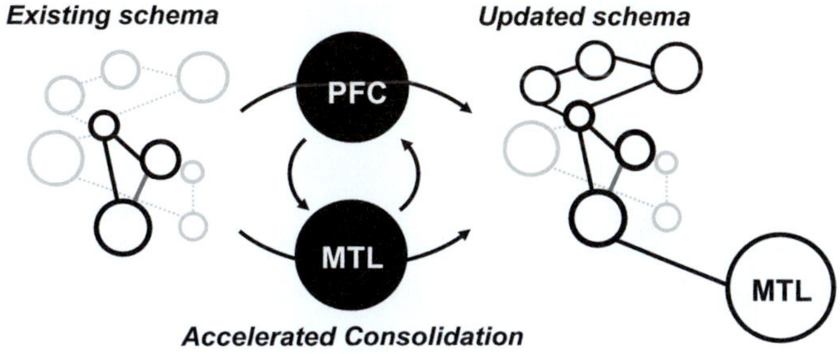

Fig. 6.5 Conceptual visualization of accelerated consolidation. An existing memory scheme enables an acceleration of the iterative consolidation through the involvement of prefrontal structures

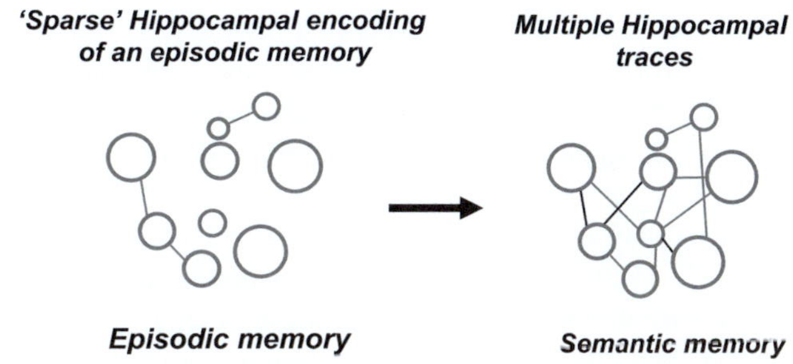

Fig. 6.6 Another theory of explicit memory formation proposes that sparse episodic memory representations are gradually being transformed into a semantic memory

semantic memories were compromised, which suggests that the MTL is less involved in recalling semantic memories.

Also, the prefrontal cortex plays a prominent role in long-term explicit memory formation. During encoding, the allocation of attentional resources is at large controlled by prefrontal areas. During recollection, the prefrontal cortex cooperates with MTL, which enables recollected information to be merged with information at hand. Novel but congruent information is swiftly fitted into an existing schema, a process mediated in a coordinated interplay between MTL and prefrontal cortex, which accelerates consolidation (Van Kesteren et al., 2012) (see Fig. 6.5).

Another theory of explicit memory formation, crudely illustrated in Fig. 6.6, proposes that episodic memories exist in an early stage as sparsely encoded ensembles of hippocampal neurons that can be attended by neocortical networks. The addition of multiple new related memories in comparable contexts gradually transformed the episode specific memory by integrating it into existing sematic knowledge that continues to reside at least in part in the MTL. This explanation aligns less with HM's ability to recall distant episodes.

6.2.6 Replay to Remember

In animals, including humans, all encoded memories decay. If efforts are not made to recall or revisit, e.g., the route to a restaurant, correct turns are typically missed at a later point in time. Fortunately, the brain is equipped with naturally occurring processes that prevent forgetting. In relation to spatial navigation, the ability to create a cognitive map of one's surroundings, and, e.g., remember the directions for a specific restaurant, is in part due to hippocampal place cells. Place cells enable the generation of cognitive spatial maps by firing only when an animal enters a specific location in its surroundings (O'Keefe & Dostrivsky, 1971). Thirty years ago, Wilson and McNaughthon (1994) discovered that hippocampal place cells in rats that systematically fired together at certain location in the cage where more likely to also fire together during subsequent slow wave sleep (SWS) (see Chap. 12). The neural activity that was present during awake encoding of a cognitive map of the cage was replayed during SWS. This finding linked SWS and replay to the concept of overnight consolidation. But how? In the up-phase of cortical slow oscillation (in humans around 0.8 Hz), a signal is sent to thalamus that in return triggers oscillatory firing (12–15 Hz), which is visible in scalp recordings (EEG) as 7–14 Hz sleep spindles. Both when entering and during the cortical up-phase, hippocampal 80–140 Hz (200 Hz in rodent) ripples occur more often. Hippocampal ripples are more frequent after tetanic induction of LTP in vitro, which points to a role in memory formation. In both rodents and human, ripples, spindles, and slow waves display a temporal correlation (Siapas & Wilson, 1998; Clemens et al., 2007). In rodents, the temporal coupling is evident even at single neuron level and likely underpins the process by which memories are consolidated from early hippocampus-based storage to neocortical representations of distant memories (Fig. 6.4). In view of the multitrace model for memory consolidation (Fig. 6.6), the role of hippocampus-neocortex communication during replay would be to organize the contextual-specific memories into semantic-like organization memories with less specific episodic traits. Later work has underlined the importance of neural replay in memory consolidation and demonstrated occurrence of this across many memory domains, during both sleep and in the awake hours after encoding. In Chap. 7, neural replay is further discussed in the context of procedural memory consolidation traditionally viewed as being MTL-independent.

Before directing the attention to implicit memory formation, a few words of caution are needed. It is pertinent to repeat that not all 'explicit' memories are the same. *Episodic* and *semantic* memories are clearly different categories underpinned by overlapping but distinct neural circuits. As it is impossible to ask a rodent to recall words or report math results, mechanisms of explicit learning are usually studied using spatial navigation tasks. It is obviously not straightforward to extrapolate network mechanisms of spatial memory formation in rodents to the formation, storage, and altering of childhood episodic memories in humans. Nonetheless, the spatial memory model has several advantages such as a clear link to the hippocampus (although, even this translation calls for caution as spatial memory is a multi-domain memory as discussed in the final section of the chapter). More importantly, the cellular and molecular events that lead to long-lasting changes in connectivity between cells are comparable between different categories of explicit learning. An overview of the cellular and molecular mechanisms, which have been studied extensively in relation to spatial memory formation in the hippocampus, is provided below. These mechanisms are also key components in the formation of implicit memories across the CNS including neocortex, basal ganglia, and cerebellum.'

Box 6.3 Hippocampal LTP

In the early 1970s, Terje Lømo and Tim Bliss discovered how repeated tetanic electrical stimulation of presynaptic cells located in the hippocampus of living rabbits (Fig. 6.7a, c) led to a long-lasting increase in postsynaptic responsiveness due to changes in synaptic efficacy. Previous demonstrations of changes in postsynaptic responsiveness following repeated activity were ascribed to increased excitability of the postsynaptic cell rather than a change in the strength of the activated synapse specifically. The increased responsiveness was transient and was never coupled to learning. In a series of experiments, Bliss and Lømo (1973) explored the properties and contingencies of what they coined long-term potentiation (LTP). A single train of high-frequency stimulation causes only short-lasting post-tetanic potentiation (PTP, Fig. 6.7b). Upon repeated tetanic stimulation, the LTP increased in magnitude and became temporarily robust. Later work demonstrated that changes in location of existing proteins and production of new proteins were the basis of the late part of LTP. The intracellular pathways that mediate these processes as well as the frequency needed to induce LTP vary across regions and the type of synapse and cells. It is noteworthy that to induce LTP, the frequency needs to be as high as 200 Hz for many types of synapses. This is higher than the natural firing rate of many neurons. The dependence on a supranatural stimulation frequency questions whether such frequency-dependent LTP is really a commonly occurring phenomenon outside of the laboratory. In fact, LTP can be induced with much lower frequencies if the postsynaptic neuron(s) is stimulated immediately after the tetanic train is delivered to the presynaptic neuron. In situ, this process of spiking-timing-dependent LTP occurs when a postsynaptic neuron is excited to the point of imitating an axon potential that then propagates back to the soma and the dendrites to thereby coincide with subsequent presynaptic activity. These two forms of LTP share the core principle of synaptic memory that were all proposed by Hebb: specificity, associativity, and co-operativity. Only synapses that are involved in the excitation of the postsynaptic cell will be potentiated, which associates two cells that fire in close temporal proximity. Most importantly for the conceptualization of cellular underpinnings of explicit memory formation is the possibility that several presynaptic neurons can cooperate to bring the postsynaptic cell to fire. This potentiates synapses between all presynaptic contributors and their postsynaptic recipient, thereby linking an ensemble of neurons that each encode different features of a stimulus (see Fig. 6.8). The specific proteins involved in frequency and spike-timing-dependent LTP differ between different types of synapses, but common features include voltage-gated calcium channels and a specialized glutamate receptor (N-methyl D-aspartate, NMDA). The NMDA receptor is a cation channel that is activated when glutamate released from the presynaptic neuron binds AND the postsynaptic cell depolarizes locally. As such, the NMDA receptors have the role as pre- and postsynaptic coincidence detectors ensuring that only active synapses are potentiated (see Fig. 6.7d).

Importantly, synaptic strength can also be reduced. This happens through mechanisms of long-term depression (LTD), which has been studied most extensively in the cerebellar and cerebral cortices but occurs throughout the central nervous system. LTD generally works in a manner opposite to that of LTP. Internalization of receptors followed by synaptic pruning underpin short- and long-term decreases in synaptic connectivity. Like LTP, LTD is typically NMDA receptor-dependent, and it is the resultant inflow of calcium ions that decides whether the postsynaptic neuron initiates the LTD or LTP machinery.

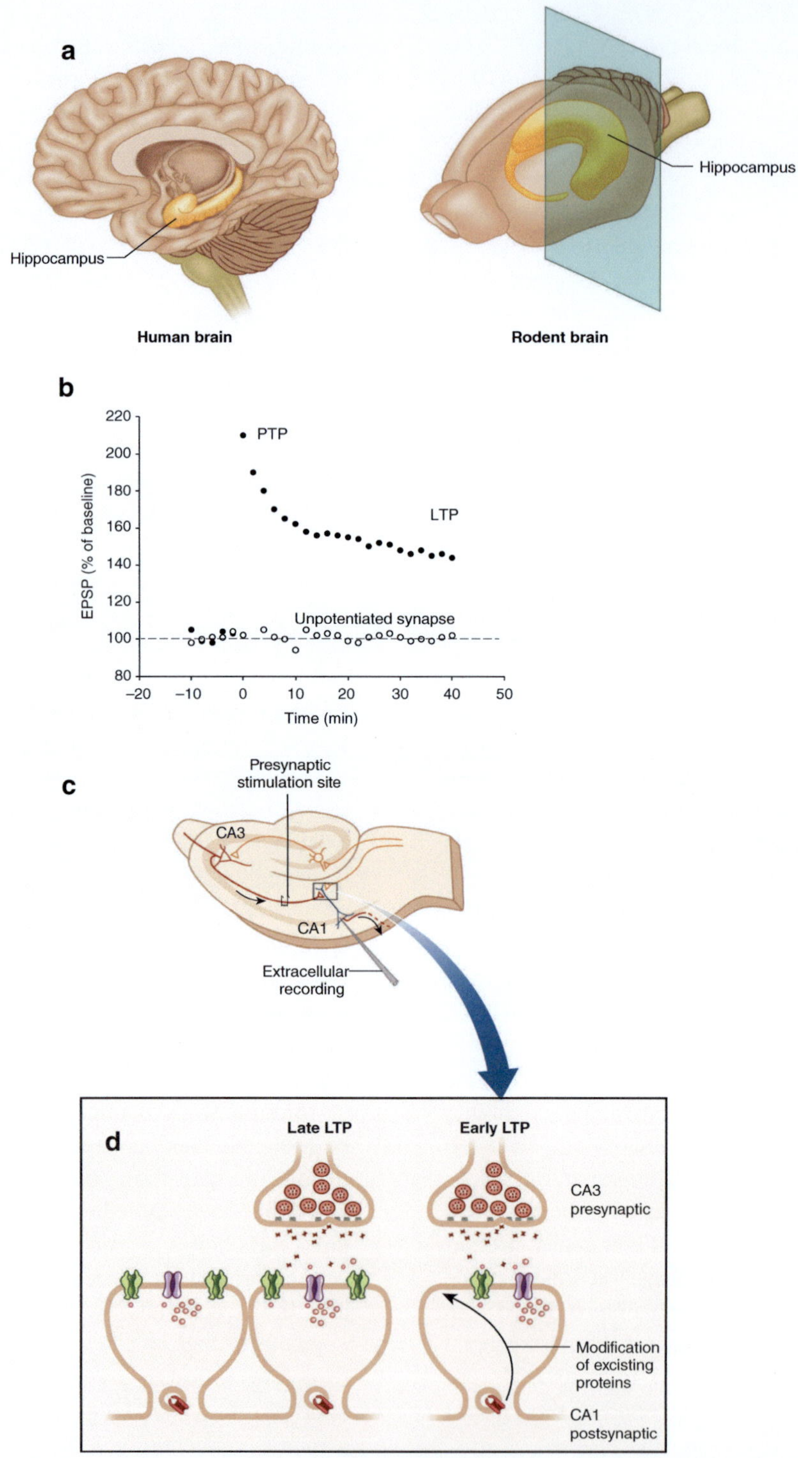

Fig. 6.7 Molecular mechanisms of hippocampal long-term potentiation (LTP). **a**) Structure of human and rodent brain. The yellow area represents the hippocampus. **b**) Simplified representation of a demonstration of LTP, showing prolonged synaptic strengthening following a high frequency pulse. EPSP means excitatory postsynaptic potential. PTP = post-tetanic potentiation **c**) Experimental setup: Long-term potentiation is typically studied in hippocampal slices by stimulating the axons of CA3 cells with a high-frequency train of action potentials. This stimulation produces

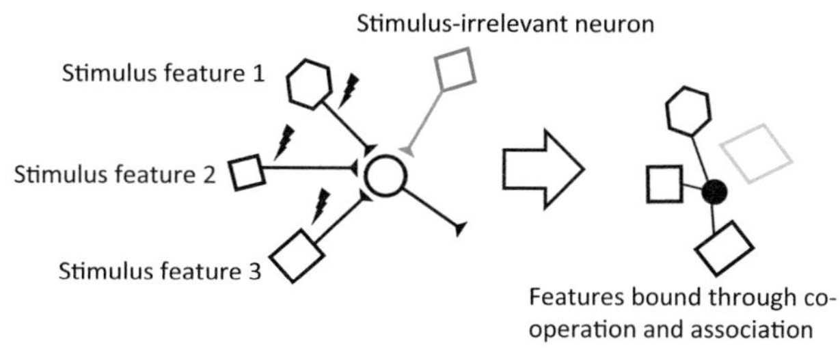

Fig. 6.8 Conceptual visualization of several presynaptic neurons that cooperate in bringing the postsynaptic cell to fire, which potentiates synapses from between all presynaptic contributor and their postsynaptic recipient and hereby linking an ensemble of neurons that each encode different features of a stimulus

6.3 Implicit, Non-declarative Memory

In contrast to the MTL-dependent, conscious, and declarable memory of episodes and semantics are several types of unconscious memory that are all unaffected in severely amnesic (to explicit memories) patients. These are implicit, non-declarative memories that typically do not require explicit awareness nor attention to be encoded and stored. As depicted in Fig. 6.1, implicit learning (or memory) encompasses the *Procedural Learning* (formation of habits and learning new skills), *Associative Learning* (learned associations between stimuli or between a stimulus and a response), *Non-associative Learning* (the gradual increase or decrease in response to a stimulus), and *Priming* (the Impact of, e.g., a sensory stimulus to subsequent stimulus).

Implicit learning is thus a category of memories, which have been joined because they share one common feature: that they are not explicit nor declarative. Implicit, non-declarative memories are consequently not located in a single region or locus of the central nervous system (like the MTL for explicit memories) although some structures appear crucial for distinct implicit categories. A thorough description of the regions mediating the various implicit memory forms is beyond the scope of this chapter, but in general procedural learning is associated with networks spanning regions in basal ganglia, cerebellum, and neocortex (see also Chap. 7 for regions and networks involved in forming motor memories). Bodily expressions of associative learning involve the cerebellum and emotional conditioning are rooted in regions of the limbic system. Finally, non-associative learning is thought to be a local phenomenon expressed in the reflex circuitry involved in a given stimulus-response behavior.

6.3.1 Non-associative Learning Keeps the Sea Hare Alive

Non-associative learning is a well-studied example of implicit, non-declarative learning. It describes how a response to a stimulus either increases or decreases upon repeated exposure. The fear response to a very lively image of a lion attenuates with repeated exposure when it is not associated with any consequences. In contrast, if the image is coupled with an unpleasant experience (it does not have to be the appearance of an actual lion), an increase in the response magnitude can be expected. From an evolutionary perspective, these two non-associative learning forms are critical for survival. Caution is warranted when experiencing a novel stimulus, but after multiple harmless exposures, the organism *habituates* and the withdrawal response from the stimulus gradually fades. Conversely, if a single

Fig. 6.7 (continued) a long-lasting increase in synaptic strength at their excitatory connections onto CA1 cells. **d**) Enlarged view of the CA3–CA1 excitatory synapse. In early LTP, brief high-frequency stimulation activates NMDA receptors, allowing calcium influx into the postsynaptic cell, which modifies existing proteins to strengthen synaptic transmission. In late LTP, repeated or stronger stimulation triggers gene expression and protein synthesis, leading to long-lasting changes such as the growth of new synapses and structural remodeling

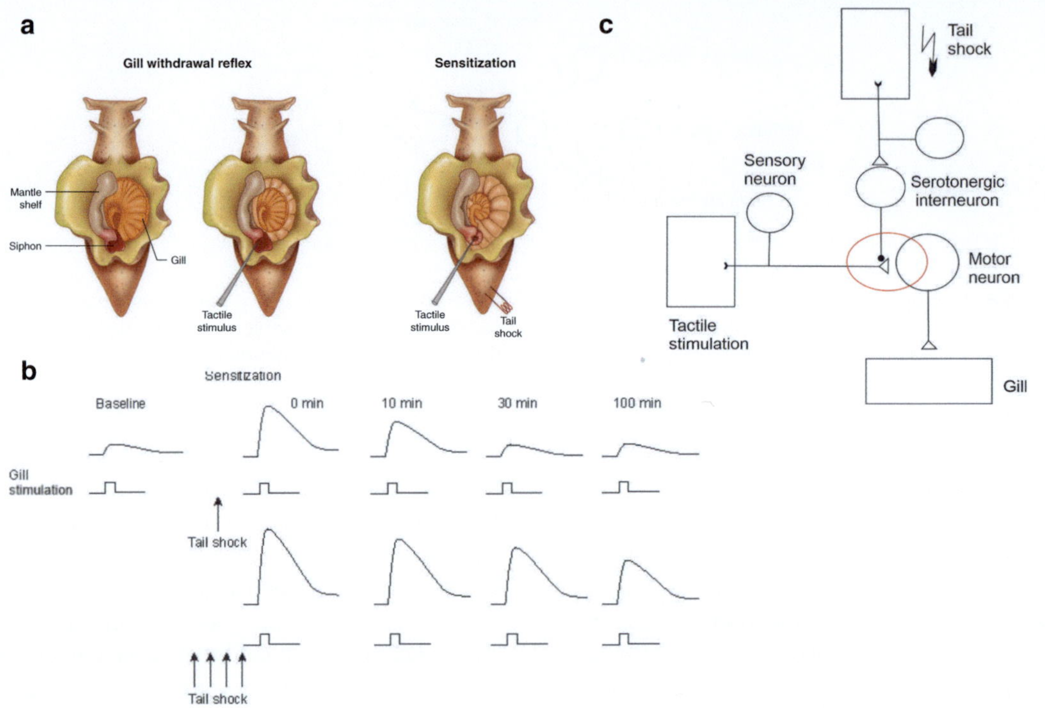

Fig. 6.9 The Aplysia and non-associative learning. (**a**) The Aplysia model. The Aplysia has an exposed gill (left), which is withdrawn alongside the siphon when the siphon or mantle is touched (middle). After an electrical shock, the reflex is much stronger (right). (**b**) This sensitization is further potentiated and prolonged when several shocks a delivered. (**c**) A simplified diagram showing the reflex circuitry. The tail shock activates a serotonergic neuron that through presynaptic mechanisms increase the synaptic potentiating leading to the increased sensorimotor reflex response or amplitude

harmful stimulus is inflicted on the organism, a stronger withdrawal response from novel stimuli is warranted even for stimuli previously learned to be safe. Consequently, such *sensitization* and *dishabituation effects* occur within very few trials. The mechanisms underlying *habituation* and *sensitization* have been studied extensively in many organisms but none more than the sea hare Aplysia Californica.

Unlike humans, the sea hare is equipped with a tail, a siphon, and a gill (see Fig. 6.9a). When the siphon is touched, the gill (and siphon) is automatically withdrawn into safety. When the siphon is repeatedly touched, the duration of the gill withdrawal decreases (*habituation*). An electrical shock to the tail abruptly reinstalls the withdrawal reflex in a habituated animal (*dishabituation*), but a tail shock will also increase the duration of the gill withdrawal response in naive animals (*sensitization*). In Fig. 6.9c, the circuitry mediating non-associative learning is depicted.

6.3.2 Associative Learning in Sea Hares, Dogs, and Humans

There are two cornerstones in behavioral conditioning: classical and operant conditioning. These are psychological concepts that emerge from the early nineteenth-century behaviorists that remain highly influential in the way the research field approached the study of learning in animals (including humans). Classical conditioning describes the process in which a conditioned stimulus (CS) that in its own is not rewarding or punishing repeatedly occurs timely paired with a rewarding or punishing unconditioned stimulus (US). The repeated pairing of the CS and US eventually leads to the organisms responding to the CS as if it was the US. In mammals, classical conditioning is best known from Pavlov's dogs, who learned to associate the sound of a bell (CS) with a food reward (US), and consequently increased the saliva secretion when the bell rang.

In rabbits (and humans), the eyeblink conditioning paradigm has been a valuable paradigm to explore mechanisms of classical conditioning. In this paradigm, a tone (CS) becomes associated with an air puff to the eye (US) that triggers an eyeblink. There is a consensus that cerebellar cortex, but also deep cerebral and cerebellar nuclei are pivotal for this learning.

The Aplysia model has been valuable in studying how classical conditioning manifests in a 'simple' circuitry. When siphon touches are repeatedly and timely paired with tail shocks, the Siphon touch (CS) is gradually being associated with the sensation of a tail shock (US). As a result, the duration of the withdrawal response to a siphon touch is consequently increased for several days, i.e., long-term memory. The circuit and molecular processes underlying long-term memory are described in the box below.

Box 6.4 Three Phases of Facilitation in the Sea Hare Aplysia

The initial sensitization after a single tail shock peaks after a few minutes. The same goes for the sensorimotor synaptic strength (*short-term facilitation*). A few shocks in sequence lead to longer lasting (hours) *intermediate facilitation*, whereas repeated shocks cause a long-lasting (days) increase in synaptic strength termed *long-term facilitation*. The initial short-lasting memory of stimuli (and associated consequences) somehow needs to be transformed into long-term memory. This consolidation process at a cellular level shares many virtues with the cellular consolidation in hippocampus. The acute short-lasting memory is expressed solely presynaptically. Presynaptic intracellular signaling results in the modification of existing proteins that yield a larger release of transmitters to the arrival of action potentials to the sensory neuron terminals(s). An example of this could be the closing of potassium channels, which 'broadens' the action potential and increases the calcium influx and thereby transmitter release. But potassium channels open again. By delivering 4 shocks, the sensitization increases in durability to a matter of hours, which is contingent on both pre- and postsynaptic modification of proteins as well as protein synthesis (see Fig. 6.9b). The initial increase in presynaptic transmitter release is massive (threefold) and acts to initiate the postsynaptic modifications and protein production. Following, and because of, the neural events that lead to short- and intermediate-term facilitation is a temporal robust facilitation that lasts days to weeks (long-term facilitation). This temporal robustness reflects the consolidation of the short-term sensitization and requires protein synthesis. For sensitization, serotonin kicks off an array of intracellular processes that eventually lead to long-term facilitation. These include synaptic growth where the number of presynaptic terminals in a sensory neuron more than doubles. At the same time, the postsynaptic spines of the gill motor neurons grow, a process that in many ways compares to the postsynaptic late LTP observed in hippocampus. Reversely, long-term memory of habituation involves the retraction of the sensory neurons. For the gill withdrawal reflex in the sea hare, the cellular consolidation that transforms a short to a long-lasting sensitization is specific to sensorimotor circuit that is involved in the sensations and motor response. In animals with more complex nervous systems, like humans, behaviors often involve multiple interconnected networks, which necessitates a less reductionistic view on the consolidation of procedural memories. Notwithstanding, the principles of long-term facilitation discovered in the Aplysia along with those of hippocampal LTP are the prime candidates for the neuroplastic changes that enable humans to expand or re-establish the sensorimotor repertoire.

Another form of associative learning is *operant conditioning* (also termed *instrumental conditioning* or *instrumental learning*). Here, an action is associated with a reward or punishment. In 1898, Edward Thorndike proposed the 'law of effect', which (in paraphrased terms) states that an action that produces a satisfying effect is likely to be repeated, whereas an action that yields discomforting effect is less likely to be repeated. He postulated this based on the observation that animals use trial-and-error rather than a carefully masterminded strategy to escape an enclosure. This is still the foundation for how animals are trained in research settings. Food or water deprivation ensures that the animal will repeat rewarded actions without understanding what part of the behavior that triggered the reward and without further exploring means to minimize the costs of the action. One example is a timing paradigm used by Olvecky and coworkers (Kawai et al., 2015), where animals are rewarded when they press a lever twice with a certain inter-press interval. Each animal fills the time gap with an idiosyncratic series of movements that (unintentionally) ensures that the animal repeat the correct timing. In support of Thorndike's original observations, each series of (unnecessary) movements becomes smoother and increasingly more like the previous series, hallmarks of motor learning, but without ever exploring the possibility of simply sitting and pressing the lever twice. It should be noted that such idiosyncratic movements can be viewed as a 'motor habit', which traditionally would be categorized as 'procedural learning' despite the clear relation to the reward system. See Chap. 7 for an introduction to the concepts of procedural learning with an emphasis on the formation of sensorimotor skills.

Operant conditioning can be subdivided into reinforcement (with the purpose of increasing behavior) and punishment (with the purpose of decreasing behavior). Reinforcement can further be positive (adding something pleasant) or negative (removing something unpleasant). In everyday terms, the carrot (positive reinforcement) is typically distinguished from the stick (punishment), but the removal of the stick (negative reinforcement) is also considered a carrot. This notion is supported by the findings that the reward system centered around the midbrain dopaminergic projection to the striatum (from substantia nigra pars compacta) and the neocortex (from ventral tegmental area, VTA) is involved in both reward-based and avoidance learning. Furthermore, dopaminergic projections from VTA to motor cortex are necessary in order for rodents to learn a skilled reaching task and for the motor cortex to reorganize to support the improved behavior. Reinforcement learning is thereby not solely a way to repeatedly choose rewarded actions, but also a pillar in the plasticity that underlies the honing of the motor execution (see also Sect. 7.5.2). Furthermore, studies in humans have revealed that reinforcing successful behavior by rewarding successful trials enhances motor skill learning by influencing consolidation processes. Reinforcement learning is thus at the core of sensorimotor rehabilitation. It provides a neurobiological basis for the use of extrinsic feedback, deliberate training, motivation, goal setting, and experiences of success in neurorehabilitation programs (see Chap. 15). Reinforcement learning also highlights two important points in relation to neurorehabilitation: Processes that take place *during* practice influence consolidation *after* practice and that lasting improvement in function relies as much on practice as the consolidation *after* practice (see Chap. 15).

6.3.3 Perception, Use, and Training Can Be Primed

A final category of implicit learning, *priming*, describes a list of psychological concepts that in some forms has application in neurorehabilitation. The idea is to prime, e.g., a sensory system with a stimulus to bias the systems perception or response to subsequent stimuli. Upon being presented with a series of images of animals, a person will be primed to identify a subsequent blurred image as an animal even though the image might as well be a motorcycle. This perceptual priming is reflected in some neurorehabilitation strategies such as context-specific virtual reality training where patients improve postural stability and locomotion as they navigate their local mall virtually. Therapists also nudge their patients to engage in rehabilitation by priming the environment with objects and cues that increase the likelihood of the patient to carry out sensorimotor actions. The motor system can also be primed in a manner that resembles *repetition priming*. This was demonstrated by Moorjani et al. (2022) who delivered repeated movement-triggered intracortical micro-stimulation to the motor cortex of non-human primates. This stimulation ensured an increased postsynaptic response in a circuit engaged by the movement. The result was an increased connectivity within the circuit but interestingly also a very clear increase in use-dependent plasticity accompanying subsequent use. In other words, the repeated activation primed the circuit to respond more to subsequent use. A similar phenomenon has been described in humans, where pathway-specific activation prior to motor practice has been demonstrated to prime the system and increase the performance gains obtained during practice (Bjørndal et al., 2024). Albeit methodologically cumbersome, this approach has demonstrated its potential to enhance motor recovery following spinal cord injury (Jo et al., 2023).

6.4 The Story of H.M: A Different Perspective and Nuanced Interpretation

By now, a revisit of H.M's case in greater detail is warranted. Seventy years ago, Wilder Penfield and Brenda Milner, both researchers at McGill University in Montreal studied humans with lesions to the temporal lobe. Penfield, Milner, and colleagues encountered several patients with MTL lobotomies who displayed various degrees of predominantly anterograde amnesia (inability to form memories) without any other intellectual losses. Milner and Penfield accredited the amnesia to the hippocampal formations in the MTL as one patient underwent MTL lobotomy in two steps, and amnesia did not manifest until the hippocampus was resected during the second step. Milner joined forces with William Scoville, a neurosurgeon, who had performed a bilateral MTL lobotomy on a patient, who now expressed severe anterograde amnesia. Milner studied HM, over several decades. As a consequence of this work, HM has become probably the most famous individual in memory research. HM suffered from very severe epilepsy, which was ameliorated after bilateral excision of the hippocampal formation, parts of the temporal cortex, and the amygdala. The MTL resections rendered HM incapable of remembering events, people, or places that he encountered after the surgery. He basically forgot what had just happened as soon as his attention was drawn away from the topic at hand. In contrast, he could recollect childhood episodes, he had well-functioning sustained attention, and could maintain information present in mind using his working memory. Altogether, these findings suggest that hippocampus is a pivotal actor in the formation of new memories. One discovery, in particular, laid the groundwork for much subsequent research into long-term memory. Over the course of 3 days, HM practiced a mirror drawing task where he traced a double-margined star while looking at the mirrored image of the target. He improved substantially over the 3 days, although he had no recollection of having tried the task before. It appeared that the MTL lobotomy only compromised the ability to form *declarative, explicit* memories that were episodic or semantic of nature. In contrast, the long-term formation of *non-declarative*, *implicit* memories such as motor skills appeared unaffected. Later investigations confirmed this distinction in that HM could learn various other motor skills and showed preserved visuo-perceptual priming but impaired visual recognition. The conclusion from the studies of HM was that general cognitive functions, including working memory, are distinct from the MTL-dependent formation of long-term memories and that the circuits involved in implicit learning (incl. motor skills) are distinct from MTL-dependent explicit learning.

However, by now it should be clear to the reader that the dichotomous view on memory based on HM (and others) symptomatology is a simplification. Decades later, after the initial investigations, HM inadvertently challenged the notion that long-term memories are formed either in an MTL-dependent 'Declarative' system or in MTL-independent non-declarative system(s) (see Corkin, 2002). Upon request, HM was able to report the exact address and draw the floor print of a house he lived in *after* the lobotomy. Despite having very little capacity to learn visual or tactile maze navigation, i.e., correct sequence of turns, HM could form a cognitive map of his house through thousands of walks through the house. This was surprising, as spatial memory is considered to be strictly explicit and hippocampus-dependent. In fact, spatial memory tasks (e.g., Morris water maze) are often used to study explicit memory in rodents that inherently have a hard time declaring experienced episodes. Later, neuroimaging and lesion studies support the existence of a topographical memory (used to draw floor plan), which is distinct from egocentric spatial memory (tasked when navigating a maze). For HM, the distinction was sharp, and interestingly, topographical and spatial memory are supported by distinct networks that include adjacent structures in the MTL. However, whereas the categorical distinctions between topographic and spatial memory along with their neural underpinnings are valuable in the laboratory and of profound scientific interest, the reality is that the ability to navigate through the streets of a city likely benefits from a combined use of both an internal map, memory of when to turn left and right, as well as visual cues.

6.5 Conclusions and Perspectives

The human ability to store information for later use enables learning of not only the names of capitals, kings, and presidents, but also the concept of multiplication as well as the sequence and magnitude of muscular activity needed to ride a bike. In broad terms, two categories of memories exist. The first spans episodic, semantic, and conceptual knowledge that can be expressed in detail, for example, the order of events and the fact that two plus two equals four. If remembered, such knowledge can easily be passed on. The second category covers all other memories that are not readily describable such as the order and extent of muscular activity needed to maintain balance and propel a bike forward.

Explicit memories are formed in networks that encompass cortical regions that are relevant to the modality of the sensory stimulus in cooperation with mediotemporal and prefrontal structures that enable long-term storage and incorporation into existing knowledge. The well-described cellular mechanisms involve increases and decreases in synaptic connectivity mediated by both changes in existing as well as the production of new proteins. Functional changes precede and are necessary for later structural changes. Similar principles govern cellular changes underlying implicit memory formation as demonstrated through extensive studies in simple invertebrate organisms. Knowledge of how the central nervous system reorganizes when encoding and consolidating new memories is of fundamental scientific interest, but importantly also valuable when optimizing the outcome of neurorehabilitation. By identifying key, structures, networks, and molecular processes involved in, e.g., relearning a sensorimotor skill, the therapist can tune training parameters to target long-lasting memory formation over short-lasting performance increments. The memory processes that are specific to sensorimotor skill learning are discussed in the next chapter.

Review Questions

- What are the core tasks of the working memory?
- How can an experience be stored as long-term memory? And why could HM not accomplish this?

References

Baddeley, A. (2010). Working memory. *Current Biology, 20*(4), R136–R140.

Baddeley, A. D., & Hitch, G. J. (1994). Developments in the concept of working memory. *Neuropsychology, 8*(4), 485.

Bjørndal, J. R., Beck, M. M., Jespersen, L., Christiansen, L., & Lundbye-Jensen, J. (2024). Hebbian priming of human motor learning. *Nature Communications, 15*(1), 5126.

Bliss, T. V. P., & Lømo, T. (1973). Long-lasting potentiation of synaptic transmission in the dentate area of the anaesthetized rabbit following stimulation of the perforant path. *The Journal of Physiology, 232*(2), 331–356.

Clemens, Z., et al. (2007). Temporal coupling of parahippocampal ripples, sleep spindles and slow oscillations in humans. *Brain, 130*(11), 2868–2878.

Corkin, S. (2002). What's new with the amnesic patient HM? *Nature Reviews Neuroscience, 3*(2), 153–160.

D'Esposito, M., et al. (1999). Maintenance versus manipulation of information held in working memory: An event-related fMRI study. *Brain and Cognition, 41*(1), 66–86.

Ferguson, M. A., et al. (2019). A human memory circuit derived from brain lesions causing amnesia. *Nature Communications, 10*(1), 3497.

Fuster, J. M., & Alexander, G. E. (1971). Neuron activity related to short-term memory. *Science, 173*(3997), 652–654.

Jo, H. J., et al. (2023). Multisite Hebbian plasticity restores function in humans with spinal cord injury. *Annals of Neurology*.

Kawai, R., et al. (2015). Motor cortex is required for learning but not for executing a motor skill. *Neuron, 86*(3), 800–812.

Moorjani, S., et al. (2022). Movement-dependent electrical stimulation for volitional strengthening of cortical connections in behaving monkeys. *Proceedings of the National Academy of Sciences, 119*(27), e2116321119.

Murray, J. D., et al. (2017). Stable population coding for working memory coexists with heterogeneous neural dynamics in prefrontal cortex. *Proceedings of the National Academy of Sciences, 114*(2), 394–399.

Nee, D. E., et al. (2013). A meta-analysis of executive components of working memory. *Cerebral Cortex, 23*(2), 264–282.

O'Keefe, J., & Dostrovsky, J. (1971). The hippocampus as a spatial map: Preliminary evidence from unit activity in the freely-moving rat. *Brain Research*.

Siapas, A. G., & Wilson, M. A. (1998). Coordinated interactions between hippocampal ripples and cortical spindles during slow-wave sleep. *Neuron, 21*(5), 1123–1128.

Van Kesteren, M. T., et al. (2012). How schema and novelty augment memory formation. *Trends in Neurosciences, 35*(4), 211–219.

Wilson, M. A., & McNaughton, B. L. (1994). Reactivation of hippocampal ensemble memories during sleep. *Science, 265*(5172), 676–679.

Skill Acquisition and Motor Learning

7

Jesper Lundbye-Jensen and Lasse Christiansen

Abstract

Throughout life, we acquire various skills essential for daily functioning. This ability is crucial for reaching adulthood. Some skills are mastered quickly, while others take years to develop. In neurorehabilitation, motor recovery happens either through relearning similar movement patterns or through compensatory recovery, using different movements to achieve the same goal. Sensorimotor skill learning is vital in both cases.

In the central nervous system, the journey from barely balancing on a bike to effortlessly maneuvering through traffic while listening to a podcast involves significant changes. Early stages of skill learning are characterized by cognitive processes, while later stages involve gradual improvements without conscious awareness. Understanding these stages and replicating real-world skills in the laboratory are key to studying skill learning.

Although skill learning is often seen as implicit, this is not entirely accurate. Early skill acquisition involves cognitive elements, while later stages consist of slow, subtle enhancements after extensive practice. The neural mechanisms behind motor skill learning follow principles like memory formation, with unique variations. Adaptations in the neocortex, basal ganglia, cerebellum, and spinal cord all play roles in acquiring, consolidating, and expressing motor skills. These complex neural processes underscore the complex nature of learning and mastering new skills.

Keywords

Motor learning · Skill learning · Skill acquisition · Motor memory · Neuroplasticity

Box 7.1 Clinical Case

A 58-year-old man, James, suffered an ischemic stroke that resulted in left-sided hemiparesis. The primary goal of his neurorehabilitation program is to recover his ability to perform daily activities independently, particularly those requiring fine motor skills and eye-hand coordination. This case underscores the importance of both acquiring new motor skills and maintaining existing ones to adapt to changing needs and sustain functional abilities.

(continued)

J. Lundbye-Jensen (✉)
Movement & Neuroscience, Department of Nutrition, Exercise & Sports, University of Copenhagen, Copenhagen, Denmark
e-mail: jlundbye@nexs.ku.dk

L. Christiansen
Danish Research Centre for Magnetic Resonance (DRCMR), Copenhagen University Hospital, Amager and Hvidovre, Hvidovre, Denmark

Department of Neuroscience, Faculty of Health and Medical Sciences, University of Copenhagen, Copenhagen, Denmark
e-mail: lassec@drcmr.dk

J. B. Nielsen et al. (eds.), *Neuroplasticity-based Neurorehabilitation*,
https://doi.org/10.1007/978-3-031-81120-3_7

Box 7.1 (continued)

James, who used to be an elite tennis player, understands the importance of targeted practice. His training includes extensive eye-to-hand exercises, essential for his sport, which is now analogous to his current rehabilitation. Just as athletes train for the Olympics or pianists practice for concerts, James' rehabilitation involves focused motor practice aimed at restoring his fine motor abilities.

During therapy sessions, James engages in repetitive, task-specific exercises designed to improve his eye-hand coordination. Activities such as throwing and catching a ball are integral to his therapy, helping to refine his motor skills and enhance his coordination. Initial improvements in his performance are noted at the end of each session, highlighting the impact of consistent motor practice.

The true measure of success in James' rehabilitation lies in the long-term retention of these improvements. It is crucial to assess his ability to perform the learned tasks at later points, such as in subsequent therapy sessions or at home, without the direct supervision of a therapist. This delayed retention indicates genuine motor skill learning and the formation of durable motor memory.

As discussed in Chap. 6, the formation of motor memories and plastic changes in the central nervous system are essential for skill acquisition and relearning. James' progress is monitored to ensure these neural adaptations occur, facilitating lasting improvements in his motor abilities. This case highlights the interrelationships between motor practice, skill acquisition, memory formation, and neural plasticity in neurorehabilitation. For James, successful rehabilitation is not only about immediate performance gains but also about ensuring these gains translate into long-term functional recovery.

7.1 Introduction—Skill Learning and Relearning in Neurorehabilitation

Improvements in sensorimotor functions in neurological disorders can be attributed to spontaneous recovery, recovery driven by motor learning, and the interaction between these. The contribution of these processes in the accumulated recovery is hard to disentangle and much of what has been accredited to spontaneous recovery may in fact be driven by continuous and improved use. As an example, non-human primates with severe spinal cord injury display marked "spontaneous" neuroplasticity in the shape of axonal outgrowth and sprouting that coincides with motor recovery (Rosenzweig et al., 2010). However, outside of planned training sessions these monkeys engage in numerous motor acts when climbing the cage, eating, grooming, and so on. The monkeys will strive to execute the motor acts with sufficient quality to achieve the goal (food, clean fur, propelling to neighboring parts of the cage). So even without *deliberate* rehabilitation (see Chap. 15), the monkeys engage in motor practice with goals, rewards, and hundreds of repetitions. The extent to which the motor recovery of the monkeys is "spontaneous" per se is consequently questionable. Albeit difficult to quantify, motor recovery and the supporting neuroplasticity are guided and in part spurred by "motor learning" and extensive motor use.

The role of sensorimotor practice in neurorehabilitation is to stimulate, steer, and hone plastic processes of the central nervous system (CNS) to optimize the outcome in the shape of long-term behavioral improvements. Whereas no single sensorimotor practice schedule fits all patients across neurological conditions, the basic principles and mechanisms of motor skill learning do indeed. These are the ones introduced and discussed in this chapter.

7.2 What Is Motor Learning?

Motor learning encompasses all internal processes aimed at optimizing behavioral outcomes and minimizing the cost of movement. This is only achieved by optimizing movements in relation to our (Newtonian) surroundings. A system is therefore required to modulate motor output based on sensory information about those surroundings. Sensory feedback enables adjustments during movement and provides information for optimizing future movements. Consequently, *sensorimotor learning* is a more appropriate term for these mechanisms that together serve as the foundation for performance improvements in sports and functional recovery or compensatory learning in patients after brain injuries. "Motor learning" is not restricted to learning a new set of new movements. Instead, motor learning comprises the ability to acquire new movement kinematics, combine known movements into new sequences, and adapt them to external perturbations. It is commonly assumed that a shift in the speed-accuracy curve with practice indicates motor learning. However, an increase in a movement's velocity accompanied by reduced accuracy does not reflect learning but rather a shift in movement strategy. The central nervous networks that underpin these two different aspects of functional improvement are not the same but are often overlapping. To complicate things further, the networks which support performance improvements during training are not necessarily the same networks, which ensure that skill learning is consolidated.

As mentioned in the beginning of the chapter, motor learning involves processes of acquisition during motor practice, but for learning to manifest as meaningful improvements in function that are relevant in real life—it is essential that the behavioral effects obtained through motor practice demonstrate permanence. During recent years, behavioral research has provided evidence for an important distinction between the immediate performance gains that accompany practice and long-term changes in motor performance that reflect retention and thus more permanent changes in the capability for the practiced skills (Kantak & Winstein, 2012). This *learning–performance distinction* is particularly important when assessing the effects of rehabilitation training. Improved in-session performance is naturally desirable—not least for motivation—but long-term retention of motor skills and transfer to real life is essential. A review of motor learning studies with a specific focus on comparing differences in performance between the end of practice and at delayed retention suggests that the delayed retention or transfer performance is a better indicator of motor learning than the performance during or at the end of practice (Kantak & Winstein, 2012). Processes of acquisition during motor practice naturally drive motor learning and lead to changes in performance and these changes in performance could be indicative of learning, but it is pivotal to stress the importance of assessing learning at delayed retention or transfer tests demonstrating long-term effects and thus memory.

7.3 Multiple Phases and Processes of Motor Learning—A Neuropsychological Point of View

Throughout history, it has been a common assumption in different conceptual models that the process of motor skill learning proceeds through different phases placing different cognitive demands on the individual. More specifically, it is often assumed that during the progression of motor learning, explicit processes and declarative memory dominate during the early phases, whereas implicit processes or procedural memory dominate during late phases. As described in Chap. 6, declarative or explicit memory represents the kind of knowledge that can be declared or explained to others, whereas procedural or implicit memory represents knowledge of "how to" without necessarily being consciously aware of it.

According to one of the early but influential models of skill acquisition, Fitts and Posner (1967) state that the process of learning progresses through three distinct learning phases that differ in cognitive demands (Fitts & Posner, 1967; see Fig. 7.1a). Fitts and Posner proposed that during early stages of learning, motor skills are attended to in a step-by-step fashion and require the involvement of declarative knowledge or memory. The application of declarative knowl-

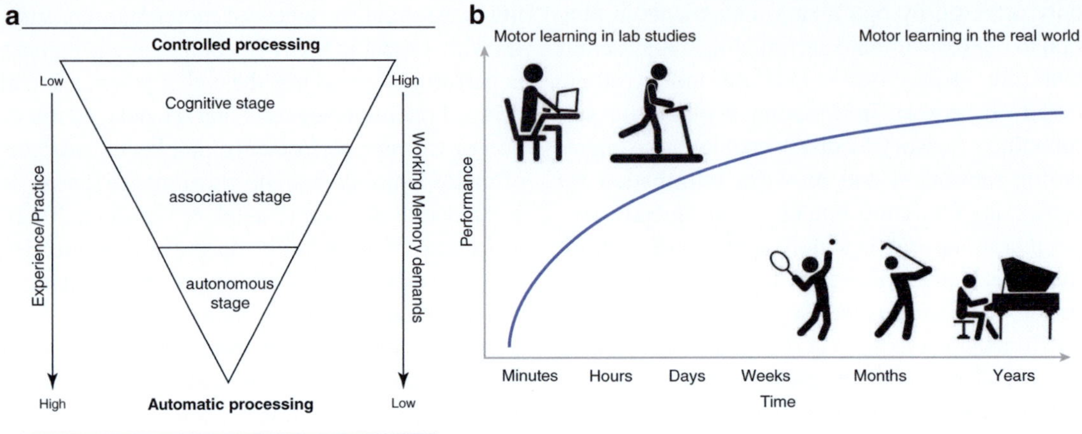

Fig. 7.1 Phases and time course of motor learning. (**a**) During the process of long-term motor learning, task performance demands change from highly cognitive controlled to automatic processing. According to the model put forward by Fitts and Posner learning goes through a cognitive, an associative, and an autonomous stage with extended practice and experience. In parallel, the task demands for working memory become increasingly lower. (**b**) During a period of motor learning, motor performance improves with increased amounts of practice. Most laboratory-based studies investigate effects in a range from minutes to weeks, whereas excellence in real-world skill requires extensive amounts of practice for several years

edge requires working memory, whereas procedural knowledge does not. Based on this, Fitts and Posner called this early phase the cognitive phase. Learning in this initial phase focuses on comprehending the task at hand, and verbal instructions offer significant opportunities for performance improvements. After this stage, learning enters the associative stage in which working memory involvement diminishes as learners begin to develop associations between specific stimuli and suitable motor actions. In the final autonomous stage, no explicit working memory resources are required for the skill execution. In this advanced stage, movement execution becomes automatic, requiring minimal influence from conscious processes. Movements are performed with precision almost every time. While the associative phase demands conscious control, motor performance in the autonomous phase is highly automated. For instance, trained pianists can direct attention elsewhere and perform complex tasks while playing the piano. The duration of the different phases varies based on task complexity. As illustrated in Fig. 7.1b, studies of motor learning in lab settings often focus on relatively simple tasks and changes within minutes to weeks, whereas it is well-known that expertise in real-world tasks such as playing the piano or being a skilled tennis player requires years of practice.

The assumption that the cognitive demand or the involvement of working memory processes decreases with continued practice is not unique to the model put forward by Fitts and Posner but common in the skill learning literature (e.g., Krakauer et al., 2019). However, the stage theories in general give a somewhat simple explanation of the involvement of working memory during motor skill learning, based on the findings that processing of declarative knowledge is not characteristic of all early stages of learning, and that skill acquisition does not have to progress from declarative to procedural memory. That said, it is important to emphasize that cognitive processes are very much part of motor learning when actions need to be selected at the right time, in the right order, or in the right combination. In all likelihood, motor skill learning involves both explicit and implicit processes with distinct dynamics and time courses and the processes may change depending on the type of practice and context (see also discussion of the model by Fitts and Posner in relation to neurorehabilitation in Chap. 15).

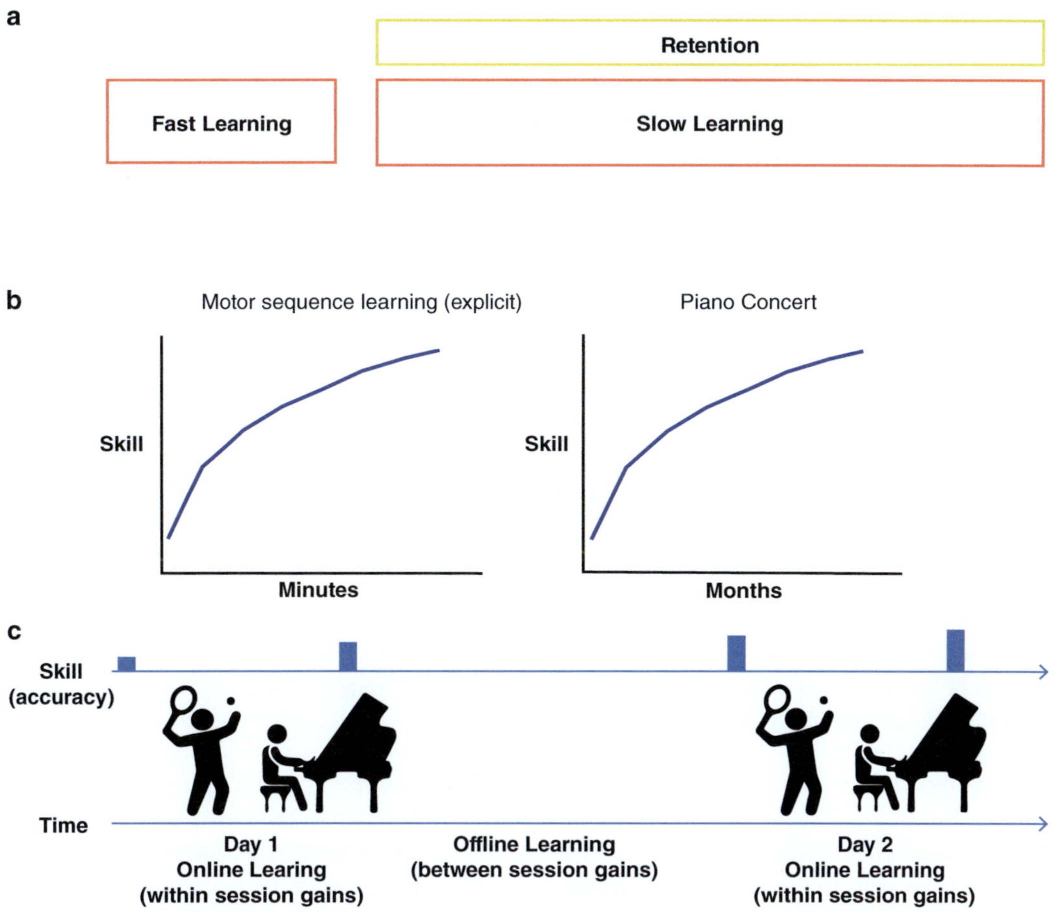

Fig. 7.2 A supplementary view on the process and phases of motor skill learning. (**a**) Motor skill learning can be divided into stages: a fast/early stage where typically significant improvements can be seen within a single training session and a later slower stage where further gains are achieved across multiple sessions of practice. Skill can be retained after a single or multiple training sessions. (**b**) The relative duration of fast and slow learning is highly task-specific. For example, the fast stage of learning an explicit sequence of key-press movements could last minutes, while the fast stage of learning to play a complex musical piece may last months. Although the shape of the learning curves for these two different tasks could theoretically be the same, the time bases of the fast stages of learning may be substantially different. (**c**) Performance improvements during skill acquisition can occur during training (online learning) but also in between sessions, with no further practice (offline learning). See Dayan and Cohen (2011).

Motor skills are typically learned over multiple training sessions until performance reaches nearly asymptotic levels. During recent years, several studies and close inspection of learning curves have typically revealed distinct time constants of motor learning: fast initial learning, followed by slower, more gradual improvements later (Krakauer et al., 2019). Across different experimental paradigms, skill acquisition develops relatively fast during the initial phase of learning, e.g., during a motor practice session (Fig. 7.2a), and more slowly over the course of continued training sessions when further gains develop incrementally (Dayan & Cohen, 2011). Note that the time course of these fast and slow learning dynamics is highly task-specific. For example, the fast stage of learning a simple keyboard sequence can have a duration of minutes, whereas the fast stage of learning to play a complex musical piece as for a piano concert may last months (Fig. 7.2b). Fast and slow skill learning processes may contribute to overall learning within sessions and over multiple sessions. While the two-state model of fast and slow learning dynamics cannot adequately describe all operations influencing the learning curve, it is a close approximation of overall sensorimotor learning, and it has since been suggested that the fast and slow processes can be equated to distinct explicit and implicit learning processes, respectively (McDougle et al., 2015).

Importantly, changes in skill levels due to practice can occur during training, i.e., within-session or online, but they can also occur after the end of training, i.e., between-session or offline (Fig. 7.2c). Offline processes involve skill stabilization and improvement and rely on motor memory consolidation processes, which serve to maintain both online and offline skill gains and form the basis of long-term retention (Dayan & Cohen, 2011).

During recent years, the neurobiological basis for motor learning has been shown to align well with the psychological literature on phases of motor learning. The following sections entail a deep dive into the neurobiological processes that subserve motor skill learning.

7.4 Sensory Predictions Guide Motor Actions: How to Handle Delay

Humans perceive the world with a delay of about 150 ms, and there is an additional 70 ms between activity in the primary motor cortex (M1) (see Fig. 7.3) and the resulting movement. These delays mean that the conscious perception of "now" is constantly a few hundred milliseconds behind real-time. Despite this, elite athletes like tennis players can perform incredible feats. For instance, a tennis player serving at over 200 km/h gives their opponent just 400 ms to react, while a handball goalkeeper has only 180 ms to respond to a 130 km/h throw.

This is possible because the nervous system predicts the future. Experienced athletes, like tennis players, use their brains to calculate where the ball will go based on experience, context, and immediate sensory information. They do not need to see the ball's full trajectory to predict its path; they rely on cues from the server's body and limb positions. This predictive ability is gained through years of training, using Bayesian inference (see further in Chap. 8) to continuously update the probabilities of the ball's destination.

The case story in the beginning of the chapter illustrates this well. The rehabilitation of James involves retraining his brain to use these predictive mechanisms, particularly in eye-hand coordination tasks like throwing and catching a ball. By comparing actual and predicted outcomes, the brain adjusts motor commands, enhancing future movements. This process is central to motor learning, where sensory predictions guide actions and corrections, ensuring that James can regain his skills through consistent practice.

7.5 Motor Learning Involves Multiple Distinct But Cooperating Learning Processes Engaging Interconnected Central Nervous Networks

Motor learning involves distinct but cooperative processes to acquire new behavioral patterns, learn new skills, or fine-tuning existing ones. These processes include error-based learning, reinforcement learning, use-dependent plasticity, and strategy-based learning (Fig. 7.4). All these mechanisms contribute to the acquisition of real-world sensorimotor skills.

This is exemplified in the case of James. Initially, he uses explicit strategies to remember how to perform tasks like throwing and catching a ball, much like a beginner memorizing the basics of driving. As he practices, he engages in error-based learning by adjusting his movements based on feedback, gradually improving his accuracy. Reinforcement learning helps him associate successful movements with positive outcomes, encouraging repetition of correct actions. Use-dependent plasticity strengthens

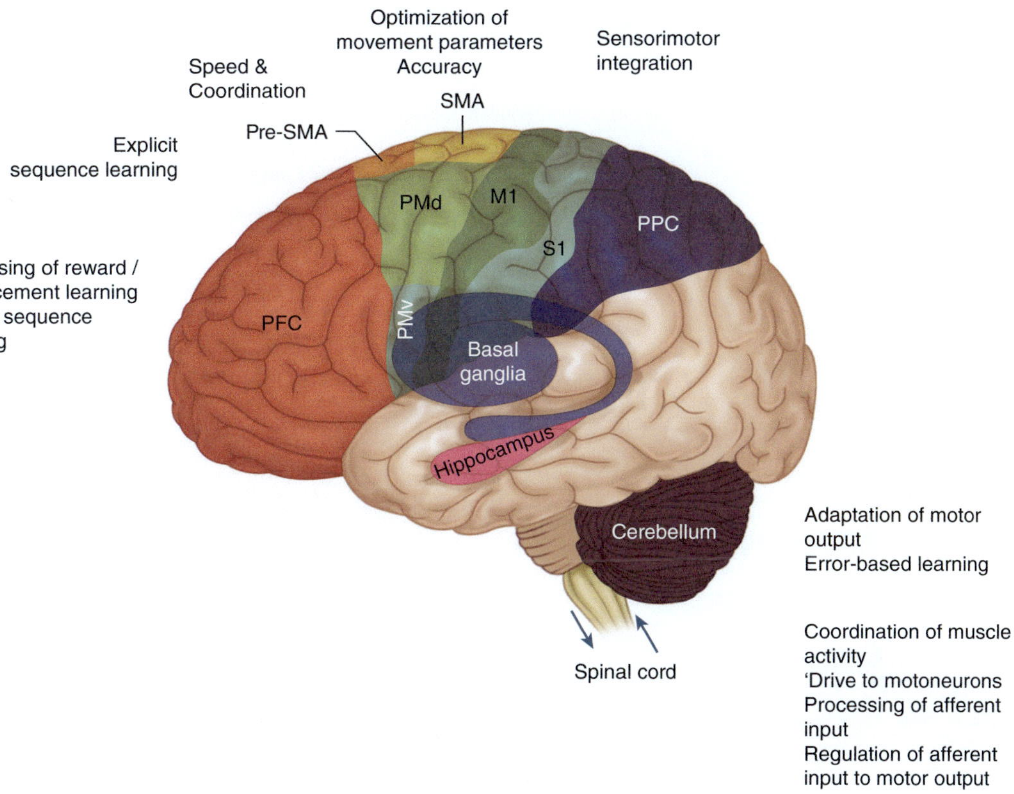

Fig. 7.3 Regions of the CNS contributing to motor skill learning. Numerous regions throughout the brain have contributing in some way to motor learning at the level of goal-setting, selection, or execution. Index to abbreviations: PFC (red): prefrontal cortex; SMA (yellow): supplementary motor area; pre-SMA (orange): presupplementary motor area; PMd (bright green): dorsal premotor cortex; PMv (cyan): ventral premotor cortex; M1 (dark green): primary motor cortex; S1 (cyan): primary somatosensory cortex; PPC (blue): posterior parietal cortex; hippocampus (pink); cerebellum (purple); basal ganglia (blue)

neural pathways through repeated use, enhancing his motor skills over time.

Over time, the discrete actions involved in these tasks become chunked into smoother, more automatic movements. Just as a driver eventually shifts gears without conscious effort, James will relearn to perform complex motor tasks seamlessly, allowing him to regain independence and functionality.

In laboratory settings, tasks used to investigate neural mechanisms subserving motor learning are conversely often reduced to target specific aspects or processes of motor learning. *Motor adaptation* paradigms study how movements are adjusted over time, when a systematic perturbation is introduced to a well-known movement. Over time, motor performance returns to baseline when the movement has adapted to the perturbation. Studies of *sequence learning* probe the speed (and accuracy) of correct responses in a specified sequence of, e.g., finger movements. Visuomotor tracking paradigms task the ability to precisely control force or position while adhering to a specific visuomotor transformation, whereas ballistic motor practice tasks the ability to maximize force development or movement acceleration. In brief, learning or relearning of a real-world sensorimotor skill combines learning processes that are underpinned by plastic changes in interconnected circuits connecting the cerebral cortex with cerebellar, subcortical telencephalic, brainstem, and spinal structures (see Krakauer et al., 2019).

The brain operates based on both predictions, feedback mechanisms and the interplay between them. Despite the CNS having access to precise

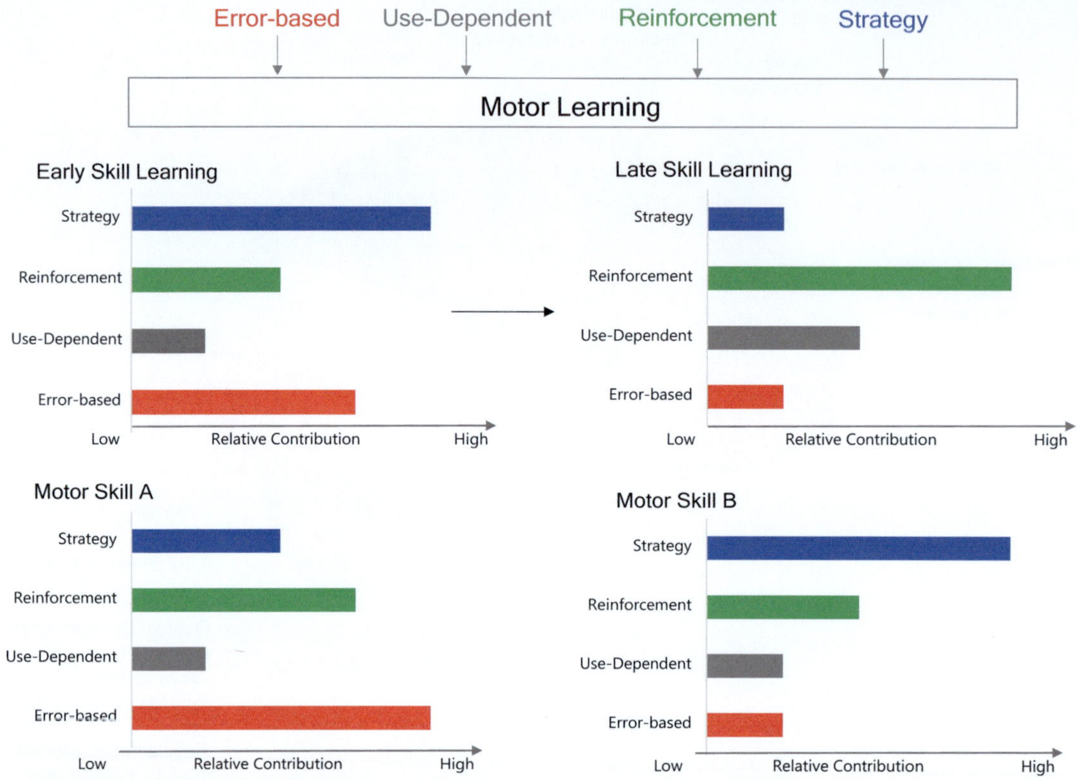

Fig. 7.4 Processes underlying motor learning. Motor learning is constituted by (i) error-based, (ii) reinforcement, (iii) use-dependent plasticity, and (iv) strategy-based forms of learning. Each of these forms of learning is continuously involved in guiding movements toward improved solutions. Although these mechanisms have a common goal in learning a skill, their relative contributions are weighed differently throughout the time course of motor skill training. The bars denote the contribution from low to high. The contributions of these mechanisms of learning may also shift depending on the specific component of the motor task that one is asked to learn. For example, to successfully hit a tennis ball, our brain must develop an understanding of how to interact with a racket/environment/ball (e.g., weight of the racket and ball, type of court), as well as to coordinate an appropriate sequence of movements (i.e., fluid serve) (Spampinato & Celnik, 2021).

information about the body's position from sensory input and the ability to send accurate instructions to muscles during movement control, the execution of reaching for an object by a test participant is very rarely identical from trial to trial. The reason lies in variability and fluctuations in the CNS—sometimes also referred to as motor noise—interacting with the many degrees of freedom, i.e., the same task can often be carried out with numerous different underlying activation patterns. The noise in the CNS introduces uncertainty into the calculations involved in the process from sensory input that informs movement planning to the motor response, including assessing the current state of the body and context, estimating the target location, and executing the movement. The following sections elaborate on the different aspects and processes of error-based learning, reinforcement learning, use-dependent learning, cognitive strategies, and possible interactions. Each of these processes is thought to involve different although interconnected neuronal substrates and computations.

To study different aspects of motor learning, different tasks and experimental paradigms are employed, based on the rationale that, the relative contributions of distinct forms of learning are likely to differ depending on the task requirements for learning to occur. Furthermore, the relative contribution of each type of learning to overall behavioral changes may change over time (Fig. 7.4). Importantly, it is unlikely that a behavioral paradigm isolates a learning process since distinct types of learning are not functionally independent and the neural basis of all types of learning may be involved at any time in the intact brain.

7.5.1 Error-Based Learning

Error-based learning plays a crucial role in the context of motor learning, and it allows us to adapt our movements by accounting for changes in our body or environment based on predictive mechanisms. An example of this may be the ability of the tennis player to adjust her groundstrokes playing in wind from the side, or in a clinical setting the ability to adjust movement parameters to a new, lightweight prosthesis replacing the former one. This type of learning relies on the modification or adaptation of an existing skill based on error signals. These error signals arise from comparing the experienced sensory consequences of a movement to the predicted ones. It is relatively fast and occurs trial-by-trial within minutes to hours of practice. Learning process is informed by sensory prediction errors, which entail vectorial information as to how a movement can be modified to reduce error, e.g., by adjusting force or direction in subsequent trials. In this way, discrepancies between predicted and experienced sensory feedback are used to (re)calibrate internal representations of body dynamics and interactions with the environment and develop forward internal models to reduce errors (Spampinato & Celnik, 2021).

Error-based (supervised) learning has been studied thoroughly in behavioral adaptation tasks. In these paradigms, participants commonly adapt their movement in response to errors caused by (predictable) perturbation introduced to the task, such as altered visual input (by wearing prism glasses or by rotation of visual feedback) or force requirements for producing a reaching movement. The nervous system strives to reduce errors and counteract disturbances by adjusting movement parameters efficiently to restore performance at baseline level or equilibrium. When the perturbation is removed, successful adaptation will be evident as behavioral after-effects and the need of readaptation. Several studies have found that cerebellum has a critical role in this type of error-based learning, and individuals with cerebellar pathologies exhibit impairments in sensorimotor adaptation, which can be attributed to a failure of learning via sensory prediction errors (see Chap. 5). Experimental work in animal models has also provided evidence that the activity of Purkinje cells in the cerebellar cortex is related to forward model learning utilizing sensory prediction errors. Successful adaptation involves cerebellar-thalamocortical activation, and it additionally involves areas of the premotor and parietal cerebral cortex (see Chap. 5). The involvement of these areas may change over time.

7.5.2 Reinforcement and Reward-Based Learning

Reducing directional errors through error-based learning can only take performance to a level where the average deviation of the selected motor program is minimal. In addition to error-based learning, another highly important type of learning is *Reinforcement learning*. This type of learning is also based on feedback mechanisms but contrary to error-based learning through a systematic bias toward choosing actions and prioritizing aspects of task performance that maximize reward. In this way, reinforcement learning refers to a success-based process in which actions leading to successful outcomes are reinforced and consequently tend to be repeated, whereas actions leading to unsuccessful outcomes are avoided. As an example, the server in tennis explores different stance positions or forearm motions to succeed with spin, speed, or position of the serve. In this way, exploration leads to learning in the way that successful behavioral modifications are reinforced and will tend to be repeated. Conversely, unsuccessful modifications will tend to be avoided.

Reinforcement learning is driven by a prediction error that encodes the probability of whether a given action or behavioral modification will result in success. This means that if the outcome of a particular action results in something unexpected, a reward prediction error signal (positive, i.e., reward or negative, respectively) will update expectations for that particular action, and this will lead to repetition or avoidance. Contrary to supervised learning, the reinforcement signal does not provide information of how behavior could be adjusted. The reward merely tells us whether the action was successful or not and does not provide information on what could have been a better choice. Interestingly, when a motor action is learned via success-based feedback, participants do not recalibrate their proprioception to match vision. This phenomenon is not seen when learning is based on sensory prediction errors as mentioned above.

It is widely acknowledged that the basal ganglia play an important role in reinforcement learning, and reinforcement is facilitated by dopaminergic neuron activity, which encodes reward prediction errors "rewarding" a positive difference between the actual outcome of the movement and the expected outcome. The reward signal is a phasic dopamine signal arising from neurons with cell bodies in (predominantly) the ventral tegmental area (VTA) of the midbrain that project to striatal and cortical targets (see Chap. 5).

Dopaminergic neurons are integral to the brain's "reward system," crucial for evolutionary success. This system likely evolved to ensure animals remember vital information, such as finding suitable food or effective problem-solving strategies. Multiple studies indicate that the dopaminergic reward system remains crucial in humans. Individuals learning a particular task also demonstrate more effective learning when provided with immediate feedback on their performance or outcomes. The brain responds to clear stimuli indicating whether the movement was an improvement over the previous one, akin to the "click" training used with dolphins and other animals. This involves consistently providing understandable stimuli that the brain can utilize to enhance its strategy and reinforce successful behaviors.

7.5.3 Repetitions and Use-Dependent Learning

Performance in different tasks can increase from mere use. *Use-dependent learning* describes this phenomenon where simple repetition of movements results in behavioral changes, regardless of whether errors are present or not. Use-dependent learning is not governed by learning algorithms per se, but rather reflects Hebbian principles of plasticity (see Chap. 6). Such *use-dependent* learning is slow and only saturates after a large number of repetitions. Use-dependent learning can be viewed as "unsupervised learning" (i.e., it does not rely on feed-forward models nor on feedback) as sensory feedback, knowledge of movement outcomes, and rewards are not a necessity. However, and of importance for sensorimotor neurorehabilitation, *unsupervised* motor learning interacts with supervised and reinforcement learning.

7.5.4 Cognitive Strategies and Sequence Learning

Strategy-based learning simply refers to utilizing cognitive strategies and explicit knowledge to solve motor problems, and it is evident that explicit, cognitive processes play an important role in motor skill learning (Krakauer et al., 2019). As described previously (remember Fitts and Posner), the literature on motor skill learning entails rich discussions on the role of implicit and explicit processes and their contribution to learning and memory.

Many skills involve sequence-based elements to complete an ordered number of subtasks. These types of sequences require learning the appropriate order of distinct, discrete actions, or steps. Sequence learning paradigms primarily investigate learning the proper order of a sequence of discrete actions such that each is selected rapidly and executed accurately, and numerous studies of motor learning have employed tasks involving sequences to study the influence of explicit (or implicit) sequence learning.

Although interesting, many factors complicate the interpretation of learning the sequential order in such tasks. It can be difficult to disentangle learning the sequence order from learning to execute the individual movement elements that make up the sequence. Additionally, it can be challenging to disentangle the contributions of explicit instructions and implicit knowledge of the sequence, which have both been hypothesized to contribute to overall changes in sequence performance (Krakauer et al., 2019). Nevertheless, recent studies have suggested that explicit aspects of learning fluctuate during early phases of learning while implicit processes occur throughout learning and are not sensitive to task instructions. Overall changes in performance reflect the joint operations of these processes.

The prefrontal cortex has been associated with cognitive processes, including planning, goal representation, and performance monitoring, and prefrontal cortical areas likely play an important role in explicit learning, especially in scenarios where task solving benefits from cognitive strategies. In particular, prefrontal contributions appear critical during early stages of learning, where prefrontal activation is high and patients with prefrontal lesions are particularly impaired during the early stages (Spampinato & Celnik, 2021). While the endpoint of learning is an implicit, procedural skill, the process of acquiring that skill is, in most cases, a richly cognitive enterprise, building on instruction, imitation, and moments of insight. Although often overlooked when investigating mechanisms of motor learning, cognition plays a key role in motor skill learning, e.g., as the ability to follow instructions and to develop new strategies. For example, the tennis player will listen to instructions from a coach to improve the position, speed, or spin of the serve as the patient will listen to the therapist. Feedback provided by an external source (e.g., a coach) is called extrinsic, augmented feedback and is further described in Chap. 15.

7.5.5 Learning Processes Interact

In real life, not unexpectedly, learning systems interact and contribute jointly when humans engage in deliberate motor practice and the acquisition of real-world motor skills. For instance, error-based and use-dependent learning can change motor behavior simultaneously. As described in Chap. 5, the activity of climbing fibers mediates information from neurons in the inferior olive to Purkinje cells in the cerebellum and provides important information on error during supervised learning, but their activity is also modulated in response to reward (Medina, 2019). Finally, the emergence of motor chunks during sequence-based motor learning is preceded by the storage of the sequence in memory. However, it is not its direct consequence. These chunks depend on, and result from, motor practice (Maceira-Elvira et al., 2022). Put in other words, when a real-world, complex motor skill like a tennis serve is practiced, different processes of learning are indeed likely to act in parallel and synergy to influence behavioral changes. The player's strategy is influenced by instructions from the coach, including information on the sequential elements of the serve and when the player practices it. These parallel learning processes, driven by error-based learning, work in tandem to acquire and refine skills, enhancing average performance and increasing the likelihood of success. The interaction between the different CNS structures involved in different aspects of motor learning is provided in Fig. 7.5 (and see also Fig. 5.6).

While the different categories of learning presented in these sections are primarily organized around the paradigms used to probe motor learning and their neural substrates, it is likely that the underlying processes that support learning in many cases overlap. As discussed, when engaging in deliberate practice of real-world motor skills, multiple forms of learning likely contribute to the observed changes in complex motor behaviors depending on conditions, context, availability of information, and phase of learning.

7.6 Mechanisms of Motor *Skill* Learning from Animals to Humans

As is the case for explicit learning, the neuroplasticity underlying motor learning can be studied on several levels from molecule to network. Generally, motor learning-related plasticity occurs in the neural circuits engaged in the trained motor tasks. These circuits may vary over the course of learning, as the same sensorimotor task is carried out through engagement of different sensorimotor systems depending on

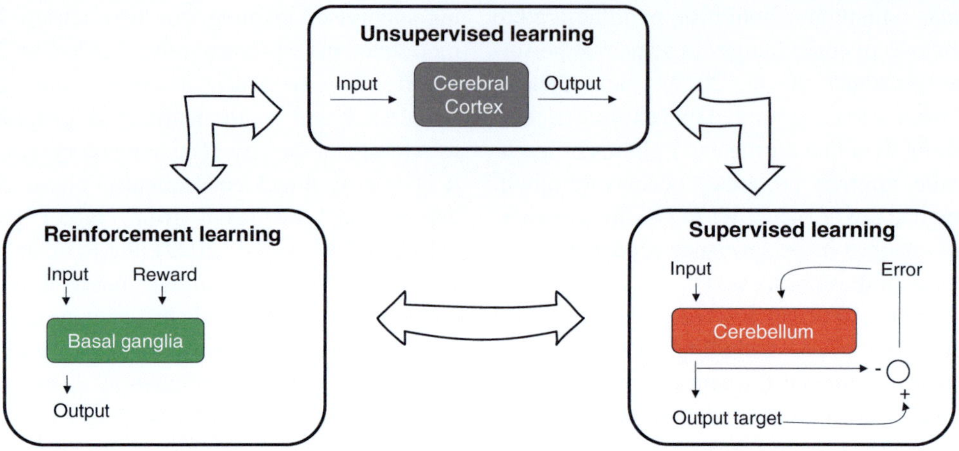

Fig. 7.5 Learning specializations of cortico-basal ganglia and cortico-cerebellar loops involved in the motor domain. The cerebral cortex, basal ganglia, and cerebellum are thought to implement distinct learning algorithms. According to this view, the cerebral cortex is specialized for unsupervised learning based on Hebbian plasticity. The basal ganglia are specialized for reinforcement (reward-based) learning, guided by the reward signals from midbrain dopaminergic neurons. The cerebellum is specialized for supervised (error-based) learning, guided by error signals from the inferior olive. The interconnections between these structures are illustrated by large arrows

whether the task is completely novel or close to being automatized. It is common for all voluntary motor tasks in humans that the motor cortex is involved. The following discussion on the network, cellular and synaptic mechanisms underlying motor learning therefore make its point of departure in the motor cortex. This is not to decry the contributions of neural adaptations in the cerebellum or the basal ganglia but rather to use illustrative and translatory examples from the primary motor cortex (M1) to emphasize the relationship between behavioral, neuronal, and neural changes accompanying motor practice.

7.6.1 Improved Performance Involves Tuning of the Activity of Populations of Corticospinal Neurons

As described in more detail in Chap. 13, reorganization of networks can be accredited to changes in the synapses connecting two neurons, which, at least in part, can be ascribed to changes in the dendritic or axonal arbor of the two neurons. Reversely, a change in behavior of an individual neuron does not necessarily arise from a neuronal adaptation but could reflect a shift in the inputs to the neuron. As such, the contributions from single neuron versus circuit plasticity can be difficult to disentangle. This intimate relation is best illustrated by the contribution of neurons in M1 to motor adaptation. The concept of population vectors of the discharge of M1 corticospinal neurons with each their preferred discharge direction is described in Chap. 5. When an external force is applied, some M1 neurons change the preferred direction to meet this perturbation, and some display a change in preferred direction even after the external force is removed (Paz & Vaadia, 2004). Cells with a directional tuning close to the practiced direction improve the information content after learning through an increase in the tuning curve. In other words, the activity of each task-relevant neuron in M1 has a higher signal-to-noise ratio and thereby entails more information about the future movement, which contributed more to the population vector of the neuronal ensemble.

7.6.2 Experts Have Larger Motor Maps

In experts such as proficient braille readers and elite racket players, motor-evoked potentials (MEPs) elicited by TMS in the task-relevant muscles can be evoked from a larger area as compared to the contralateral hemisphere or in less proficient individuals (see also Chaps. 5 and 13). In a similar manner, the gain and plateau level of the input-output relationship between stimulation intensity and MEP amplitude is higher in expert musicians compared to non-musicians (Rosenkranz et al., 2007). This is likely not related to their better performance per se, but rather to continued daily practice (Christiansen et al., 2020). Motor maps increase in area and stay increased as long as the individual is actively engaged in acquiring skillful behavior. Basic motor skills, like riding a bike down a straight road, are maintained even without practice but skillful behavior and even more so expertise calls for continuous deliberate practice.

7.6.3 "Motor Maps" Expand with Learning Through Mechanisms Resembling Hippocampal LTP

A wealth of animal work has investigated the mechanisms underlying the larger motor area observed in "experts," i.e., animals trained in skilled movements such as reaching for food pellets through a small window (Adkins et al., 2006). These experiments have shown that the motor cortex displays similar plastic and metaplastic properties as the hippocampus (see Chaps. 6 and 13); i.e., synaptic connections can increase or decrease in strength through synaptic LTP and LTD based on synaptic activity reflecting experiences. Weeks of practice of a skilled reaching task, thus, leads to expansion of the forelimb area in rat M1, whereas such changes are not seen following simple repetition of movement or strength training (Adkins et al., 2006). Similar to the hippocampus, high-frequency stimulation may potentiate excitatory synapses in the M1 (Hess & Donoghue, 1996). Interestingly, this requires that the network is rendered in a susceptible state through disinhibition by administration of Bicuculine, a GABA antagonist. A disinhibition is also the prevailing theory of how other "cortical representations" invade representations of unused or denervated limbs (see Chap. 13). Formation of new synapses also follows the rapid unmasking of connections in M1 through disinhibition and ensuing potentiation of excitatory connections (Adkins et al., 2006).

7.6.4 Long-Term Learning and Maintenance of Skilled Movements Depend on Protein Synthesis

Very few skills (if any) outside the laboratory can be acquired with a single or a few practice sessions. Motor memories take time to form but are also resilient to the passage of time. This is related to strengthening of existing synapses and formation of new synapses both of which require protein synthesis. When protein synthesis is blocked, motor learning cannot take place and maintenance of skilled movements and expansion of motor maps are compromised (Adkins et al., 2006). The motor maps are dynamic and undergo continuous adjustments contingent on protein synthesis within M1 to uphold integrity and support formation of skilled movement. Removal of stimuli to the trained M1 network either by lack of inputs to and/or outputs from the networks will cause a motor map underlying skilled behavior to fade. Here, it is important to note that many human movements, which may not intuitively be categorized as *skills*, are in fact highly trained and skilled movements. The larger M1 in the dominant than the non-dominant hemisphere is a result of the extensive fine motor use and learning encountered and endured over a lifetime of engaging in progressively more dexterous actions. In this perspective, all fine motor actions executed daily, e.g., cooking, cleaning, grooming, and walking up the stairs, should be considered "skilled" movements, which are underpinned by dynamic networks that need to be used to be maintained. The long-term impairments in fine motor function observed following lesions to the pyramidal tract and corticospinal pathway therefore likely reflect both lesion and learned non-use.

7.6.5 Monoamines Are Necessary for Expansions of Motor Maps and Motor Learning

The fact that mere *use* does not increase the motor maps in M1 may be that (at least in rodents) repetition of stereo-typical movement trajectories relies on subcortical structures associated with habit formation such as the basal ganglia. Additionally, repetition of over-learned movements is unlikely to evoke a strong dopaminergic response from the midbrain to the M1. In agreement with this, dopamine has been shown to be necessary for M1 LTP and motor learning. This demonstrates not only that dopaminergic innervation of the motor cortex is a necessity for the functional and structural neuronal and network plasticity underlying motor learning, but also provide a mechanistic link between use-dependent plasticity and reinforcement learning in the interneuronal circuits and output neurons of the motor cortex.

7.6.6 Below the Cortex: Does It Matter?

Human and animal studies have documented that neural circuitries in the spinal cord show adaptive changes caused by altered supraspinal and/or afferent input to the spinal circuitry in relation to learning, immobilization, injury, and neurorehabilitation. Reversible adaptations following, e.g., the acquisition or refinement of a motor skill, rely heavily on the functional integration between supraspinal and sensory inputs to the spinal cord networks. The spinal circuitry relays descending influences on α-motoneurons—the final common pathway to muscle activation. Simultaneously, the spinal circuits also process inputs sensory inputs from afferents influencing motoneurons directly or indirectly through interneurons, and relays afferent input to ascending pathways. Accordingly, what is frequently conceived as a change in the spinal circuitry may be a result of changes in either descending or afferent input or in the relative integration of these, i.e., a change in the neuronal weighting. This is evident from findings documenting only task-specific functional changes after periods of altered inputs, whereas resting responses remain unaffected. In fact, the proximity of the spinal circuitry to the outer world may demand a more rigid organization compared to the highly flexible cortical circuits.

As it turns out, spinal cord circuitries adapt throughout life to enable the brain (or CNS as a whole) to control a changing body, to control movements, and hence to interact optimally with surroundings. The understanding of the complex functions of spinal circuits is important for understanding mechanisms of motor learning and hence neurorehabilitation.

7.7 Consolidation, Retention, Interference and Transfer in Motor Skill Learning

In humans, consolidation of procedural memories is not a single process but rather multiple processes that happen both during encoding and even more during the hours after motor practice and overnight following encoding (see, e.g., Robertson, 2004). For new skills, the consolidation process is susceptible to interfering and modulatory activities. Practice of skills that share neural resources, i.e., are dependent on the same structures and networks, can interfere with each other. It is noteworthy that during the hours following practice, the newly formed memory is susceptible to not only interfering but also promoting stimuli.

7.7.1 Consolidation and Interference in Motor Learning

A crucial aspect of learning a task is the stabilization of encoded information, a process known as consolidation. Although the term consolidation was coined more than 100 years ago, during recent decades, neurophysiologists, neuropsychologists, and clinicians have had an increased focus on understanding processes of consolidation. Sensorimotor skills are typically retained over a long period, but for long-term memory to be established, consolidation in the nervous system is necessary. Consolidation is closely tied to retention, the amount of information available when previously encoded information is recalled. Although performance improvements can typically be observed during motor skill practice, in order for these improvements to be retained, consolidation processed serve to form long-term memory through plastic processes in the involved circuits of the CNS. As such, consolidation is a prerequisite for learning and memory and or retention of skill the day after initial motor practice, and the average error at re-testing (Day 2) would then be substantially lower than the average error at Day 1 (Fig. 7.6a).

Recent research has highlighted the importance of the hours following task learning for consolidation and subsequent recall. This consolidation process continues after the learning period to secure and solidify the learned information (Fig. 7.6b). In the early post-learning period, motor memory is fragile and can be disrupted if other motor tasks are trained before consolidation processes have proceeded. Molecular and cellular changes, particularly protein synthesis, are essential for consolidation, and this process takes time. The timing of introducing potential disruptors plays a crucial role. Experimental factors like pharmacological substances or cortical stimulation, as well as practical activities requiring plastic changes in overlapping networks, can disrupt consolidation. In essence, practicing different motor tasks activating the same neural network in succession can cause both anterograde and retrograde interference. Practicing task B after task A can cause retrograde interference by disrupting ongoing consolidation processes but also have anterograde effects limiting recall of A when returning to this task later (Fig. 7.6c). Other studies have demonstrated that these interfering effects are timing-sensitive in the sense that interference can be catastrophic if there is no break in between tasks A and B, i.e., there is no retention of task A, whereas this effect decreases with longer breaks between tasks A and B (Fig 7.6d). Therefore, there is a relation between retention and negative transfer (Brashers-Krug et al., 1996). Studies indicate that the primary motor cortex (M1) plays a critical role during early consolidation, and brain scans post-learning show increased activity in certain brain areas during motor task recall. Frontal areas and M1 are involved in early motor learning and consolidation. In contexts where different motor tasks activating the same muscle groups need to be practiced within the same session, practice schedules can be worked out to reduce the risk of interference effects. For instance, practicing different motor tasks not in blocks but in randomized order can have the advantage that risk of interference is lower, and this practice schedule leads to beneficial retention effects. Blocked motor practice conversely leads to steeper performance gains during motor practice but also risk interference effects and lower retention (Robertson, 2004).

7.7.2 Sleep Is Important for Consolidation of Memory

As for explicit memory, sleep plays a prominent role in the consolidation of motor or procedural memories. Results from experiments in rodent have demonstrated that the neural activity in the rodent homologue of motor cortex is replayed during non-REM sleep (Ramanathan et al.,

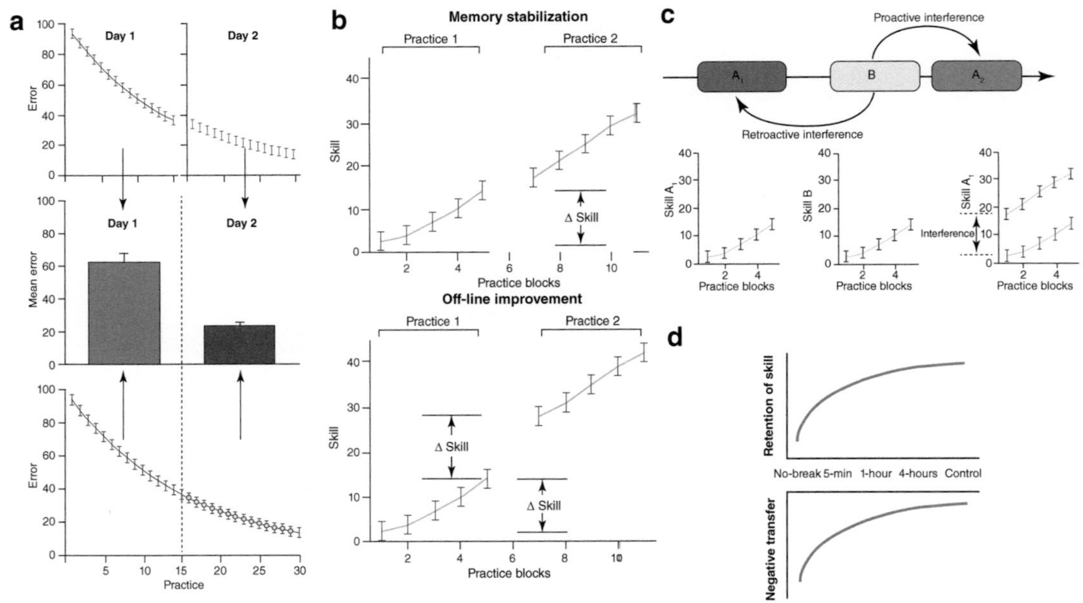

Fig. 7.6 Online and offline motor learning, consolidation, and interference effects. (**a**) Practice in a novel motor task leads to a reduction in error. These reductions can take place over several days. During practice, there are considerable improvements in performance, whereas between practice sessions, improvements can take several hours to emerge. If the testing and re-testing sessions were combined into one single practice session, and the average error of the first half of practice ("testing" session) were compared with the second ("re-testing" session), a substantial difference would emerge. This reduction, however, did not take place "offline" but can be accounted for by the effects of practice. (**b**) For offline learning, consolidation processes serve to stabilize memory and thereby motor performance. In some instances,—for some tasks offline learning can involve behavioral improvements. These can take several hours to emerge. (**c**) If different motor tasks are practiced in close temporal proximity, this can cause proactive or retroactive interference, e.g., if tasks are practiced and tested in the order task ABA. Retroactive interference is responsible for disrupting the memory, whereas proactive interference is responsible for disrupting the retrieval of the memory. The lower panels show the skill improvements expected during each task. Over five practice blocks, there are similar skill improvements in both task A and task B. When returning to task A, it might reasonably be expected that participants' skill (skill A2) would be similar to the skill achieved at the end of the first practice (skill A1). This is shown as a turquoise curve in the third graph. Contrary to this expectation, only a naive level of skill might be present, shown as the orange curve in the third graph. The interference responsible for this skill impairment can have either a proactive or a retroactive source. See Robertson et al. (2004). (**d**) Interference and time between motor practice sessions. Retention of the task A motor skill and transfer to task B as a function of temporal distance between tasks A and B. Controls did not perform task B. Retention was calculated as the difference between the mean performance in task A on days 2 and 1. Transfer was calculated as the difference between mean performance in task B and task A, both on day 1. The concomitant decline of negative transfer and retrograde interference seen in the group data suggests a relation between the two phenomena. Inspired by Brashers-Krug et al. (1996)

2015). Changes in neocortical-hippocampal coupling appear to be mediating this process (Kim et al., 2023). In humans, neural replay during sleep has been directly demonstrated in a spinal cord injured patient with electrodes implanted in motor cortex. Interestingly, patterns of activity of both single and ensamples of neurons in motor cortex were replayed with up to four times original speed during slow wave sleep (Rubin et al., 2022). The possibility of targeting neural replay during sleep to promote, e.g., sleep-dependent consolidation of procedural memories in the context of motor recovery is intriguing but remains to be demonstrated.

7.7.3 Consolidation Takes Place Already During Practice

There is an evident difference when comparing the time course of explicit and implicit memory formation. Whereas explicit working memory lasts seconds or perhaps minutes with rehearsal, motor memory is labile for hours after a practice session. Consequently, consolidation of procedural memories has been viewed as strictly "offline" processes that take place in hours after practice. However, consolidation appears to occur already during practice (Bonstrup et al., 2019), in the form of so-called micro-consolidation. The velocity and accuracy of key-presses in a motor sequence learning task (learning to play the piano) is thus evident early in practice. The neural mechanisms underlying this micro-consolidation are still largely unexplored, but recent findings suggest that replay of neural activity in pathways linking the hippocampus and sensorimotor cortex during short rest periods interspersed with active training may play a role (Jacobacci et al., 2020). Whereas these intriguing findings challenge the exclusive coupling of hippocampus to declarative memory and suggest targets to enhance effect of practice in, e.g., neurorehabilitation, there are a few notable limitations. Micro-consolidation appears to operate predominantly in the very early phase of practice, which questions how well the findings translate to the numerous hours needed to regain meaningful functions after injuries to the central nervous system. In addition, the participants were aware of the trained sequence, so the hippocampal involvement could reflect an *explicit* element of the task and it therefore remains to be demonstrated that hippocampal replay is a general feature of procedural learning and not solely explicit sequence learning. Upcoming research can shed light on these outstanding questions.

7.7.4 Transfer of Motor Learning

In addition to potential interference, positive effects in the form of transferability or transfer can be observed. Between-task transfer involves the phenomenon in which learning of one task can be applied or utilized—at least in part to performance or learning of another task. This phenomenon refers to positive transfer between similar skills or tasks, while interlimb (or intermanual) transfer occurs between, for example, the right and left hand, i.e., for the same individual. Also, for interlimb transfer, progressive practice promotes motor learning (Christiansen et al., 2017). The degree of transfer is clinically significant. Near transfer, such as transitioning from walking on a treadmill to walking on the ground, is important for rehabilitation of patients with impaired walking function. Interlimb transfer can be beneficial for patients with a severely affected arm and hand function after a stroke, as training effects for exercises performed with the less affected arm and hand can be transferred. This may also be the case during immobilization. Combining this with mirror therapy, where the patient observes the less affected hand's movement in a mirror can enhance interlimb transfer.

The degree of transfer is influenced by the learning phase, with greater transferability observed in the early phase. As discussed before, learning movement sequences is proposed to occur in two separate but parallel systems. Initially, the movement is encoded in external coordinates, reflecting the environment. In the associative/motor phase, encoding shifts more toward internal coordinates, such as muscle kinetics and joint angles. The dominance of these systems can be examined during unimanual tasks, revealing that training primarily encodes in external coordinates and is most transferable in the early phase. Transferability diminishes as the movement becomes more automated and is coded more in internal coordinates. Various cortical and subcortical structures are suggested as involved in the neural basis of transfer. Supplementary motor areas (SMA) in both hemispheres are strong candidates (Chap. 5). SMA activity during learning is related to the degree of intermanual transfer. Disruption of SMA reduces subsequent transfer to the contralateral hand. The ipsilateral primary motor cortex has also been suggested to be involved in intermanual transfer.

7.8 What Motor Skill Learning Is All About

In essence, motor skill learning concerns expanding the motor repertoire whether it be when engaging in unfamiliar task learning new skills, improving existing skills, or regaining motor skills as in the case of rehabilitation training. The aim of motor learning is to improve performance during execution of motor tasks in absolute terms, e.g., reduce error and increase speed non-reciprocally, but also to reduce variability and reduce the metabolic cost of movements, i.e., make them more affordable. As evident from this chapter (and Fig. 7.3), many different parts of the CNS contribute to this during motor learning.

Certain motor skills may take years to master, because of the number of interacting factors that must be considered when movements are trained. For example, in tennis, selecting the type of stroke based on body position, movements, and the entire context will vary greatly. This complexity leads to a combinatorial explosion, resulting in a large, multidimensional space, and optimal actions must be found for each state in it. This also goes for tasks relevant to practice in rehabilitation training like walking in different conditions or reaching and grasping different objects from different positions.

How can knowledge of motor skill learning and memory enhance recovery in patients? As discussed during the chapter, learning and performing everyday tasks likely involves all the presented processes of learning. If these processes of learning remain intact following injury or illness, they can be targeted to enhance motor skill learning or relearning in patients. For example, patients with cerebral stroke maintain the ability to adapt to environmental changes, likely through error-based learning, leading to improved gait step-symmetry (Reisman et al., 2007). Similarly, providing reinforcement feedback to stroke patients during motor practice can enhance learning rates (Quattrocchi et al., 2017). Patients who practiced with reinforcement conditions were also faster to adapt their movements when exposed to a similar perturbation on a subsequent day, suggesting that reinforcement can have longer-lasting beneficial effects in motor practice after stroke. Importantly, motor skill learning does not only arise from deliberate practice but may result from all experiences. In the context of rehabilitation training, deliberate practice is, however, highly relevant (see Chap. 15). Numerous studies have shown that it is possible to augment specific processes or aspects of learning of reductionist lab-based tasks. This is promising since it provides proof-of-principle that these different processes of learning can be targeted and enhanced. It is however more difficult to investigate the impact when targeting complex motor behaviors that engage multiple forms or learning in parallel. Nevertheless, it is important to keep in mind that different processes of learning can be at stake at different times and in different contexts for the learner, and this is also an important notion for therapists working in rehabilitation.

Review Questions

- What are the different stages of motor learning?
- How are different parts of the CNS involved in motor skill learning?
- What do the terms consolidation, retention, interference, and transfer mean?
- How can skill acquisition and memory be assessed?

References

Adkins, D. L., Boychuk, J., Remple, M. S., & Kleim, J. A. (2006). Motor training induces experience-specific patterns of plasticity across motor cortex and spinal cord. *Journal of Applied Physiology (Bethesda, MD: 1985), 101*(6), 1776–1782. https://doi.org/10.1152/japplphysiol.00515.2006

Bonstrup, M., Iturrate, I., Thompson, R., Cruciani, G., Censor, N., & Cohen, L. G. (2019). A rapid form of offline consolidation in skill learning. *Current Biology, 29*(8), 1346–1351. e1344. https://doi.org/10.1016/j.cub.2019.02.049

Brashers-Krug, T., Shadmehr, R., & Bizzi, E. (1996). Consolidation in human motor memory. *Nature, 382*(6588), 252–255. https://doi.org/10.1038/382252a0

Christiansen, L., Larsen, M. N., Grey, M. J., Nielsen, J. B., & Lundbye-Jensen, J. (2017). Long-term progressive motor skill training enhances corticospinal excitability for the ipsilateral hemisphere and motor performance of the untrained hand. *The European Journal of Neuroscience, 45*(12), 1490–1500. https://doi.org/10.1111/ejn.13409

Christiansen, L., Larsen, M. N., Madsen, M. J., Grey, M. J., Nielsen, J. B., & Lundbye-Jensen, J. (2020). Long-term motor skill training with individually adjusted progressive difficulty enhances learning and promotes corticospinal plasticity. *Scientific Reports, 10*(1), 15588. https://doi.org/10.1038/s41598-020-72139-8

Dayan, E., & Cohen, L. G. (2011). Neuroplasticity subserving motor skill learning. *Neuron, 72*(3), 443–454. https://doi.org/10.1016/j.neuron.2011.10.008

Fitts, P. M., & Posner, M. I. (1967). *Human performance*. Brooks/Cole.

Hess, G., & Donoghue, J. P. (1996). Long-term potentiation and long-term depression of horizontal connections in rat motor cortex. *Acta Neurobiologiae Experimentalis (Wars), 56*(1), 397–405. https://doi.org/10.55782/ane-1996-1143

Jacobacci, F., Armony, J. L., Yeffal, A., Lerner, G., Amaro, E., Jr., Jovicich, J., et al. (2020). Rapid hippocampal plasticity supports motor sequence learning. *Proceedings of the National Academy of Sciences of the United States of America, 117*(38), 23898–23903. https://doi.org/10.1073/pnas.2009576117

Kantak, S. S., & Winstein, C. J. (2012). Learning-performance distinction and memory processes for motor skills: A focused review and perspective. *Behavioural Brain Research, 228*(1), 219–231. https://doi.org/10.1016/j.bbr.2011.11.028

Kim, J., Joshi, A., Frank, L., & Ganguly, K. (2023). Cortical-hippocampal coupling during manifold exploration in motor cortex. *Nature, 613*(7942), 103–110. https://doi.org/10.1038/s41586-022-05533-z

Krakauer, J. W., Hadjiosif, A. M., Xu, J., Wong, A. L., & Haith, A. M. (2019). Motor learning. *Comprehensive Physiology, 9*(2), 613–663. https://doi.org/10.1002/cphy.c170043

Maceira-Elvira, P., Timmermann, J. E., Popa, T., Schmid, A. C., Krakauer, J. W., Morishita, T., et al. (2022). Dissecting motor skill acquisition: Spatial coordinates take precedence. *Science Advances, 8*(29), eabo3505. https://doi.org/10.1126/sciadv.abo3505

McDougle, S. D., Bond, K. M., & Taylor, J. A. (2015). Explicit and implicit processes constitute the fast and slow processes of sensorimotor learning. *The Journal of Neuroscience, 35*(26), 9568–9579. https://doi.org/10.1523/JNEUROSCI.5061-14.2015

Medina, J. F. (2019). Teaching the cerebellum about reward. *Nature Neuroscience, 22*(6), 846–848. https://doi.org/10.1038/s41593-019-0409-0

Paz, R., & Vaadia, E. (2004). Learning-induced improvement in encoding and decoding of specific movement directions by neurons in the primary motor cortex. *PLoS Biology, 2*(2), E45. https://doi.org/10.1371/journal.pbio.0020045

Quattrocchi, G., Greenwood, R., Rothwell, J. C., Galea, J. M., & Bestmann, S. (2017). Reward and punishment enhance motor adaptation in stroke. *Journal of Neurology, Neurosurgery, and Psychiatry, 88*(9), 730–736. https://doi.org/10.1136/jnnp-2016-314728

Ramanathan, D. S., Gulati, T., & Ganguly, K. (2015). Sleep-dependent reactivation of ensembles in motor cortex promotes skill consolidation. *PLoS Biology, 13*(9), e1002263. https://doi.org/10.1371/journal.pbio.1002263

Reisman, D. S., Wityk, R., Silver, K., & Bastian, A. J. (2007). Locomotor adaptation on a split-belt treadmill can improve walking symmetry post-stroke. *Brain, 130*(Pt 7), 1861–1872. https://doi.org/10.1093/brain/awm035

Robertson, E. M. (2004). Skill learning: Putting procedural consolidation in context. *Current Biology, 14*(24), R1061–R1063. https://doi.org/10.1016/j.cub.2004.11.048

Rosenkranz, K., Williamon, A., & Rothwell, J. C. (2007). Motorcortical excitability and synaptic plasticity is enhanced in professional musicians. *The Journal of Neuroscience, 27*(19), 5200–5206. https://doi.org/10.1523/JNEUROSCI.0836-07.2007

Rosenzweig, E. S., Courtine, G., Jindrich, D. L., Brock, J. H., Ferguson, A. R., Strand, S. C., et al. (2010). Extensive spontaneous plasticity of corticospinal projections after primate spinal cord injury. *Nature Neuroscience, 13*(12), 1505–1510. https://doi.org/10.1038/nn.2691

Rubin, D. B., Hosman, T., Kelemen, J. N., Kapitonava, A., Willett, F. R., Coughlin, B. F., et al. (2022). Learned motor patterns are replayed in human motor cortex during sleep. *The Journal of Neuroscience, 42*(25), 5007–5020. https://doi.org/10.1523/JNEUROSCI.2074-21.2022

Spampinato, D., & Celnik, P. (2021). Multiple motor learning processes in humans: Defining their neurophysiological bases. *The Neuroscientist, 27*(3), 246–267. https://doi.org/10.1177/1073858420939552

Computational Neuroscience and Neurorehabilitation

8

Mark Schram Christensen

Abstract

Neurorehabilitation builds on the principle that the central nervous system (CNS) is plastic and adapts to the situations the CNS is exposed to. Cases of acquired injury (stroke, traumatic, SCI, concussion), progressive disorders (MS, PD, dementia), or congenital injury (CP) are clinical situations where neuroplasticity becomes relevant. Regardless of how these clinical conditions are treated, the CNS will adapt through physiological processes to the conditions in the different situations. Environmental, clinical, medical, psychological, social, and physical factors all have an influence on how the CNS adapts to neurological injury. This is where clinical personnel become relevant. Because how a person with a lesion to the CNS is treated, has an impact on the plastic changes in the CNS. This chapter will describe some of the possible computational mechanisms that underlie this principle of central nervous plasticity, and how descriptions of both behavior and physiological processes can be formalized with the help of a computational mindset.

Keywords

Computational neuroscience · Homeostatic balance · Degrees-of-freedom problem · Internal models · Bayesian inference

M. S. Christensen (✉)
Department of Psychology, University of Copenhagen, Copenhagen, Denmark
e-mail: markc@psy.ku.dk

Box 8.1 Case Story

A physiotherapist specializing in stroke rehabilitation works with Luke, a 58-year-old stroke survivor who experiences difficulties with balance, often stumbles, and has an increased risk of falling following his stroke. The therapist begins by assessing Luke's motor function, paying close attention to his balance control. She identifies that Luke tends to look at his feet while walking, walking slowly and co-contracting the lower leg muscles when asked to increase walking speed. He tells the therapist that he has a lot of difficulty stepping over things, such as stepping over a doorstep.

At the rehabilitation center, they have a long hallway. The therapist puts tape strips on the floor and tells Luke he must walk from one end to the other without touching the tape. The tape offers Luke clear visual feedback while providing a task where Luke can feel safe during initial practice. Moreover, the tape is sticky on both sides meaning that when Luke steps on the tape, he can feel and hear his shoe sticking shortly to the tape, providing an immediate error signal.

At first, Luke can perform the task by stopping in front of each piece of tape. His body stiffens and he slowly steps over while looking directly at his feet. They keep on practicing the task and Luke's job is to step over the obstacles without making a full stop. Through repeated practice, Luke

(continued)

J. B. Nielsen et al. (eds.), *Neuroplasticity-based Neurorehabilitation*,
https://doi.org/10.1007/978-3-031-81120-3_8

Box 8.1 (continued)
slowly becomes better. He makes fewer errors; his movements seem less stiff; and after a week of practice, Luke begins talking to the therapist during the task. He often looks at her in between obstacles and can glance at the ground in front of him to evaluate how far he needs to step over the tape. The fact that Luke no longer has to stop and look at his feet and that he can talk while performing the task leads the therapist to decide that the task has become more automatized requiring less conscious effort. She evaluates that Luke has efficiently integrated the sensory feedback he is provided and can use it predictably without paying the task much attention.

Over the next months, the therapist keeps making the task more difficult by constraining time or introducing more difficult obstacles and the process continues. Luke slowly gains confidence in his ability to execute movements with greater accuracy and efficiency, enabling him to participate more actively in daily activities. The therapist continues to monitor his progress and adjust the rehabilitation program as needed, ensuring ongoing stimulation to support long-term recovery.

8.1 Introduction to Computational Approaches

Why consider neurorehabilitation as a computational problem? The benefit of using a computational perspective provides researchers and clinicians with a theoretically solid foundation for making predictions about the impact of specific rehabilitation initiatives. It is possible in certain domains of scientific description, to observe behavior or physiological processes, and then, founded in computational principles, make predictions on how a given rehabilitation program will impact an individual based on the observed behavior, physiological processes, and the individuals' motivations. This can be used to tailor-make rehabilitation initiatives for individuals without having to test different procedures and then evaluate whether they had a clinical impact. Using computational models of either movement or cognitive control require a level of knowledge and insight into the principles of computational neuroscience and a vocabulary that allow clinicians and researchers to communicate about very specific behaviors and neurophysiological mechanisms that can be impacted by treatments, training, and practice.

This chapter will introduce some of the principles that allow clinicians to understand neurorehabilitation as a computational task, which can impact different levels of description of the CNS. Some of the principles allow explanations for neuroplastic changes at a neurotransmitter level, others at a cellular level, and others again at a systems level of description.

What is the problem, that computational neuroscience in relation to neurorehabilitation wants to address, that cannot be addressed just by verbal explanations but requires computational models? Computational neuroscience tries to describe the principles that underlie the behavior and thoughts of humans or other species with a central nervous system using neurophysiological explanations.

Two overall principles are important to keep in mind when addressing neurorehabilitation as a computational neuroscience problem, these are on the one hand the homeostatic balance of the organism and on the other hand, the degrees-of-freedom (DoF) problem (Bernstein, 1967; Bizzi et al., 1991).

8.1.1 Homeostatic Balance

The homeostatic balance (Cannon, 1929) is a way to describe how an organism, in this case, a person with a neurological disorder, can maintain physiological states such that the person can function. This could for instance be how to become sated when hungry or rested after being tired. By maintaining a homeostatic balance, it is possible to account for goal-directed behavior, where the person wants to be placed in a desired state. This problem can be extended to include situations where it is required that the person avoids being further injured, i.e., it can also account for behavior that is made to avoid harmful stimuli to the person. Maintaining homeostatic balance is therefore one of the starting points for computational approaches to neuroscience.

8.1.2 Degrees-of-Freedom Problem

The other principle that needs to be investigated is how the body in practice solves the problem of maintaining the homeostatic balance, when the body of a person has many possible actions it can take. At the surface this may seem a trivial problem; if a person is thirsty, the person will reach for a bottle of water, and if none is within reach, the person will go and grab a glass and turn the tap, and so on. Depending on the complexity of the desired task and the possibilities available, solving the desired task may require different degrees of planning. However, the problem is less trivial, if all possible ways a person can reach for a bottle of water are considered; one can start by lifting the arm, then stretching the arm, and then opening the hand. But one can also start by opening the hand, then lifting the arm, and then stretching the arm toward the bottle of water. There are in principle an infinite number of possible combinations to how the simple task of reaching a bottle of water can be solved. How the central nervous system decides which movements to make with the different limbs to accomplish the task is considered the "degree-of-freedom problem" of computational and behavioral motor neuroscience.

Solving the DoF problem is by no means an easy task. An inherent question in the DoF problem is to figure out whether solving the DoF problem requires optimization of a specific movement parameter. There have been, and still are, ongoing debates related to this question, and it is still not known whether solving the DoF problem requires minimizing the jerk of the movement or minimizing the amount of energy spent. To solve the DoF problem, it is necessary to consider the biomechanical constraints of the body under investigation.

8.1.3 Biomechanical Optimization

Biomechanics is the study of the movements of organisms, based on the mechanical properties of the moving bodies. Using biomechanics, it is possible to derive mathematical equations of the forces and loads that the moving body is exposed to during a movement. Using these mathematical equations, it is possible to optimize the relevant movement parameter (e.g., energy (Alexander, 2002), jerk, load, speed, accuracy, etc.) and then observe the actual movement behavior of the person, that is investigated. This makes it possible to compare the real movements with a "model" of the movements that are based on the optimization of a specific movement parameter.

The link between biomechanics and neuroscience is the next difficult step that needs to be considered. Bottom line is that movement of the body is made by the interplay between the contraction of the muscles and the external forces that influence the body, these include forces such as gravity but also ground reaction forces, which all influence the way movements are performed. Contraction of muscles is governed by motor neurons in the spinal cord. The motor neurons in the spinal cord are under constant influence of signals from the parts of the central nervous system that controls movements as well as under the influence of sensory signals from the peripheral nervous system. This topic will be covered later in this chapter.

8.1.4 Circular Interaction of Sensations and Movement

Already at this stage of description, one important feature of the computational approach to motor neuroscience becomes apparent. Movements take place in a constant interaction between the observed person and the environment the person moves in. Movements can both take place based on the person's desire to be in a specific state (safe, sated, rested, excited) or due to external factors (harm avoidance, reaching for food). However, every movement will almost never only be determined by either the desire to be in a specific state or react to external factors, but always be a mixture of internal desires and external factors. There is no single place within the person, where you can identify that the movement originates from.

8.1.5 Temporal Delays of Signals

The next element that needs to be taken into consideration, when trying to describe movements as a computational problem, is an inherent feature of the fact that humans have a physical size. Having a physical size means that neural signals from the periphery take some time before they are processed in the central nervous system. So how does the CNS take that delay of signal processing into account, when it plans a movement?

Consider the example of grasping a cup from Chap. 5. The time it takes for the signals from the skin receptors of the fingertips and proprioceptors of the finger muscles to reach the spinal cord and then excite the motor neuron, which then can send action potentials to contract the muscles of the fingers, is in the order of 30–50 ms. This does not sound like as much time, but this is the time it would take for the nervous system to produce a simple reflex response, without much-advanced adjustment. If the signal from the periphery would have to undergo cortical processing, the time it takes for the signal to result in a more coordinated movement is in the order of 100–120 ms. By the time 120 ms have passed, a cup that falls free, would have traveled 7 cm, and would no longer be graspable. If control of movements were to rely solely on reactions to external stimuli, such as the slipping of a cup between the fingers, before one started to hold more firmly, humans would be highly incapable of acting in an environment that constantly changes. Humans (and other animals) would simply be too far behind in time.

Based on all these considerations, there are good reasons to believe that the CNS does something else than just react to sensory feedback.

8.1.6 Internal Models

The concept of internal models (Kawato, 1999; Wolpert & Ghahramani, 2000) is probably the most prevailing mechanic through which the CNS can account for goal-directed movements, and thereby maintain homeostatic balance, and at the same time, overcome the difficulties that delays in sensory feedback give. The overall idea of internal models is that they provide the CNS with an internal representation of a prediction of the sensory consequences of any given movement. The representation of the predicted sensory feedback is made by a computational module of the CNS called a forward model. By using the predicted sensory feedback as a guideline for an ongoing movement, it is possible to perform the movement according to the goal or intention that one has set up for the movement. If unexpected events then give rise to actual sensory feedback that is different from the predicted sensory feedback, there are now reasons to adjust the ongoing movement, given the present sensory feedback, and act accordingly. An example could be that someone moves the cup you are reaching for, and when you are at the position with your hand where you expected the cup would be, you realize that the cup is no longer there.

In addition to the forward model, internal models also comprise a module known as the inverse model. The task of the inverse model is to use the present state of a person and the intended state, or goal of the movement, to calculate how the person can get from the present state to the intended state. Hence, the name "inverse model" (see Fig. 8.1).

8.1.7 Motor Learning and Error Correction

Internal models have been suggested to be *the* part of the CNS that undergoes change when a person learns new motor skills (Wolpert et al., 2011). What happens is that the deviation

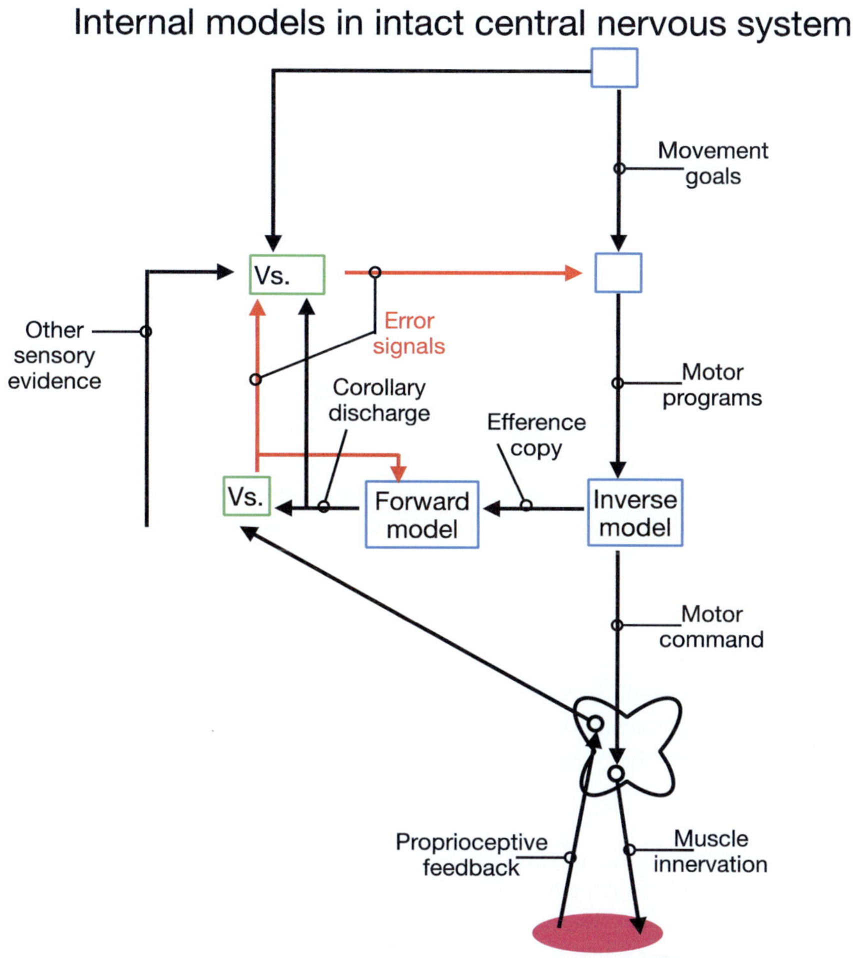

Fig. 8.1 Internal model. Internal models are a way to describe the different signals and computational elements involved in movement control. At the top right corner, a blue box depicts a higher-order brain region that computes the goal of a movement. The goal of the movement is signaled to lower-order brain regions that compute the motor program which in the end solves the problem of how the body reaches the desired goal state based on its initial positions. This task is accomplished by the so-called inverse model. The inverse model generates a motor command signal, which is sent to the muscles, and at the same time a copy of the motor command, known as an efference copy is sent to the so-called forward model that computes a prediction of what sensory consequences, known as a corollary discharge, which the movement that one is performing will lead to. The corollary discharge signal can be compared with the intended goal of the movement. If there is no difference between the two signals, the intended and predicted sensory feedback, the movement will just be performed as initially planned. If there is a difference, for instance, caused by a displacement of the goal detected by other sensory evidence or a change of mind, an error signal is computed by the top green box that can be used to adjust the ongoing movement. The corollary discharge signal can also be compared with the actual proprioceptive feedback from the movement, and if that is different from the predicted feedback, as indicated by an error signal from the lower green box, there is reason to adjust the movement. It is believed that this latter signal is essential for error-based motor learning. The figure is inspired by Jeannerod (2006).

between the predicted sensory feedback (e.g., "I am now going to throw the dart in the bull's eye") and the actual feedback (e.g., "Oops, that was just inside the dartboard way to the right") is used to update the internal model. The deviation between the predicted (intention) of the throw and the actual position of the dart is then incorporated into an adjustment of the next throw. Therefore, the deviation between the predicted and actual sensory feedback is essential for the ability to adjust and improve one's movements, and thereby it becomes an essential ingredient in the ability to learn new motor skills as described in Chap. 7.

8.1.8 Uncertainty and Noise in Sensorimotor Processing

Uncertainty comes in many flavors. The example provided above with the deviation between the predicted sensory feedback and the actual sensory feedback during dart throwing illustrates one aspect of uncertainty in sensorimotor processing, which is that movements are performed with an uncertain outcome. In other words, the motor system is noisy, and all movements are performed with a degree of uncertainty (Körding & Wolpert, 2004).

Uncertainty can also be expressed in relation to how the senses process stimuli from the external environment. The senses may not be accurate. Perhaps the vision becomes blurry when getting older.

Uncertainty also plays a role when it comes to external factors that change the environment. These can be highly detrimental to the performance of a specific task, and something these changes need to be considered when performing a task. E.g., when moving around in the landscape, one might encounter a situation where yesterday it was possible to cross the creek by simply stepping over it. However, due to heavy rain during the night, the creek has turned into a small river, and therefore one must find another place to cross the creek. In general, when external factors must be taken into consideration during a sensorimotor interaction task, understanding how these external factors may impact the environment is also necessary. These considerations may require a cognitive understanding of the relationship between the external factors and how they impact the environment and are therefore beyond what purely sensorimotor models may encompass.

Motor learning, as described in the previous section where one tries to reduce the difference between the predicted and actual sensory consequence of a movement, is one way to improve and learn a new skill. But another way of improving a motor skill is to reduce the uncertainty of the motor system, i.e., reduce the noise of the movements. However, reducing the uncertainty or improving the precision of the motor output can be done in many ways, and the easiest way is often to reduce the speed of the movement and improve the precision. This improvement of precision at the cost of reducing speed is not considered a true improvement of skill, but rather a trade-off between speed and precision. This is also discussed in Chap. 7.

When both motor signals and sensory signals are under the influence of uncertainty, the process of making precise predictions about the sensory consequences of movements is not a simple task. One way to incorporate uncertainty about the motor and sensory signals when predicting sensory consequences of movements is to use Bayesian integration.

8.2 Bayesian Inference

Bayesian integration or Bayesian inference is a mathematical approach to calculate conditional probabilities, which has found its way into neuroscience as a way to understand how the CNS makes sense of the world that it moves around in. The idea builds upon the principle that the perceptual system is designed in such a way that it makes sense of the world by testing hypotheses of what causes the sensory percept that is received. The hypotheses build upon prior knowledge, and that received sensory information, is compared with prior knowledge, i.e., testing the hypotheses that what is sensed is what is believed perceived. The posterior knowledge is then a precise mathematical combination of the prior and the sensory information.

Bayesian inference builds upon the principle of combining the probability of prior information with the probability of the present sensory information into an integrated posterior probability.

Bayesian inference has been proposed as a mechanism central to the function of the CNS based on behavioral studies and neuroanatomical arguments. Neuroscientific evidence has started to emerge within the last 5–10 years.

Central to Bayesian inference are the three probability distributions displayed in Fig. 8.2: the prior, the likelihood, and the posterior. The prior is the already-established knowledge about the sensory stimuli that the body receives. The likelihood is the new sensory information that is received from the sensory system. The posterior is the updated best estimate of what has caused the sensory stimuli, that is received, and is a mathematical combination of the prior and likelihood. The strength of the Bayesian inference approach is that it incorporates the probability *distribution* of the three elements: prior, likelihood, and posterior. So not only can the procedure account for the most likely value of the prior, likelihood, and posterior of a certain sensory stimulus, but also the uncertainty of the respective measures. This means that the method allows us to take into consideration the uncertainty of both sensory information and movements when the CNS tries to derive the cause of sensory events. Figure 8.2a shows an example of strong (meaning low uncertainty) prior information. This means that the posterior estimate of the sensory information is more influenced by the prior information than the likelihood information. Alternatively, Fig. 8.2b shows an example of strong sensory information (low uncertainty of the likelihood compared to the prior), which gives a posterior estimate of the sensory information that is more influenced by the likelihood information.

One of the first behavioral examples of Bayesian integration was a motor adaptation study by Körding and Wolpert (2004). Here they asked participants to make line-drawing movements from a starting position to an end goal. To begin with, the participants trained the movement, so their perceived end-positions were displayed slightly off to one side, but the displacement was done with a probability following a normal distribution, so on average the displacement was 1 cm to the side with a specific uncertainty determined by the distribution of the training feedback. When an average displacement of 1 cm to the side was established after 1000 training trials subsequently, test trials were performed. Here the displacement was now added to the opposite side, and this was done with different degrees of uncertainty. Using Bayesian integration, it was then possible to calculate and predict, how participants would perform the line drawing task when it was first imposed with a prior in one direction with a specific uncertainty, and then exposed to a new set of feedback trials with different uncertainties. The experiment showed that the actual behavior followed exactly what was predicted by Bayesian integration.

Two important lessons in relation to Bayesian integration to learning and updating motor behavior are also worth mentioning. One relates to the uncertainty of the likelihood, i.e., the sensory information. If the uncertainty of the likelihood is small compared with the uncertainty of the prior, one will see that the posterior is more likely to align with the likelihood than the prior (see Fig. 8.3a). On the other hand, if the uncertainty is smaller for the prior than the likelihood, the posterior will align more with the prior (see Fig. 8.3b). This means that to learn fast and adjust one's prior toward the sensory evidence, the process will be facilitated by either low sensory uncertainty, i.e., clear feedback, or alternatively, as high prior uncertainty. These patterns have been observed in behavioral experiments, where fast learning was present when the uncertainty of the likelihood was low (Wei & Körding, 2010). Alternatively, as studies have shown if participants to begin with had high trial-to-trial variability, they would learn faster compared with participants with low variability (Wu et al., 2014).

8.3 Reward-Based Learning/ Reinforcement Learning

The last topic covered in this chapter concerns how tasks, actions, and behavior can be learned when certain behaviors are rewarded. This type of learning is often called reinforcement learning (Niv, 2009; Dayan & Daw, 2008) because the presence of rewards will reinforce the type of behavior that is rewarded. As described in the section on motor learning, error-based updating of internal models can also be considered as a type of reward-based learning, just with opposite

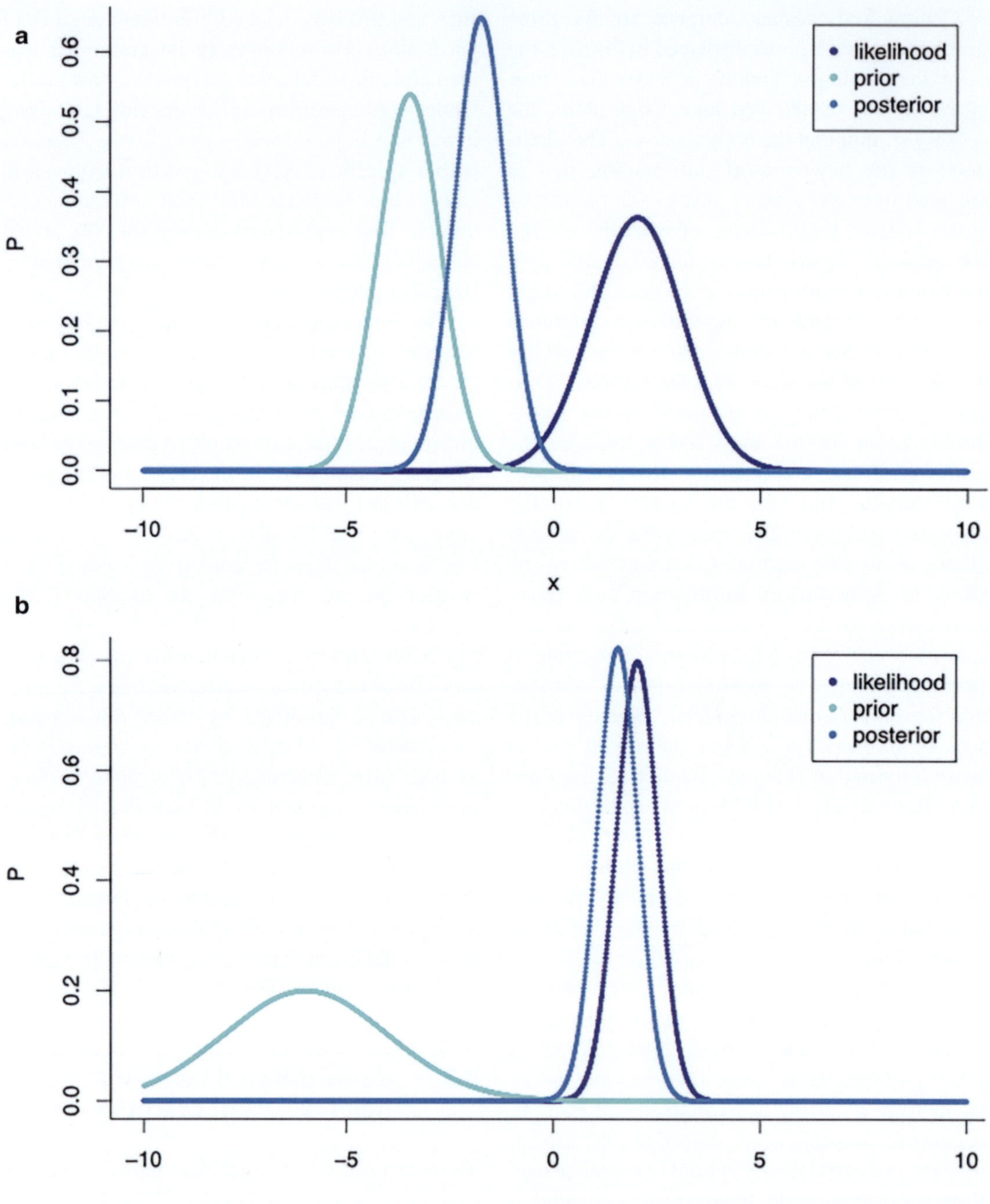

Fig. 8.2 The figure depicts two examples of Bayesian inference. Figure (**a**) is an example of a probability distribution of the prior information centered around $x = -4$ with a relatively low uncertainty that is combined with a likelihood distribution centered around $x = +2$ with relatively larger uncertainty. These distributions are combined by Bayes law as the posterior best-estimate that is closer to the prior distribution than to the likelihood due to the lower uncertainty of the prior probability distribution. Figure (**b**) is an example of a probability distribution of the prior information centered around $x = -6$ with a relatively high uncertainty that is combined with a likelihood distribution centered around $x = +2$ with low uncertainty. The posterior best-estimate is now very close to the likelihood distribution due to the low uncertainty of the likelihood

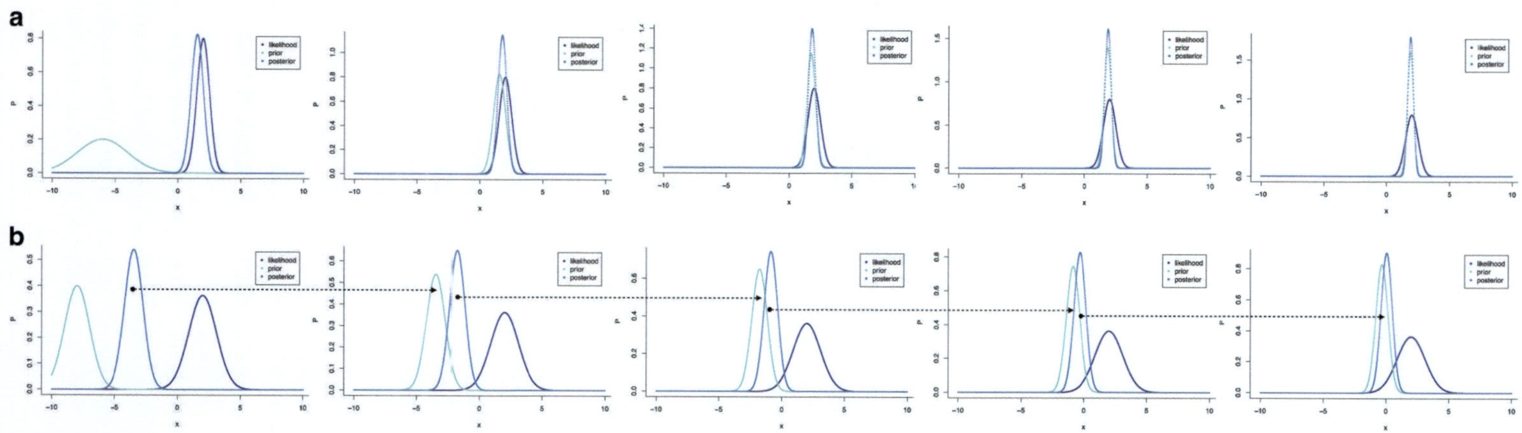

Fig. 8.3 This figure shows two examples of Bayesian updating. In example A, the prior initially (furthest to the left) has large uncertainty compared with the likelihood. This means that the posterior best-estimate is close to the likelihood. In the second step, the posterior distribution calculated in the first step becomes the prior information in the second step. When the likelihood has lower uncertainty than the prior, the update of the posterior approaches the likelihood very fast. In example B, the prior initially (furthest to the left) has lower uncertainty compared with the likelihood. This means that the posterior best-estimate is closer to the prior than the likelihood. In the second step, the posterior distribution calculated in the first step becomes the prior information in the second step. When the prior has lower uncertainty than the likelihood, the update of the posterior approaches the likelihood much slower than in example A

sign, so large error means small rewards. When there is a large deviation between the predicted and actual feedback, there is a low reward, but on the other hand, a high reward prediction error. Reward prediction errors play an important role in guiding instrumental behavior. Instrumental behavior is the type of behavior that is observed, when a person performs, supposedly random actions, and at some point, a specific action leads to the appearance of a reward. The idea with reinforcement learning is that a reward prediction is associated with a given action, here indexed as action *i*. For each action you can then calculate the difference between the reward prediction (RP_i) and the actual reward (R_i) obtained from doing that action. If the actual reward is larger than the predicted reward, you can then ascribe an updated value (V_{i+1}) associated with that action that is larger than the previous expected value (V_i), and thereby the associated reward increases, and the action is reinforced. On the other hand, if the actual reward is smaller, the action will be associated with a smaller reward than previously and hence be less likely favored. The degree to which the calculated reward prediction error is used in updating the associated reward value with the action is called the learning rate (α). This can be

$$V_{i+1} = V_i + \alpha\left(R_i - RP_i\right)$$

Reinforcement learning is a very strong tool in the toolbox of computational neuroscience since it is very simple to implement and intuitively easy to understand. It differs from the internal model formulations of computational approaches to motor control in that it is only rewards that drive the dynamics of the changes in the behavior. Therefore, reinforcement learning approaches to motor learning are often called "model free" in contrast to the internal model approach to motor learning, that is called "model based," because the internal models both require a model that calculates the predicted sensory feedback (i.e., the forward model) and a model that calculates how you get from the present state of the body to the desired state (i.e., the inverse model). The use of different approaches to motor learning is further discussed in Chap. 7.

Reinforcement learning models have also been used to understand gambling behavior and risk aversion both in healthy participants and clinical populations.

8.4 Computational Approaches to the Understanding of Cognition

Computational neuroscience is not only relevant for neurorehabilitation in relation to control movements but also as a tool to investigate cognitive impairment for instance after a stroke.

One approach is to investigate the ability to identify visual stimuli and use the modeling of performance parameters to identify processing speed and capacity, spatial bias, and perceptual threshold. This approach has successfully been employed in studies of neglect, pure alexia, dyslexia, MCI in AD, Huntington's disease, and ADHD (Habekost, 2015).

Another computational approach is to investigate neural processes as dynamical systems. Dynamical systems theory is a branch of mathematical modeling that describes properties of physical systems as a set of coupled differential equations of the relevant variables and how they evolve over time. The modeled variables could be neurophysiological measures. This approach has successfully been used to describe; the relationship between seizure and nonseizure states in epilepsy, the relationship between dopamine and neural functions in PD, mood fluctuations in bipolar disorder, the relationship between dopamine and working memory function in schizophrenia, and decision-making (Roberts et al., 2017).

8.5 Practical Use

The computational approach to neurorehabilitation could be used in several ways. Let us assume you as a professional work together with a stroke survivor and must come up with a rehabilitation program for this person. If the stroke survivor has sensorimotor deficits, you might want to use the internal models sketched in Fig. 10.1 to work out what parts of the circuitry involved in voluntary motor control are affected by the stroke. One first step might be to identify whether simple sensory tasks or simple motor tasks are affected. If sensory feedback seems to be more affected than motor signals, one approach could be to help the person by providing clearer sensory feedback, letting the person use other sensory modalities such as vision to guide their movements. Another approach adopted from the Bayesian updating example might be to help a person who moves in very stereotypical ways, by challenging them to do movements slightly outside their comfort zone and still provide them with clear feedback on how well they are doing. This may help them adopt the ability to change their movement patterns. Finally, the idea of reinforcement learning as guidance to change behavior in patients could be a tool to consider if you as a therapist might not see the improvements in a patient that you are working together with. Perhaps, you should reconsider the type of reward that you focus on for this specific patient, and in collaboration with the patient, find the type of reward that may motivate them more than what previously has been provided.

Review Questions

- How does computational neuroscience contribute to understanding neurorehabilitation, and why is it considered essential in tailoring rehabilitation initiatives?
- Explain the concepts of homeostatic balance and the degrees-of-freedom problem in the context of neurorehabilitation. How do these principles influence rehabilitation strategies?

References

Alexander, R. M. (2002). Energetics and optimization of human walking and running: The 2000 Raymond Pearl memorial lecture. *American Journal of Human Biology, 14*, 641–648. https://doi.org/10.1002/ajhb.10067

Bernstein, N. A. (1967). *The coordination and regulation of movements*. Pergamon Press.

Bizzi, E., Mussaivaldi, F. A., & Giszter, S. (1991). Computations underlying the execution of movement— A biological perspective. *Science (New York, N.Y.), 253*, 287–291.

Cannon, W. B. (1929). Organization for physiological homeostasis. *Physiological Reviews, 9*, 399–431.

Dayan, P., & Daw, N. D. (2008). Decision theory, reinforcement learning, and the brain. *Cognitive, Affective, & Behavioral Neuroscience, 8*, 429–453. https://doi.org/10.3758/cabn.8.4.429

Habekost, T. (2015). Clinical TVA-based studies: A general review. *Frontiers in Psychology, 6*, 290. https://doi.org/10.3389/fpsyg.2015.00290

Jeannerod, M. (2006). *Motor cognition*. Oxford University Press.

Kawato, M. (1999). Internal models for motor control and trajectory planning. *Current Opinion in Neurobiology, 9*, 718–727.

Körding, K., & Wolpert, D. M. (2004). Bayesian integration in sensorimotor learning. *Nature, 427*, 244–247. https://doi.org/10.1038/nature02169

Niv, Y. (2009). Reinforcement learning in the brain. *Journal of Mathematical Psychology, 53*, 139–154. https://doi.org/10.1016/j.jmp.2008.12.005

Roberts, J. A., Friston, K. J., & Breakspear, M. (2017). Clinical applications of stochastic dynamic models of the brain, part I: A primer. *Biological Psychiatry: Cognitive Neuroscience and Neuroimaging, 2*, 216–224. https://doi.org/10.1016/j.bpsc.2017.01.010

Wei, K., & Körding, K. (2010). Uncertainty of feedback and state estimation determines the speed of motor adaptation. *Frontiers in Computational Neuroscience, 4*, 11. https://doi.org/10.3389/fncom.2010.00011

Wolpert, D. M., & Ghahramani, Z. (2000). Computational principles of movement neuroscience. *Nature Neuroscience, 3*(Suppl), 1212–1217. https://doi.org/10.1038/81497

Wolpert, D. M., Diedrichsen, J., & Flanagan, J. R. (2011). Principles of sensorimotor learning. *Nature Reviews Neuroscience, 12*, 739–751. https://doi.org/10.1038/nrn3112

Wu, H. G., Miyamoto, Y. R., Castro, L. N. G., et al. (2014). Temporal structure of motor variability is dynamically regulated and predicts motor learning ability. *Nature Neuroscience, 17*(2), 312–321. https://doi.org/10.1038/nn.3616

Executive Functions

9

Frederik Have Dornonville de la Cour
and Laila Øksnebjerg

Abstract

Executive functions are a set of higher-order cognitive processes that monitor and regulate other systems in purposive and goal-directed behavior. The prefrontal cortex is the primary seat of executive functions, and the lateral, orbital, and medial aspects of the prefrontal cortex and their networks are associated with different subprocesses of executive functioning. Several neurological conditions affecting prefrontal networks, including cortical and subcortical circuits, may result in mild to severe executive impairment. The neuropsychological examination may help identify the nature of these impairments and provide a basis for increased self-awareness and a case formulation of assets and deficits to guide treatment and rehabilitation. Two approaches to managing executive impairment are presented. The first is concerned with improving or subsuming the function of the executive system by training metacognitive strategies that support executive attention and control in everyday life. The second is concerned with compensating for the impaired executive system by modulating the environment or establishing new behavioral routines using errorless learning.

Keywords

Dysexecutive syndrome · Supervisory attentional system · Prefrontal cortex · Frontal-subcortical circuitry · Neuropsychological assessment · Ecological validity · Neurorehabilitation · Goal-management training · Errorless learning · Neurobehavioral disorder

F. H. Dornonville de la Cour (✉)
Department of Neuroscience, University of Copenhagen, Copenhagen, Denmark

Neurorehabilitation Research and Knowledge Centre, Copenhagen University Hospital—Rigshospitalet, Copenhagen, Denmark

The Elsass Foundation, Charlottenlund, Denmark
e-mail: flc@sund.ku.dk

L. Øksnebjerg
Department of Psychology, University of Copenhagen, Copenhagen, Denmark
e-mail: Laila.Oeksnebjerg.02@regionh.dk

Box 9.1 Case Story

Ben, a 48-year-old man, worked as a carpenter and lived with his wife and two teenage children. He suffered a head trauma when he slipped and fell from a scaffold. Initially he was unconscious, but when the paramedics arrived after 10 min, he was conscious, and they reported a Glasgow Coma Scale score of 12 (see Box 12.3). He reacted to stimuli but acted confused. At the emergency department, an acute cerebral CT scan showed multiple bifrontal contusion lesions, but no signs of bleeding. He was bruised but had no skull or face fractures, and he showed no signs of focal neu-

(continued)

J. B. Nielsen et al. (eds.), *Neuroplasticity-based Neurorehabilitation*,
https://doi.org/10.1007/978-3-031-81120-3_9

Box 9.1 (continued)
rological symptoms. He was admitted for observation where he gradually recovered, but he had posttraumatic amnesia for the day of the accident. He was discharged after three days to a program of outpatient examinations. At three weeks, a control cerebral MR scan confirmed the bilateral prefrontal contusion lesions, mainly dorsolateral and orbitofrontal. After two months, a neuropsychological examination was conducted. His wife accompanied him to this appointment, and she described that her husband's behavior had changed significantly after the accident. Most often he lacked interest and initiative, and when he did chores around the house, his behavior was generally disorganized, he was often distracted, and he did not finish the tasks. He was still on sick leave, and he showed no interest in the invitations to visit his workplace and colleagues. He did not seem to care much about this, and his wife was greatly worried about his future employment. Results from neuropsychological tests showed that his performance on basic tests of learning and recall, language, abstract thinking, and visuo-perceptual and visuo-constructive skills were normal. However, his psychomotor and cognitive speed was generally slow, and in some tests, his performance was marked by distractibility, disorganized or perseverative behavior, and lack of inhibition, as demonstrated in Fig. 9.1, thereby supporting the observation of severe executive dysfunction.

9.1 Executive Functions Regulate Cognitive Processes in Intentional and Goal-Directed Behavior

Navigating everyday life puts great demands on the ability to plan, monitor, and regulate behavior. Many situations involve routines and follow a familiar and predictable series of events. Often, however, people need to consider unexpected elements of a situation as they go about their daily activities to carry out their intentions, plans, and obligations. An apparently plain activity such as shopping for groceries requires several cognitive processes, including planning and decision-making to determine what groceries to buy and where to get them, the ability to search for the specific goods among a large number of items on the shelves, and the ability to inhibit impulses and resist the temptation of buying things that are not on the list. If some items are missing or sold out, judgment is required to determine if the item can be replaced or left out, if a stop is needed at another store, or if the plan needs to be adjusted altogether. The ability to navigate a situation like this—and much more complex and difficult situations in everyday life—relies on a range of cognitive processes collectively termed executive functions. These processes are higher-order cognitive abilities that serve to supervise and regulate other abilities such as attention, memory, and motor skills when carrying out goal-directed behavior. Several abilities are usually associated with the term executive functions such as problem-solving skills, abstract thinking, and inhibitory control, but there is no clear consensus on the distinction, classification, or organization of these functions. When executive functions are impaired, behaviors tend to be disorganized, rigid, impulsive, or socially inappropriate, as was exemplified in the case of Ben.

In this chapter, the role of executive functions in neurorehabilitation will be characterized using Norman and Shallice's model of information processing in action control (Fig. 9.2) (Norman & Shallice, 1980; Shallice, 1982; Shallice & Cooper, 2011). In this model, human action and thought are organized in a set of processes called schemas. A schema is an overlearned sequence of actions or mental operations, which effectively utilizes the resources of neural subsystems such as visuospatial, memory, language, and motor systems to achieve a specific goal when activated. Recall in Chap. 5 on sensorimotor control, all the neural processes involved in grasping a cup of coffee. This simple movement requires yet fine coordination of cognitive, perceptual, and motor systems to locate, grasp, move, and drink from

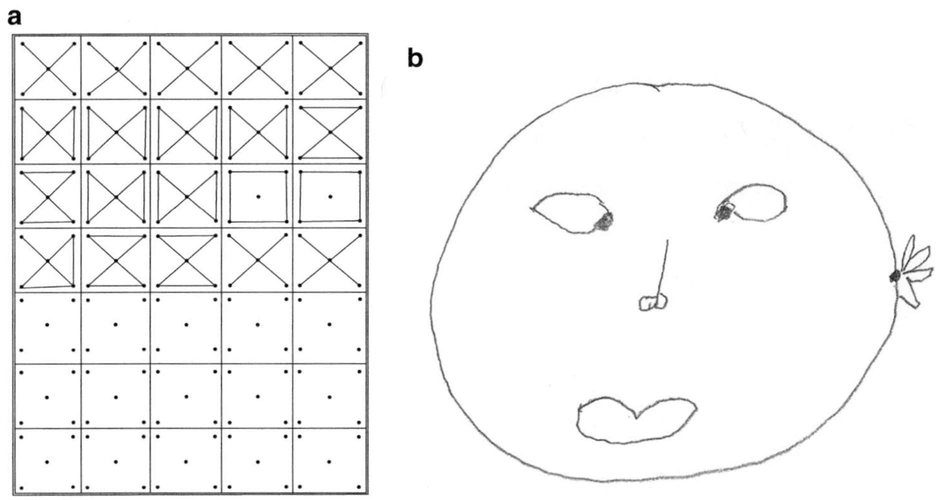

Fig. 9.1 Ben's performance on two neuropsychological tests. (**a**) The Five-Point Test: Ben was to produce as many different figures as possible, but he repeated the same figure many times, illustrating his perseverative behavior. This test is described in more detail in Box 9.4. (**b**) The Clock Drawing Test: Ben was to draw a clock, but he got triggered by the round shape and could not inhibit the impulse to draw a face

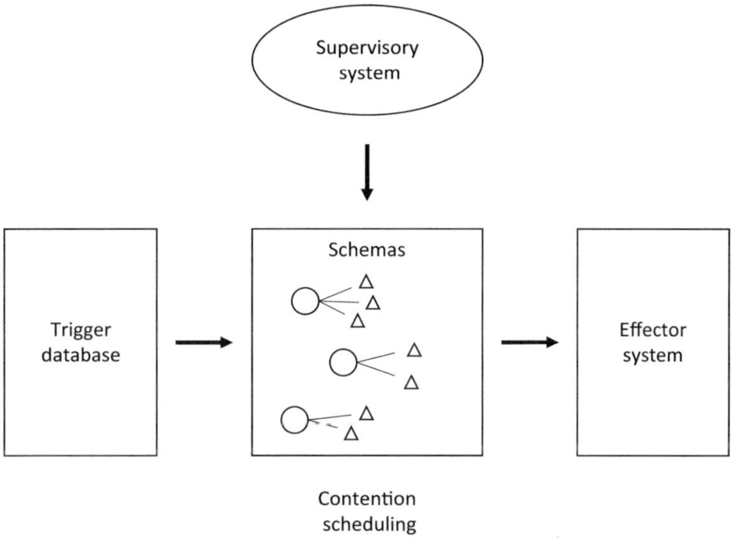

Fig. 9.2 A simplified representation of the Norman-Shallice model (1980). The activation of schemas is triggered by inputs from the trigger database, including perceptions and the output of other schemas. The supervisory system modulates the activation of schemas in contention scheduling. Circles represent source schemas (superordinate), and triangles represent component schemas (subordinate). Schemas activate specific purpose-processing units of the effector system, which are involved in the operation of action and thought schemas and initiation of behavior

the cup. These subprocesses are overlearned and automatized by repetitions to enable one to grasp the cup without having to think deliberately about how to position, move, and angle the hand, etc. (see also Chap. 7 on motor learning about the mechanisms involved in the automatization of overlearned actions). These well-rehearsed sequences of both actions and cognitions are called schemas within the model of Norman and Shallice. Schemas are hierarchically organized, and more complex schemas may activate other lower-level schemas. For example, the schema of driving a car involves several subroutines such as steering the wheel, controlling the pedals, shifting gears, checking mirrors, signaling, etc.

According to the Norman-Shallice model, behavior is initiated by the activation of certain schemas. Two systems control which schemas are being selected at any moment in time, namely a contention-scheduling system and a supervisory system (Shallice & Cooper, 2011). Contention scheduling involves the rapid and automatic selection of learned schemas that will realize the task demands in any given situation. For example, approaching a red traffic light while driving automatically excites the activation of the braking schema. When the level of activation exceeds a given threshold, the schema will be triggered to initiate the associated behavior (braking), and it will stay active until it attains its goal or is inhibited by a competing or superordinate schema. The contention-scheduling system is analogous to an "autopilot," enabling people to carry out routine activities without having to think through every single step. In novel situations, however, this automatic selection process is insufficient. Thus, a higher-level supervisory system modulates the contention-scheduling system in a deliberate fashion by inhibiting or exciting certain schemas or constructing new temporary schemas that normally would not be activated in that situation (Shallice & Cooper, 2011). The supervisory system corresponds to the willed control of behavior and enables people to adopt flexible strategies when facing novel problems or an unexpected turn of events, when dealing with dangers or high-stakes situations, and when strong impulses, temptations, or habitual responses need to be overcome. The supervisory system involves several subprocesses such as strategy generation and application, error monitoring, and verification processes. The problems that characterized Ben at the beginning of this chapter resemble behavior that relies predominantly on the processes of the contention-scheduling system without adequate top-down modulation from the supervisory system.

9.2 The Prefrontal Cortex Mediates the Executive Control of Cognitive, Emotional, and Motivational Processes

Executive functions are associated with the prefrontal cortex (PFC) and its vast connections with the rest of the brain. The PFC lies in the anterior frontal lobes, situated in front of the motor and premotor cortex on the lateral surface. It constitutes about one-third of the neocortex and is involved in higher-order processing of information. The PFC can be subdivided grossly into three major regions based on their main neuropsychological functions: The lateral, the orbital, and the medial PFC (see Box 9.2) (Szczepanski & Knight, 2014; Fuster, 2015). Broadly speaking, the lateral PFC is mainly involved in cognitive processes, the orbital PFC is critical to many of the brain's emotional circuits, and the medial PFC is important for social behavior and the "energization" of volitional thoughts and actions. The functions of these regions are, however, substantially overlapping and interactive, and many executive functions are supported by widespread neural networks across the brain (Szczepanski & Knight, 2014). Each of the three major regions is described in the following paragraphs.

Box 9.2 Gross Anatomy of the Prefrontal Cortex (PFC)

The PFC can be subdivided by its lateral, orbital, and medial aspects (Fig. 9.3). The lateral PFC includes the rear part of the PFC on the lateral surface, extending from the premotor cortex to the frontal pole. In the inferior part of the PFC, the orbitofrontal cortex is positioned, just above the orbits, in which the eyes are situated. Finally, the medial PFC includes the medial surfaces of the PFC and overlaps with the anterior cingulate cortex, which arches around the corpus callosum. The lateral and medial regions are often subdivided by their dorsal (upper)

(continued)

Box 9.2 (continued)
and ventral (lower) aspects. The ventromedial PFC overlaps with the orbitofrontal cortex, and these regions are closely connected to limbic structures, including the amygdala, hypothalamus, and limbic and temporal cortices. In the front of the brain, extending across the lateral and medial PFC is an area called the rostral PFC, which is particularly involved in "metacognitive" processes such as multitasking, introspection, and prospective memory (the ability to remember to carry out an intended act in the future). This region is proportionately larger in humans than in any other animal (Burgess & Wu, 2013).

The lateral PFC is involved in a wide range of cognitive processes such as working memory (see Box 9.3), attention, language, and active thought, including reasoning, abstraction, deduction, flexibility, planning, problem-solving, etc. (Szczepanski & Knight, 2014; Shallice & Cipolotti, 2018). The ventral aspect of the left and right lateral PFC is critical for language production and spatial attention, respectively. Lesions to the dorsal aspect are mainly associated with impairments in attention and working memory, leading to increased distractibility and difficulties keeping information in mind. Patient studies show that the left side is primarily involved in the generation and application of strategies to solve nonroutine problems, which is equivalent to the top-down modulation of the supervisory system in the Norman-Shallice model (Shallice & Cooper, 2011). Meanwhile, the right side is more specialized in self-monitoring and checking processes to detect errors and use feedback to update problem-solving strategies. Lack of self-monitoring and inflexibility in strategy switching can lead to rigid and perseverative behaviors, as illustrated by the test performance of Ben in Fig. 9.1.

Box 9.3 The Executive Component of Working Memory
Working memory is the ability to keep information in mind while performing mental operations using that information. It is a basic component of many executive functions (Shallice & Cipolotti, 2018). Baddeley and Hitch (1974) proposed a multicomponent model of working memory, which is elaborated upon in Chap. 6. In its basic form, the model involves a central executive component and a number of short-term memory "buffers," which are dedicated to specific modalities, e.g., verbal and visuospatial processing (Fig. 9.4). The short-term memory "buffers" maintain information in

(continued)

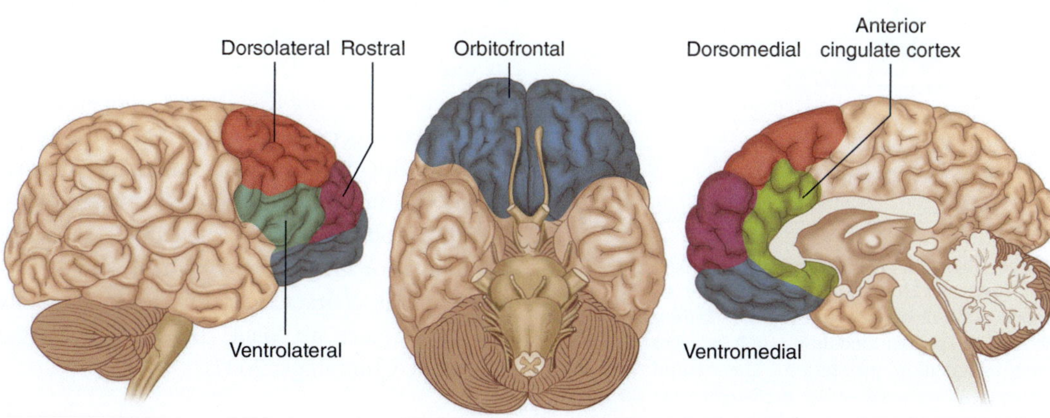

Fig. 9.3 The lateral (left), orbital (middle), and medial (right) aspects of the human prefrontal cortex. Approximate anatomical locations of common subdivisions of the prefrontal cortex are color-coded and labeled

Box 9.3 (continued)
memory temporarily, while the central executive component is responsible for performing mental operations on the information retained in short-term memory. As such, the central executive component is equivalent to the supervisory system of the Norman-Shallice model. The capacity of working memory is limited, and the amount of information that can be processed at a time is referred to as cognitive load. Patients with prefrontal lesions rarely have problems simply retaining information in working memory, but they typically have trouble related to the central executive component/the supervisory system (Shallice & Cipolotti, 2018). For example, they may simply repeat a sequence of numbers without problems but have substantial difficulties repeating a sequence of numbers in the opposite order (backwards), as this task requires one to maintain information in mind while having to carry out mental operations with an executive load. Decreasing the executive load of the operations that need to be carried out while retaining information in mind can increase working memory capacity.

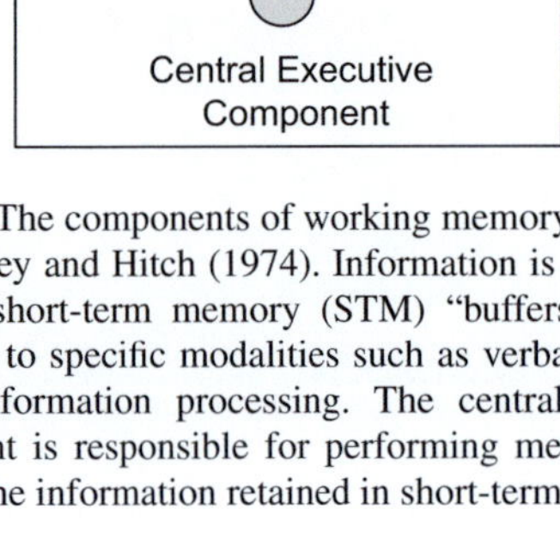

Fig. 9.4 The components of working memory according to Baddeley and Hitch (1974). Information is retained in separate short-term memory (STM) "buffers" that are dedicated to specific modalities such as verbal or visuospatial information processing. The central executive component is responsible for performing mental operations on the information retained in short-term memory

The orbital and medial PFCs are primarily involved in emotional, motivational, and energizing processes. The orbitofrontal cortex is particularly important for the integration and regulation of emotional and motivational processes in social behavior and value-based decision-making. In other words, it is critical for determining appropriate behavioral responses at any given time and place. Lesions in the orbital and ventromedial PFCs are associated with disinhibition, emotional lability, and reduced social cognition, e.g., reduced ability to mentalize and lack of empathy. Some patients may appear with an increased propensity for impulsive and socially inappropriate behaviors, and excessive risk-taking. In cognitive tasks, patients tend to perform errors related to a lack of care and a failure to remain on task (Shallice & Cooper, 2011), and they exhibit poor feedback-based learning.

The dorsal aspect of the medial PFC is primarily involved in energization, including volitional effort, drive, and motility. Referring to the Norman-Shallice model, the dorsomedial PFC is critical for energizing and initiating the operations of the supervisory system, which is the prerequisite for volitional thoughts and actions and the ability to sustain attention over time (Shallice & Cipolotti, 2018). Accordingly, lesions in the dorsomedial PFC and its circuits are associated with apathy, abulia, hypokinesia, a loss of initiative, intention, and spontaneity, and diminished motor activity. The lack of energization affects both willed movement, speech, and thinking, and patients generally perform slower in neuropsychological tests, even simple reaction time tasks, and present with a wide range of executive deficits due to the global function of energization in executive functioning (Shallice & Cooper, 2011). Diminished supervisory control makes behaviors more stimulus-dependent and vulnerable to interference, leading to perseverations, stereotypies, and utilization behavior. Massive bilateral lesions of the anterior cingulate cortex can lead to akinetic mutism, characterized by profound apathy and indifference to pain, thirst, and hunger (Bonelli & Cummings, 2007).

9.2.1 The Networks of the Prefrontal Cortex with Other Regions Are Critical to Executive Functioning

The PFC is the most richly connected of all cortical regions, including both cortico-cortical and cortico-subcortical circuits (Fuster, 2015). Each of the three main regions described above connects with subcortical structures in parallel circuits, including the striatum, globus pallidus, substantia nigra, and thalamus (see Fig. 9.5) (Bonelli & Cummings, 2007). Damage to any of these subcortical structures, including the white matter tracts connecting them with the PFC, can produce executive deficits, even if the PFC is spared. Likewise, executive impairments can also be due to disruptions of the neural connectivity of the PFC with other cortical regions. These deficits are commonly termed disconnection syndromes.

9.3 Neurological Conditions Affecting Prefrontal Networks Produce Executive Deficits

Various brain pathologies involve the PFC and its circuitry and may result in executive impairments. In closed-head trauma (Chap. 23), the PFC is exposed to injury due to the impact of the brain on the bony ridge of the front of the skull. The orbital surface, just above the base of the skull, is particularly vulnerable, and disinhibition and neurobehavioral disabilities are common sequelae of moderate and severe traumatic brain injury. Head trauma may also cause diffuse axonal injury affecting distributed neural networks, adding to the consequences of injury. Stroke (Chap. 17), infections, and tumors may also affect the PFC. Most strokes involve the middle cerebral artery, which supplies the lateral PFC among other cortices, leading to hallmark symptoms of hemiparesis, aphasia, or hemispatial neglect (see Box 4.3). The medial aspect of the frontal lobe is supplied by the anterior cerebral artery, which is less frequently affected by stroke. Subcortical strokes affecting distributed networks of the PFC can also produce executive deficits. Intracranial tumors, e.g., gliomas and meningiomas, frequently affect the frontal lobes and can lead to progressive behavioral and cognitive impairments.

Neurodegenerative disorders such as Parkinson's (Chap. 21) and Huntington's disease affect subcortical structures in the frontostriatal circuits. Consequently, executive functions and social cognition in addition to motor symptoms deteriorate as the striatum gradually degenerates (Larsen et al., 2015). A specific type of dementia (Chap. 22), the behavioral variant of frontotemporal dementia, is characterized by degeneration

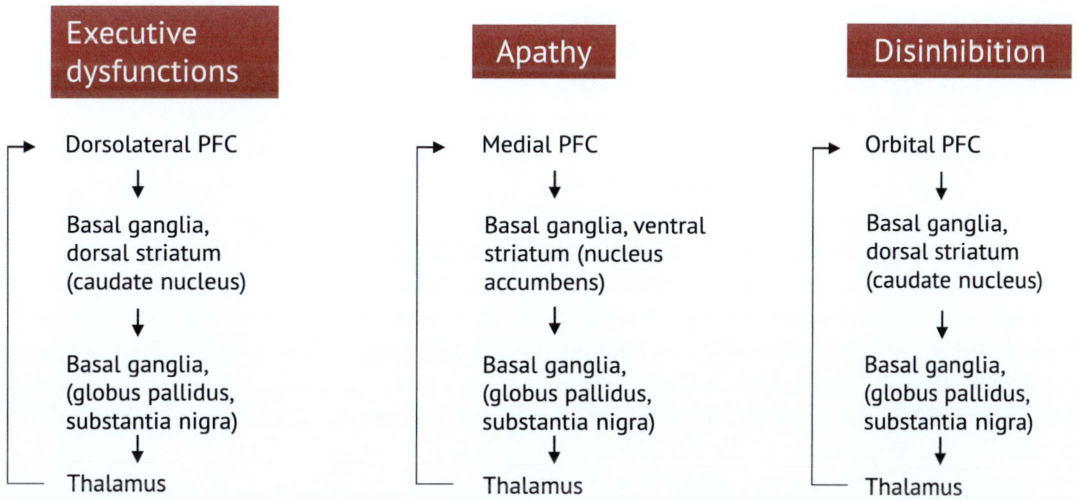

Fig. 9.5 Three main frontal-subcortical circuits facilitating executive functions. Damage to any of the structures involved in each circuit may lead to different types of executive deficits

of primarily the PFC, leading to progressive impairments in executive and social functioning. In addition to neurological conditions, several psychiatric and developmental disorders such as schizophrenia and attention-deficit/hyperactivity disorder (ADHD) are characterized by executive deficits and associated with changes in frontal-subcortical circuitry.

9.4 Assessment Is Important to Identify the Nature of Executive Problems

A neuropsychological examination can help identify the nature of executive deficits in relation to the subprocesses of the supervisory system. A detailed assessment and understanding of both deficits and assets can increase self-awareness and guide appropriate treatment and management approaches to improve everyday life functioning. In addition to cognitive deficits, neuropsychological examinations can yield an account of social and emotional functioning in relation to executive impairment. Several sources of information are utilized in the examination, e.g., formal tests, clinical observations, rating scales, medical records, and history-taking from the patient and other informants. Collecting information from close relatives and taking proxy measures is particularly important with pediatric patients or when patients have poor self-awareness or insight into their own functional level. Patients with dys-executive problems typically lack insight into the consequences of their deficits and fail to take them into account as they go about their day, as exemplified in the case of Ben.

Tests of executive functions put demands on the supervisory system, and different tests may load on specific subprocesses of the supervisory system. For example, strategy generation and planning can be addressed by the Tower of London (Shallice, 1982), flexibility in thinking can be addressed by the Wisconsin Card Sorting Test (Berg, 1948), and response initiation, organization, and self-monitoring can be addressed by fluency tests such as the Five-Point Test (Regard et al., 1982) (see Box 9.4). In addition, a broad range of executive functions can be assessed using large test batteries such as the Delis-Kaplan Executive Function System (D-KEFS) (Delis et al., 2001). However, subjects may fail tests for different reasons. Executive functioning depends on the integration of multiple subprocesses of the supervisory system, and a profound deficit in inhibition, for example, may impact several other functions, leading to different kinds of executive problems. Additionally, performance on tests of executive functions also relies on more basic cognitive, sensory, and motor skills that are to be utilized by the supervisory system. Tests usually require general language or visuospatial abilities, which may be compromised by the neurological insult. This concern is referred to as "task impurity," meaning that no executive task is a pure test of any single executive function. Knowing the state of other abilities, and careful observations of how the subject responds to different tests, are integral to determine the nature of executive problems, as illustrated in the examination of Ben. Executive impairments may also affect other cognitive abilities, e.g., memory, where disorganized behavior during learning or lack of interest in remembering irrelevant information can be mistaken for amnesia. Finally, it is important to take into account the effect of fatigue and performance fatigability and plan regular breaks during the examination, because fatigue significantly impacts executive performance (see Box 9.5).

Box 9.4 Regard et al.'s Five-Point Test

The Five-Point Test (Regard et al., 1982) was designed to examine nonverbal response fluency. The test consists of a page with 40 squares, and each square contains five symmetrically arranged dots (see Fig. 9.1a). The examinee is instructed to produce as many different figures as possible within 5 min by connecting any number of dots with straight lines, without repeating any figure. The test is scored by counting the number of unique figures produced at the end of the test. The efficient solution requires the test taker to establish some

(continued)

Box 9.4 (continued)
structure to the production of figures, e.g., by rotating or making small variations to a figure. However, patients with executive impairment may have trouble coming up with any ideas for a figure or keeping track of what kind of figures they have made already. They may violate the rules of the task, or they may repeat the same figure over and over again, an example of perseverative behavior, as seen in the case with Ben in Fig. 9.1. As such, this rather simple test may reveal various kinds of executive problems by observing how test takers solve the task.

At the same time, neuropsychological examination is also challenged by situations where patients perform normally in a structured examination despite exhibiting executive problems in everyday life (Lezak et al., 2012). Formal testing is often conducted in a highly structured setting with the examiner telling the subject what to do. However, the supervisory system is mainly taxed in ill-structured situations requiring the subject to direct and organize goal-directed behavior for oneself. In other words, formal tests may not be sensitive to subtle yet disabling executive deficits. Likewise, executive deficits may not manifest themselves in the well-structured clinical setting of a hospital department or a 24-h residential rehabilitation unit until the patient returns to independent living. In this context, clinical observations, and proxy reports of how the subject manages everyday situations are critical to the overall assessment.

Many traditional tests of executive functions are derived from experimental research and were not originally designed for clinical purposes. Consequently, many traditional tests are criticized for not being "ecologically valid," i.e., the tasks are artificial in the sense that they do not adequately represent real-world situations or generalize to real-life functioning. Some tests such as the Multiple Errands and the Six Element tests (Shallice & Burgess, 1991) were designed to correspond more closely to the demands of real-world situations to demonstrate real-life planning problems and increase the clinical utility of test results. More recently, virtual reality-based instruments have been developed to mimic real-world situations in a standardized clinical assessment of executive functions (Borgnis et al., 2022).

Box 9.5 Fatigue and Performance Fatigability
A constant lack of energy or feeling of tiredness and need for rest (fatigue), which is exacerbated in response to tasks that require physical or mental focus (performance fatigability), is very common in people with a neurological disorder. This experience of fatigue is often coupled with failing memory and emotional control and is not related to lack of sleep. Even after a good night's sleep, severe fatigue may be experienced in relation to relatively minor mental or physical efforts. Daily fatigue is reported more often among individuals with Parkinson's disease, multiple sclerosis, stroke, traumatic brain injury, and cerebral palsy compared to the general population, and is a significant problem that interferes with usual and desired activities. It is frequently a factor preventing individuals from fully adhering to a neurorehabilitation program, even though, purely in terms of physical capability, they should be able to do so.

Performance fatigability should not be confused with muscle fatigue, which is caused by the reduced capacity of a muscle to generate force following repeated activation. Reduced muscle strength and increased fatigability of muscles following brain injury probably contribute to reduced ability to overcome things in daily life and thereby to an increased experience of fatigue, but it is important to understand that performance fatigability is caused by central mechanisms in the nervous system distinct from muscle fatigue. In line with this, performance fatigability may also be

(continued)

Box 9.5 (continued)
seen in relation to both physical and mental efforts. There is considerable overlap between the two, but there are also clearly domain-specific failures in networks involved only in mental processes or in sensorimotor control. Certain patients primarily report mental fatigue, while others emphasize physical fatigue or a combination of both. This is probably linked to the specific areas of the brain and networks affected in each individual patient as well as secondary factors such as comorbidities or psychological processes that may contribute to the subjective experience of fatigue.

Fatigue and performance fatigability, whether in a mental or physical context, likely represent a diminished ability to process information rapidly and efficiently with minimal conscious awareness in the relevant cortical and subcortical circuits. In essence, fatigue can be seen as the mental equivalent of a brain with a reduced capacity to automate processes, ensuring that the person's attention and awareness don't have to oversee every detail. This is a direct response to an underlying lesion or disturbance, which hinders the establishment of an optimal internal model for the individual's interaction with the environment (discussed in Chap. 8). Consequently, the individual must continue expending significant conscious and mental efforts in tackling relatively straightforward tasks. In connection with the automation inherent in motor learning (as discussed in Chap. 7), fatigue can be viewed as the outcome when an individual fails to optimize control of a movement (or a cognitive task) adequately to automate the process. This results in the individual remaining in the cognitive or associative stage of learning, necessitating substantial mental resources.

The severity of fatigue usually diminishes as (cognitive and motor) functions recover, but there are several reasons to specifically address fatigue in rehabilitation. Fatigue is distressing and burdensome to patients and caregivers and is associated with disability and poor vocational outcomes. Fatigue and performance fatigability may also prevent or greatly diminish the efforts that need to be put into training and learning sessions and may therefore prevent an optimal effect of the rehabilitation program. Self-management therapies which help the individual to anticipate when fatigue or performance fatigability occurs and to recognize early signs and find ways of coping with them have shown good results in several patient groups and should be considered as an aid for the patient in order to manage daily activities or accomplish a challenging training program during rehabilitation.

9.5 Targeted Rehabilitation Can Improve Executive Functions and the Management of Executive Problems in Everyday Life

Rehabilitation needs to be planned according to personal goals based on a formulation of the problem behaviors and how impairments in executive functions are expected to contribute to those problems. A theoretical framework such as the Norman-Shallice model is helpful in forming a coherent understanding of the nature of the problems and how to address them (Burgess & Alderman, 1994; Evans, 2009). Based on this model, two overall approaches to managing executive difficulties are described below. The first is a top-down approach concerned with training or remediating the impaired processes of the supervisory system. The second is a bottom-up approach focused on compensating for the deficits.

First, treatment can be targeted toward increasing the effectiveness of the supervisory system in modulating the automatic selection of schemas

Table 9.1 The five self-instructional steps in goal management training (Levine et al., 2000)

Stage	Name	Self-verbalization
1	STOP!	"What am I doing?"
2	DEFINE	"What is the main task?"
3	LIST	"What are the specific steps?"
4	LEARN	"Do I know the goal and the steps?"
5	CHECK	"Am I doing what I planned to do?"

(Burgess & Alderman, 1994). This may include any of the subprocesses of the supervisory system such as strategy application, self-monitoring, or set-shifting. Metacognitive strategy training such as Goal Management Training (Levine et al., 2000) is an effective treatment for improving planning and problem-solving skills and managing problems with impulsivity, self-monitoring, and emotional self-regulation (Cicerone et al., 2019). The program teaches a mental-checking routine, involving five self-instructional steps, which aim to interrupt the automatic processing of contention scheduling and direct attention toward the overall intended goal. The five steps are presented in Table 9.1.

These steps are rehearsed and practiced in real-world situations to mitigate disorganized behavior. However, metacognitive strategy training requires adequate cognitive ability to be able to learn, apply, and generalize the strategies in everyday life, and patients with severe deficits or compromised awareness, poor motivation, or initiation difficulties are less likely to benefit from metacognitive strategy training (Cicerone et al., 2019). External promptings such as alerts, cues, or text messages can help people remember to do the mental-checking routine in everyday life, and a protocol has been adapted for children with acquired brain injury and spina bifida (Stubberud et al., 2021). Referring back to the case of Ben, his presumptive lack of care and interest may impede any attempts of improving his executive behavior through metacognitive strategy training. At least, he will likely need detailed information about his impairments to increase his awareness and insight into his difficulties and their implications. Further, he would need a large degree of support for implementing any strategies at home, in close collaboration with his wife, based on any personal goals of his that may be identified in a value-based goal negotiation process. Perhaps, a second approach to the management of his problems may be more fruitful, depending on the severity and nature of his impairments.

The second approach to managing executive impairment is to reduce the demand for the supervisory system to select the appropriate schemas in everyday situations. Treatment may be targeted toward structuring or modifying the features of the environment that triggers the problem behaviors, or the aim may be to modify the contention-scheduling process to establish new behavioral routines and habits in place of the problematic responses (Burgess & Alderman, 1994). For example, checklists can be provided to help remember the steps of complex tasks. Skill-specific training such as errorless learning is recommended for patients with severe cognitive impairment or limited capability of using metacognitive strategies (Cicerone et al., 2019). Errorless learning is a principle of minimizing or eliminating errors to reinforce the correct response in the process of learning specific information or procedures, in contrast to trial-and-error learning (Haslam & Kessels, 2018). So, rather than relying on the impaired supervisory system to learn from mistakes, the correct selection of schemas is routinized or "overlearned" in the contention-scheduling system by constraining the possibility of errors during learning. This learning is highly task-specific and is unlikely to be transferable to other tasks or situations as that would involve the supervisory system to make that generalization. However, learning specific knowledge or skills that improve the quality of life can be highly valuable even if it does not generalize across different contexts (Haslam & Kessels, 2018). In the case of Ben, therapies based on errorless learning may be initiated to help him manage his chores around the house in a structured manner.

Review Questions

- How does the supervisory system influence human behavior?
- What methods can be used to assess executive functions?
- What treatments can be used for executive impairments and when should one or the other be used?

References

Baddeley, A. D., & Hitch, G. (1974). Working memory. In G. A. Bower (Ed.), *Recent advances in learning and motivation* (pp. 47–89). Academic Press.

Berg, E. A. (1948). A simple objective technique for measuring flexibility in thinking. *The Journal of General Psychology, 39*, 15–22. https://doi.org/10.1080/00221309.1948.9918159

Bonelli, R. M., & Cummings, J. L. (2007). Frontal-subcortical circuitry and behavior. *Dialogues in Clinical Neuroscience, 9*, 141–151. https://doi.org/10.31887/dcns.2007.9.2/rbonelli

Borgnis, F., Baglio, F., Pedroli, E., et al. (2022). Available virtual reality-based tools for executive functions: A systematic review. *Frontiers in Psychology, 13*, 833136. https://doi.org/10.3389/fpsyg.2022.833136

Burgess, P. W., & Alderman, N. (1994). Rehabilitation of dyscontrol syndromes following frontal lobe damage: A cognitive neuropsychological approach. In R. L. Wood & I. Fussey (Eds.), *Cognitive rehabilitation in perspective* (1st ed., pp. 183–203). Routledge.

Burgess, P. W., & Wu, H.-C. (2013). Rostral prefrontal cortex (Brodmann area 10): Metacognition in the brain. In D. T. Stuss & R. T. Knight (Eds.), *Principles of frontal lobe function* (2nd ed., pp. 524–544). Oxford University Press.

Cicerone, K. D., Goldin, Y., Ganci, K., et al. (2019). Evidence-based cognitive rehabilitation: Systematic review of the literature from 2009 through 2014. *Archives of Physical Medicine and Rehabilitation, 100*, 1515–1533.

Delis, D. C., Kaplan, F., & Kramer, J. H. (2001). *Delis-Kaplan executive function system*. The Psychological Corporation.

Evans, J. J. (2009). Rehabilitation of executive functioning: An overview. In M. Oddy & A. Worthington (Eds.), *The rehabilitation of executive disorders* (pp. 59–73). Oxford University Press.

Fuster, J. M. (2015). *The prefrontal cortex* (5th ed.). Academic Press.

Haslam, C., & Kessels, R. P. C. (Eds.). (2018). *Errorless learning in neuropsychological rehabilitation*. Routledge.

Larsen, I. U., Vinther-Jensen, T., Gade, A., et al. (2015). Assessing impairment of executive function and psychomotor speed in premanifest and manifest huntington's disease gene-expansion carriers. *Journal of the International Neuropsychological Society, 21*, 193–202. https://doi.org/10.1017/S1355617715000090

Levine, B., Robertson, I. H., Clare, L., et al. (2000). Rehabilitation of executive functioning: An experimental-clinical validation of goal management training. *Journal of the International Neuropsychological Society, 6*, 299–312. https://doi.org/10.1017/S1355617700633052

Lezak, M. D., Howieson, D. B., Bigler, E. D., & Tranel, D. (2012). Executive functions. In *Neuropsychological assessment* (5th ed., pp. 666–711). Oxford University Press.

Norman DA, Shallice T (1980) Attention to action: Willed and automatic control of behavior. San Diego, CA, USA

Regard, M., Strauss, E., & Knapp, P. (1982). Children's production on verbal and non-verbal fluency tasks. *Perceptual and Motor Skills, 55*, 839–844. https://doi.org/10.2466/pms.1982.55.3.839

Shallice, T. (1982). Specific impairments of planning. *Philosophical Transactions. Royal Society of London, 298*, 199–209.

Shallice, T., & Burgess, P. W. (1991). Deficits in strategy application following frontal lobe damage in man. *Brain, 114*, 727–741.

Shallice, T., & Cipolotti, L. (2018). The prefrontal cortex and neurological impairments of active thought. *Annual Review of Psychology, 69*, 157–180. https://doi.org/10.1146/annurev-psych-010416-044123

Shallice, T., & Cooper, R. P. (2011). *The organisation of mind*. Oxford University Press.

Stubberud, J., Holthe, I. L., Løvstad, M., et al. (2021). The feasibility and acceptability of goal management training of executive functions in children with spina bifida and acquired brain injury. *Neuropsychological Rehabilitation, 31*, 601–620. https://doi.org/10.1080/09602011.2020.1723649

Szczepanski, S. M., & Knight, R. T. (2014). Insights into human behavior from lesions to the prefrontal cortex. *Neuron, 83*, 1002–1018. https://doi.org/10.1016/j.neuron.2014.08.011

Speech, Language, and Communication

10

Iben Christensen, Lise Randrup Jensen, Sonia Brownsett, and Jytte Kjærgaard Isaksen

Abstract

Communication is a highly complex human task depending on a neurologically widespread and simultaneous interplay between a range of sensory, motor, and cognitive functions. This makes the neurobiological basis of communication sensitive and vulnerable to brain injuries, and therefore communication disorders after a brain injury are common. After a short introduction to brain areas involved in the intact function of speech, language, and communication, three frequent and distinct communicative disorders are presented: dysarthria affecting motor speech production, aphasia affecting language at the linguistic levels of phonology, semantics, and grammar, and cognitive-communication disorders affecting adequate communication in social interaction. Definitions, anatomical localization, and clinical symptoms of each of these disorders as well as the distinctive features across them are described. Furthermore, specific interventions based on principles of neuroplasticity are highlighted. These include therapies that harness the brain's capacity to reorganize and adapt, thereby improving communication abilities in individuals with communication disorders. The insights provided are crucial for clinicians providing neurorehabilitation for people with communication disorders following brain injury.

Keywords

Speech · Language · Social interaction · Dysarthria · Aphasia · Cognitive-communication disorders

Box 10.1 Case Story

Micky, a 62-year-old male accountant, suffered an ischemic stroke in the left frontal lobe 2 months ago. After 3 days at the acute stroke ward, he was transferred to an inpatient rehabilitation unit where he is about to be discharged home and continue community-based rehabilitation. Micky has a hemiparesis in his right arm, fingers, and leg as well as a facial paresis. He also has unilateral upper motor neuron dysarthria affecting phonation (harsh vocal quality) and articulation (imprecise consonants). Furthermore, Micky has nonfluent aphasia, Broca's aphasia, resulting

(continued)

I. Christensen (✉) · L. R. Jensen
Department of Nordic Studies and Linguistics, University of Copenhagen, Copenhagen South, Denmark
e-mail: i.christensen@hum.ku.dk; randrup@hum.ku.dk

S. Brownsett
School of Health and Rehabilitation Sciences, University of Queensland, St. Lucia, QLD, Australia
e-mail: s.brownsett@uq.edu.au

J. K. Isaksen
Department of Culture and Language, University of Southern Denmark, Odense, Denmark
e-mail: jisa@sdu.dk

J. B. Nielsen et al. (eds.), *Neuroplasticity-based Neurorehabilitation*,
https://doi.org/10.1007/978-3-031-81120-3_10

Box 10.1 (continued)
in moderate word-finding difficulties (anomia). His anomia makes it hard to express most things, as nouns and verbs are hard to retrieve, as are many words from other word classes. Additionally, Micky has difficulties understanding longer, more complex sentences. Micky is also unable to functionally read or write. The multidisciplinary staff in the two hospital wards has been supporting Micky's communication in daily conversations and meetings by employing strategies such as slowing down their speaking pace, using less complex sentence structures, asking yes/no questions, maintaining eye contact, writing down keywords, and providing pictorial materials to support decision-making. During his in-patient rehabilitation, Micky has received intensive individual and group-based speech-language therapy. The therapy was based on goals set by Micky with this speech-language therapist (SLT). These goals were meaningful to Micky and his life situation (e.g., practicing vocabulary related to numbers and his leisure activity, stamp collection). The group therapy was based on the Constraint-Induced Aphasia Therapy (CIAT) approach (Pulvermüller et al., 2001). Given that his dysarthric speech difficulties were less prominent in Micky's communication, the SLT and Micky chose to focus therapeutic efforts on his aphasia. Micky's speech-language therapy has been underpinned by a number of theoretical concepts of neuroplasticity: "use it or lose it," "use it and improve it," specificity, and "repetition, intensity, time, and salience matters" (see Chap. 15).

10.1 Communication Is a Multilevel Highly Complex Activity

Communication is a highly complex activity requiring the successful integration of general cognitive and social abilities, linguistic competence, and motor, visual, and auditory skills. This chapter initially provides a short introduction to brain areas involved in the intact function of speech, language, and communication followed by a focus on acquired disorders of production and comprehension of spoken communication. The written language modalities (reading and writing) depend on many of the same components and processes as spoken communication but also require additional functional components and skills. Much of the knowledge obtained within the field of speech, language, and communication is derived from acquired injuries within involved brain areas.

It is important to distinguish between **speech, language, and cognitive levels** in the production (or comprehension) of spoken communication. **Speech** is a predominantly motor activity, in which the speaker transforms a linguistic message into finely tuned movements of the muscles relevant for speech, i.e., the muscles controlling our respiration, phonation, velopharyngeal function, jaw, tongue, and lips. The complex coordinated activation of all these muscles requires participation of a large network of interconnected cortical and subcortical areas. Some of these areas are predominantly localized in the left hemisphere, whereas others are bilaterally represented (see Box 10.2).

Language is to be understood as the core linguistic system shared by speakers. It enables them to use and understand symbols (typically words), to refer to objects or concepts, and to apply grammatical rules to construct or comprehend phrases and sentences with those symbols. At the level of language processing, word forms and word meanings are retrieved or recognized, and morphological and syntactic structure is planned or decoded. Language processing relies predominantly on the left hemisphere for most right-handed adults.

The use of language in social interactions i.e., to communicate, involves many different and interacting **cognitive processes**, as well as intact speech and language functions. Furthermore, social interaction involves the knowledge of, and adaptation to, a given con-

Box 10.2 Anatomical Structures Involved in Speech, Language, and Communication
The organization of speech, language, and communication within the human brain entails a distributed network of specialized regions, each playing a distinct role. The motor system for speech production engages various anatomical structures, including primary and association cortices, basal ganglia, thalamus, cerebellum, and the neuromuscular junction. These components interact to execute the physical act of speech production. Language processing is controlled by structures in the left hemisphere for the majority of right-handed people. Traditionally, the processing of language has been attributed to three brain structures: Broca's and Wernicke's areas and the Arcuate Fasciculus (Fig. 10.1). Broca's Area is placed in the left frontal lobe and controls speech production. Wernicke's Area is placed in the left temporal lobe and orchestrates language comprehension. The Arcuate Fasciculus acts as a neural conduit, connecting Wernicke's and Broca's areas and facilitating communication between language perception and production. In the last decades, the newer dual-stream processing model of language has become more widely acknowledged. This model delineates distinct dorsal and ventral pathways responsible for mapping sound to motor articulation and meaning, respectively. The model is based on functional imaging and diverse etiological evidence that have implicated additional brain regions such as the inferior parietal regions, superior temporal regions, and frontal regions in language processing. The processes involved in communicating in social interaction (i.e., pragmatics) rely on multiple extended neural networks in both hemispheres. Frontotemporal regions are associated with executive functions, social cognition, and pragmatic language use, including language planning. Specifically, the right hemisphere's fronto-parietal and temporal structures are implicated in expressing and perceiving emotions through vocal tone and facial expressions.

versation's specific and general context. For example, talking about one's illness is carried out differently if speaking to a friend or a medical doctor. The speaker or listener also relies on his or her memory of what has already been said in a conversation, they must plan how to unfold a coherent narrative of an event and attend to the conversation partner's "on-line" reactions or responses. The brain regions involved at this level include frontal as well as several bilateral cortical areas involved in social and cognitive functioning.

Thus, for successful communication to occur, all the abovementioned functions are involved in a highly complex, neurologically widespread, and simultaneous interplay, which makes the neurobiological basis of communication sensitive and vulnerable to brain injuries. Therefore, communication disorders following acquired brain injury are common, and the type of disorders vary depending on the etiology of the brain injury. The three communication disorders described in this chapter (dysarthria, aphasia, and cognitive-communication disorders) may occur

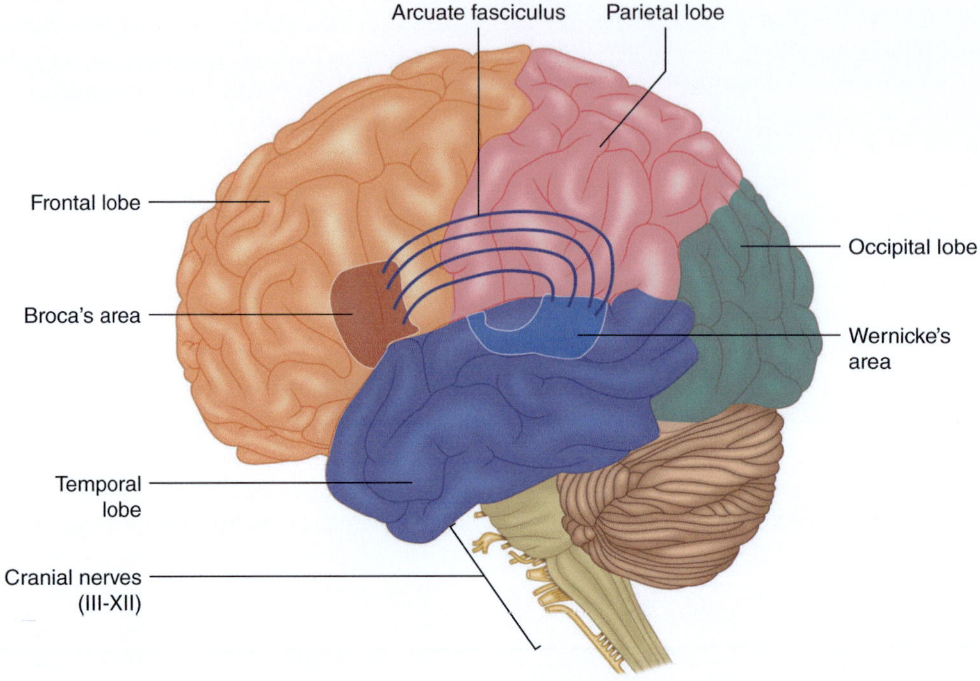

Fig. 10.1 Brain areas involved in speech, language, and communication

in isolation or cooccur with each other. Box 10.2 below provides further information on the brain areas involved in speech, language, and communication.

10.2 Damage to Different Brain Areas Results in Distinct Communication Disorders

As described above, the different levels involved in producing and comprehending spoken communication require the interaction of several distinct brain areas. Damage to these areas or their interconnective tissue gives rise to quite distinct communicative disorders: **dysarthria** (affecting speech), **aphasia** (affecting language), and **cognitive-communication disorders** (affecting social interaction).[1] Dysarthria is a disorder of the motor system supporting speech. Aphasia is a disturbance to components of the core system of language. Cognitive-communication disorders are disturbances of the cognitive processes required for language use.

Differentiating between these diagnoses is an important basis for selecting an appropriate approach to rehabilitation, which is the task of a

[1]The diagnosis *verbal apraxia* (or *apraxia of speech*) is not described in the current chapter due to prioritizing of more in-depth focus on the three major diagnoses affecting communication following acquired brain injury: dysarthria, aphasia, and cognitive-communication disorders. See Freed (2020) for an introductory description of verbal apraxia. Since the motor *planning* of speech is associated with apraxia of speech, this chapter will only focus on motor *execution*, which is associated with dysarthria.

Table 10.1 Overview of the three diagnoses: dysarthria, aphasia, and cognitive-communication disorders

Diagnosis	Primary level of disorder	Primary localization of disorder	Significant problems	Estimated incidence
Dysarthria	Motor speech	The motor system in the central and peripheral nervous systems: Association cortex, basal ganglia, cerebellum, thalamus, primary motor cortex, extrapyramidal and pyramidal systems, cranial nerves, and neuromuscular junctions	The physical realization of speech: Respiration, phonation, resonance, articulation, and prosody	20–60% of people with stroke and traumatic brain injury Note: Some types of dysarthria are caused by progressive etiologies (e.g., Parkinson's disease)
Aphasia	Language	Perisylvian area and underlying connective tissue of left hemisphere (for right-handed adult individuals)	The structure of language: Sound structure (phonology), meaning structure (semantics), and grammatical structure (syntax)	32–38% of people with stroke and traumatic brain injury
Cognitive-communication disorders	Cognition	Frontotemporal regions and multiple extended neural networks in both hemispheres	The use of language in social interaction (pragmatics) and in the management of information and verbal reasoning	50–75% of people with stroke and traumatic brain injury

speech-language therapist. Table 10.1 provides an overview of the main characteristics of dysarthria, aphasia, and cognitive-communications disorders. In the following sections, the specific nature of each of the diagnoses will be described in terms of clinical symptoms, assessment, and neural localization.

10.3 Dysarthria Is a Motor Speech Disorder Affecting the Listener's Comprehension of the Intended Message

Dysarthria is defined as a collective group of motor speech disorders that reflects abnormalities in the strength, speed, range, steadiness, tone, or accuracy of movements required for speech production. Dysarthria is purely a collection of motor speech disorders and is to be distinguished from language disorders (aphasia) and communication disorders caused by cognitive disorders (cognitive-communication disorders and dementia) (Freed, 2020).

Speech production includes respiration, phonation, articulation, resonance, and prosody. All, some, or one of these speech production components can be affected. Each of the components is associated with a range of speech characteristics that can be affected depending on what is the underlying cause of the damage and localization hereof (see Table 10.2) (Freed, 2020). A large range of deviant speech dimensions are seen in dysarthria. Each of these speech dimensions can be ascribed to affected speech components, e.g., imprecise consonants and distorted vowels are articulatory disturbances, whereas distorted pitch level, pitch breaks, and monopitch are associated with phonatory and/or respiratory disturbances.

There are seven types of dysarthria: flaccid, spastic, unilateral upper motor neuron, ataxic, hypokinetic, hyperkinetic, and mixed (Freed, 2020). Each type, apart from mixed dysarthria, is associated with different locations and in some cases specific disorders (e.g., Parkinson's Disease

Table 10.2 Overview of localization, etiologies, and common speech production errors in the dysarthria subtypes. Based on Freed (2020)

Subtype	Flaccid	Spastic	Unilateral upper motor neuron	Ataxic	Hypokinetic	Hyperkinetic	Mixed
Localization	Lower motor neuron in spinal nerves or cranial nerves	Upper motor neurons of the pyramidal and extrapyramidal systems (bilateral damage)	Upper motor neurons (unilateral damage, either left or right hemisphere)	Cerebellum or its control circuits	Basal ganglia control circuit (extrapyramidal system)	Basal ganglia and major pathways (extrapyramidal system)	Neurological damage to two or more parts of the motor system
Etiologies (nonexhaustive)	Physical trauma Brainstem stroke Myasthenia Gravis	Stroke Amyotrophic Lateral Sclerosis Traumatic brain injury	Stroke Tumors Traumatic brain injury	Degenerative diseases like various forms of cerebellar ataxia and Friedrich's ataxia Stroke Toxic conditions Traumatic brain injury	All types of parkinsonism Traumatic brain injury Stroke	Chorea including Sydenham's and Huntington's Chorea Stroke Tardive Dyskinesia Traumatic brain injury	Stroke (single or multiple) Tumors Multiple Sclerosis Amyotrophic Lateral Sclerosis Traumatic brain injury
Five most common speech production errors	Hypernasality Imprecise consonants Breathiness Monopitch Nasal emission	Imprecise consonants Monopitch Reduced stress Harsh voice quality Monoloudnes	Imprecise consonants Slow alternation motion rates (AMRs) Harsh voice quality Imprecise AMRs Irregular AMRs	Imprecise consonants Excess and equal stress Irregular articulatory breakdown Distorted vowels Harsh voice quality	Monopitch Reduced stress Monoloudness Imprecise consonants Inappropriate silences	Imprecise consonants Prolonged intervals Variable pitchy Monopitch Harsh voice quality	Depends on which motor systems are affected

causes hypokinetic dysarthria, cf. Table 10.2). The examination of dysarthria particularly focuses on how intelligible and natural the patient's speech is and how that affects the listener's overall comprehension of the speech. The latter is based not only on the physiological and perceptual evaluation but also takes nonverbal cues into consideration to give a full description of the person with dysarthria's speech and communicative ability in a natural context, sometimes described as the person's comprehensibility.

10.3.1 Dysarthria Is Caused by Neuromotor Damage to the Nervous System (Localization of Dysarthria)

Damage to any of the components or levels of the motor system can cause movement disorders, and if these movements are related to speech production, the result will be dysarthria. As described by Yorkston et al. (2010), motor execution is a range of complex processes referring to how motor plans result in the execution of the muscle contractions contributing to speech. Accordingly, in a highly simplified manner, the execution phase of motor control can be viewed as a system of "neuroelectrical lines" in which the motor control signals pass from the primary motor cortex to the lower motor neuron pool, activating peripheral nerves in such a way that peripheral fibers wrap around one or more muscle fibers and release acetylcholine, causing the muscle fibers to contract. Furthermore, motor execution also involves refinement of the neuromotor signal providing feedback and coordination for the movements and hence the sounds to be precisely as intended to be understood correctly. Each of the dysarthric subtypes is associated with specific locations in the nervous system and for some of the subtypes, there is a close relationship also with certain etiologies, although stroke and traumatic brain injury can be the cause of all subtypes. Also, progressive etiologies like Multiple Sclerosis, Parkinson's Disease, Amyotrophic Lateral Sclerosis, and Huntington's Chorea can cause dysarthria. Table 10.2 presents an overview of localization, etiologies, and common speech production errors in the dysarthria subtypes.

10.4 Aphasia Is a Communication Disability Due to an Acquired Impairment of Language at the Linguistic Levels of Phonology, Semantics, and Grammar

Aphasia is a communication disability due to an acquired impairment of language at the linguistic levels of phonology, semantics, and grammar. The most common symptom of aphasia is anomia i.e. word-finding difficulties (Goodglass & Wingfield, 1997). Anomia affects meaning-bearing words, such as nouns, verbs, and adjectives as mentioned in the case example above. Another indication of anomia is paraphasia, where the person unknowingly produces another word than the intended target word (e.g., chair for bed). So-called neologisms (unrecognizable wordforms or nonwords) may also occur (e.g., bibi for bed). Neologisms or word forms with phonological errors (sound substitutions) should not be confused with the articulatory distortion of word pronunciation, which is the main feature of dysarthria. In a clinical evaluation, anomia is typically assessed with picture naming tests.

The person with aphasia may also have symptoms at the level of sentence construction, such as difficulty with combining words to construct grammatical sentences. This may take the form of agrammatism, where the person is not able to combine meaning-bearing words into grammatical sentences using word order and supportive grammatical words, such as prepositions and pronouns. Paragrammatism is another such symptom, in which syntactic structure and grammatical words are present in the spoken language of the patient, but they are erroneously used. A clinically meaningful distinction can be made between so-called nonfluent and fluent speech in aphasia based on the average length of utterance produced by the person with aphasia: One to four words per utterance is defined as nonfluent

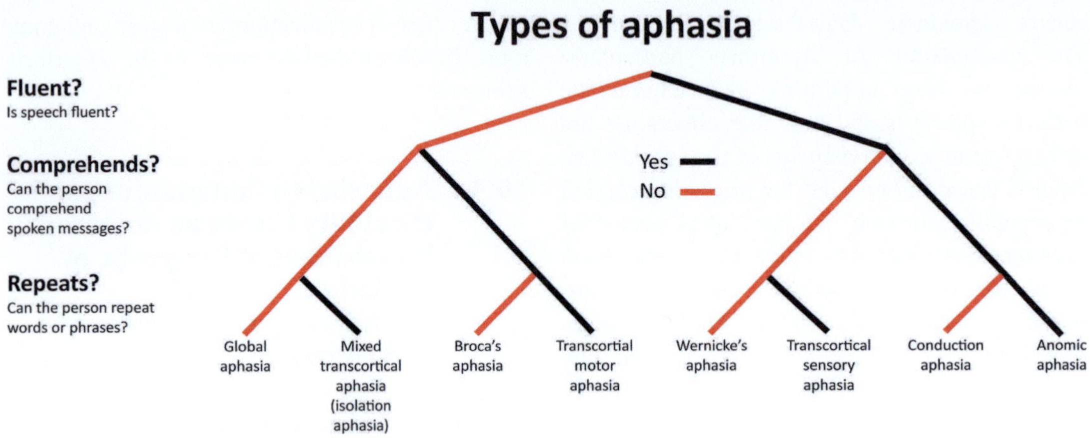

Fig. 10.2 Classical syndromes of aphasia according to the Boston School approach (reprinted with permission from National Aphasia Association)

speech, whereas five or more words define fluent speech. Other characteristics of nonfluent speech are labored, slow speech, agrammatism, and latency or failure in word retrieval. For fluent speech, other characteristics are normal or even fast speech, paragrammatism, and paraphasic errors in word retrieval. In the clinic, fluency is typically evaluated in free conversational speech or through the use of a picture description task.

Aphasia also affects other language modalities than spoken language production i.e., comprehension, reading, and writing. Assessment batteries provide subtests on all language modalities. In addition, assessments traditionally include subtests of repeating words or sentences, because preservation or loss of repetition skills was considered important in distinguishing different forms of aphasia. The most widely used classification of aphasia types is the Boston School approach, which is based on the classical nineteenth-century Wernicke-Lichtheim model attributing language processing to Broca's and Wernicke's areas and the Arcuate Fasciculus. As can be seen in Fig. 10.2, the aphasia types are differentiated from each other based on the relative preservation or loss of fluency, comprehension, and repetition skills. Whilst the aphasia types are often considered a useful shorthand for interdisciplinary communication, classifying aphasia into different types risks mislabeling the impairments and reinforcing misperceptions of the true impact of a person's stroke on their ability to communicate. Thus, classification of aphasia neither assists the clinician in setting goals or choosing relevant and effective therapy methods nor has research provided support for a type-based approach to rehabilitation.

An alternative approach to assessing aphasia is to evaluate functional communication i.e., the person's ability to convey and understand messages if aided by the use of gesture, drawing, writing, or other resources to supplement language. From a clinical perspective, a functional communication assessment is a useful starting point for therapy aiming to increase the communicative resources of the person by teaching compensatory strategies or by developing personally relevant supportive picture tools.

10.4.1 Aphasia Results from Damage to Extended Language Networks in the Brain (Localization of Aphasia)

The classifications of the Wernicke-Lichtheim model have remained in clinical use today, with clinicians across disciplines endeavoring to characterize the disruptions of language observed, using these labels to classify the presentation of aphasia. This is likely because the infarction of these neural regions is restricted by the vasculature anatomy supplying them, and therefore leads to patterns of impairment emerging depending on the vascular structures affected. However, language localization in the brain is not fully accounted for by the Wernicke-Lichtheim model. Despite patterns emerging, the extent and location of a stroke are invariably different across individuals, given that different structures may be blocked at different locations, cortical regions can receive innervation from different blood vessels, allowing blood to flow with differing degrees of efficiency. These variations likely explain some of the variability in impairments observed across individuals.

In addition, functional imaging studies have suggested that in the presence of pathology leading to aphasia, neural networks other than the language network may also contribute to language and communication. The ability to switch between thoughts and task requirements is termed "cognitive control," and is likely essential to learning, and re-learning. For example, participation in aphasia therapy requires attention to the task, the therapist, and the stimuli. It also requires the filtering of distractions including thoughts and external noises, and simultaneous monitoring for the most salient aspects of the task requirements to guide and monitor responses. Two major nonlanguage, "domain-general" networks are thought to be responsible for this task-based monitoring and action initiation. The frontal-parietal network is involved in initiating and adjusting task-relevant information (including the dorsolateral prefrontal cortex, inferior frontal cortex, and intraparietal sulcus) (Dosenbach et al., 2006); and the cingulo-opercular, or "saliency" network involved in task switching (including bilateral anterior cingulate cortex, anterior insula, and anterior prefrontal cortex) (Seeley et al., 2007). Whilst distinct from the language network, these networks have been shown to be recruited when speech and language are difficult, such as in aphasia, or during explicit language learning tasks in healthy controls (Brownsett et al., 2014). Paus (2001) suggests that the dorsal anterior cingulate region within the saliency network is engaged when deliberate behavior is required and when rehearsed actions are insufficient to guide behavior. So, whilst healthy adults may not require these domain-general networks to support their everyday communication, people with communication impairments may upregulate these networks during communicative acts that have become difficult and require effort.

10.5 Cognitive-Communication Disorders Are Communication Impairments Arising from Underlying Cognitive Disorders

Cognitive-communication disorders are caused by an acquired deficit in cognition e.g., attention, memory, executive functions, and social cognition. These cognitive functions are all involved in successful communication, and depending on how they are affected by an acquired brain injury, different symptoms of cognitive-communication disorders may occur.[2]

Frequently, symptoms of cognitive-communication disorders manifest as difficulties processing and comprehending large amounts of information or information presented in a fast pace without sufficient time for processing. Moreover, complex conversation topics or complex linguistic constructions (e.g., lexical ambiguity) may cause a lack of understanding or misunderstandings for people with cognitive-communication disorders. Disturbances in the production of discourse are also a frequent symptom presenting as challenges in the management of the conversation topic (i.e., initiating, maintaining, and shifting the topic) or as disorganized discourse with repetition of words and phrases, lack of overall cohesion, tangential discourse (i.e., digressions from the current topic), leaving out important information, and/or providing irrelevant information. Finally, in terms of social interaction, people with cognitive-communication

[2] In recent decades, there has been an emerging use of the term social communication impairments. However, as the term cognitive-communication disorders is internationally agreed upon in guidelines and practice recommendations, this term is preferred in this chapter.

disorders may be challenged in adapting their discourse to the conversational context and topic, which may include the use of inappropriate or egocentric language. Challenges understanding the mimics and emotional prosody of conversation partners as well as adhering to conversational rules of turn-taking (i.e., being either too assertive or too passive) are frequent symptoms too.

Assessment of cognitive-communication disorders is a complex process as this must integrate both formal and informal approaches to fully understand the specific communicative symptoms and their variation associated with the context in which the communication takes place. To ensure a systematic approach to assessment, it should be guided by theoretical models emphasizing the interaction between numerous neural functions in successful social interaction. One such model is the Model of cognitive-communication competence (MacDonald, 2017), which is based on the well-known International Classification of Functioning, Disability, and Health framework by the World Health Organization (Fig. 1.1). The model depicts how a complex interplay between cognitive, communicative, physical, emotional, individual, and contextual factors is required to obtain a successful cognitive-communication competence.

Accordingly, an assessment of cognitive-communication disorders must carefully investigate the neural functions of cognition and communication using formalized testing of executive functions, social cognition, attention, memory, verbal inferences, verbal reasoning, and information processing. Furthermore, the model implies an assessment of the influence of contextual factors on communication through observations of different types of discourse production such as narratives, instructions, and conversations with both close relatives and unfamiliar conversation partners. As communication style in social interaction may be highly individual even for people without an acquired brain injury, a consideration of the individual's premorbid communication competence including the sociocultural background is also imperative.

10.5.1 Cognitive Communication Disorders Are Associated with Multiple Lesion Sites (Localization of Cognitive-Communication Disorders)

As cognitive-communication disorders are caused by disturbances of a range of different cognitive functions, several lesion sites may be associated with this type of communication disorder. The many areas of the brain involved in pragmatics and communication competence make this competence highly vulnerable to changes in neural connectivity as seen for instance following diffuse axonal injuries in individuals with traumatic brain injuries (Rigon et al., 2016) or focal damage to white matter tracts central to pragmatic functions as for instance the arcuate fasciculus, which is suggested to be involved in the processing of theory of mind (the ability to understand other people's mental states) (Catani & Bambini, 2014).

This is coherent with studies associating a direct connection between damage to the prefrontal cortex with disorders in the regulation of verbal behavior, challenged comprehension of inferences and lexical ambiguity, disturbed general pragmatic knowledge, and impairment of story comprehension and narrative discourse production. In addition, spared frontotemporal white matter has been associated with intact social communication skills in people with traumatic brain injury (Rigon et al., 2016).

10.6 Speech and Language Therapy for Communication Disorders

People with communication disorders are at great risk of experiencing stigma. For example, people with dysarthria are often perceived as drunk, people with aphasia as unintelligent, and people with cognitive-communication disorders as socially inappropriate. Speech and language therapist members of the multidisciplinary team are specialized in communication disorders and in assessing and treating dysarthria, aphasia, and cognitive-communication disorders as well as addressing the psychosocial consequences of the different communication disorders.

However, all multidisciplinary team members need to communicate with people with dysarthria, aphasia, or cognitive-communication disorders in order to engage them in care and rehabilitation. Over the past decades, several communication partner training programs for staff have been developed, tested, and implemented with the purpose of training staff in supported communication with good evidence of improving communicative behavior for trained staff (Simmons-Mackie et al., 2016). Provision of supported communication for all staff members is also emphasized in clinical guidelines. When communication between multidisciplinary staff and people with communication disorders does not function well, a range of negative consequences are likely to happen (e.g., lack of health information, poorer rehabilitation outcomes, and adverse events). From a neuroplasticity perspective, supported communication holds the potential to increase the communicative participation of the patient and thereby harness the principle of "use it and improve it." However, further research across diagnoses is required to fully understand the potential of communication partner training programs.

10.6.1 Principles from Motor Learning Is Foundational to Interventions for Dysarthria

Interventions for dysarthria should be underpinned by accepted principles from motor learning (Yorkston et al., 2010). The exercises are often drills, that are carried out after instructions from a speech and language therapist, who also provides feedback. Working on modifying speech is a complex motor learning task with movements that can be characterized as both continuous and discrete and requires as many repetitions as other motor tasks. The exact guiding principles will depend on the goals of the exercises (e.g., static vs. dynamic exercises). Another guiding principle is that exercises should be task-specific and modeling what the person with dysarthria needs to learn. Mistakenly, oral motor exercises are sometimes recommended to people with dysarthria, although, no evidence for this is present (Freed, 2020). The principles of neuroplasticity described in the dysarthria literature are: "use it or lose it," "use it and improve it," and "specificity, intensity, timing, and salience matters" (see also Chap. 15).

10.6.2 Intensive Aphasia Therapy Can Improve Verbal Communication in Chronic Aphasia

The overall goal of speech and language therapy is to improve functional communication for persons with aphasia, so that they may participate in everyday life activities of their own choice. With this end goal in mind, speech and language therapists teach augmentative nonverbal communication strategies to the person with aphasia (using gestures, drawing, picture materials, and communication aids) and provide communication partner training to family members and health professionals.

A growing body of evidence demonstrates that verbal language can be improved in chronic aphasia with speech and language therapy. This has also been demonstrated in large-scale clinical trials providing intensive therapy (Breitenstein et al., 2017). For subacute aphasia, the limited research conducted to date has not been able to establish if language therapy improves function beyond the natural course of recovery after stroke. Some therapy approaches have been studied more comprehensively than others, and one example is briefly presented here: Constraint-Induced Aphasia Therapy (Pulvermüller et al., 2001) takes the form of a guided group card game with 2–5 persons with aphasia. The cards depict objects with a suitable degree of difficulty. Participants must request cards from other participants by naming an object or producing a sentence. Use of gesture or pantomime is prevented by placing a "constraint," a screen, on the table (inspired by constraint-induced movement therapy, see Box 15.2). The game is played for 2–3 hours every day for 5 days for two consecutive weeks and has been found effective in improving the functional communication of the participants. The driving principles related to neuroplasticity are thought to include the constraint on using nonverbal language, the intensity of training and shaping of responses, and the use of language for purposeful social interaction. However, a recent study suggests that better outcomes may be obtained for persons with moderate or severe aphasia by lifting the constraint on nonverbal language and integrating gesture, writing, and drawing in the card game to facilitate word retrieval (Rose et al., 2019).

10.6.3 Social Competence Can Be Improved Through Structured Group Interventions for People with Cognitive-Communication Disorders

Throughout the last decades, the evidence base for interventions aimed at cognitive-communication disorders has expanded significantly. In terms of the use of language in social interaction, interventions aim to provide the person with brain injury with social competences to participate adequately in communicative interactions. Thus, interventions may focus on enhancing the skills of social communication (e.g., starting a conversation) or using compensatory strategies to overcome the underlying challenges (e.g., bringing a list of possible topics for an upcoming conversation) (MacDonald, 2017).

Many intervention programs have been suggested, especially one that has been studied extensively in different study designs including small-scale randomized-controlled trials: the Group Interactive Structured Treatment (GIST) (Hawley & Newman, 2010). This program aims to improve social competence through structured training of the cognitive, communicative, and emotional skills underpinning this competence and incorporates both skills training and compensation techniques. The program consists of 13 group sessions and two follow-up sessions postintervention. Each session covers a certain topic (e.g., "Keeping Conversations Going and Using Feedback") through structured discussions, tasks, and real-life practice to ensure generalization. In terms of neuroplasticity, the GIST program is founded on the principles of "use it and improve it" and "repetition, salience, and intensity matters." The program has been shown to significantly improve the social competences of people with cognitive-communication disorders in chronic stages (at least 12 months postinjury). The intervention program is not originally recommended for use in acute or subacute stages since it requires the participants to have gained a certain amount of awareness of their communicative challenges.

Review Questions

- What level of spoken language production and comprehension is affected in dysarthria, aphasia, and cognitive-communication disorders, respectively?
- What is the most common symptom of aphasia?
- What approach to rehabilitation is common to dysarthria, aphasia, and cognitive-communication disorders?

References

Breitenstein, C., Grewe, T., Floel, A., Ziegler, W., Springer, L., Martus, P., et al. (2017). Intensive speech and language therapy in patients with chronic aphasia after stroke: A randomised, open-label, blinded-endpoint, controlled trial in a health-care setting. *Lancet, 389*, 1528–1538. https://doi.org/10.1016/S0140-6736(17)30067-3

Brownsett, S., Warren, J., Geranmayeh, F., Woodhead, Z., Leech, R., & Wise, R. (2014). Cognitive control and its impact on recovery from aphasic stroke. *Brain, 137*, 242–254. https://doi.org/10.1093/brain/awt289

Catani, M., & Bambini, V. (2014). A model for social communication and language evolution and development (SCALED). *Current Opinion in Neurobiology, 28*, 165–171. https://doi.org/10.1016/j.conb.2014.07.018

Dosenbach, N., Visscher, K., Palmer, E., Miezin, F., Wenger, K., Kang, H., et al. (2006). A core system for the implementation of task sets. *Neuron,*

50(5), 799–812. https://doi.org/10.1016/j.neuron.2006.04.031

Freed, D. (2020). *Motor speech disorders: Diagnosis and treatment* (3rd ed.). Plural Publishing.

Goodglass, H., & Wingfield, A. (1997). *Anomia: Neuroanatomical and cognitive correlates* (1st ed.). Elsevier Science.

Hawley, L., & Newman, J. (2010). Group interactive structured treatment (GIST): A social competence intervention for individuals with brain injury. *Brain Injury, 24*(11), 1292–1297. https://doi.org/10.3109/02699052.2010.506866

MacDonald, S. (2017). Introducing the model of cognitive-communication competence: A model to guide evidence-based communication interventions after brain injury. *Brain Injury, 31*(13–14), 1760–1780. https://doi.org/10.1080/02699052.2017.1379613

National Aphasia Association (n.d.). *Types of Aphasia*. https://aphasia.org/what-is-aphasia/

Paus, T. (2001). Primate anterior cingulate cortex: Where motor control, drive and cognition interface. *Nature Reviews Neuroscience, 2*, 417–424. https://doi.org/10.1038/35077500

Pulvermüller, F., Neininger, B., Elbert, T., Mohr, B., Rockstroh, B., Koebbel, P., et al. (2001). Constraint-induced therapy of chronic aphasia following stroke. *Stroke, 32*(7), 1621–1626. https://doi.org/10.1161/01.str.32.7.1621

Rigon, A., Voss, M., Turkstra, L., Mutlu, B., & Duff, M. (2016). Frontal and temporal structural connectivity is associated with social communication impairment following traumatic brain injury. *Journal of the International Neuropsychological Society, 22*(7), 705–716. https://doi.org/10.1017/S1355617716000539

Rose, M., Copland, D., Nickels, L., Togher, L., Meinzer, M., Rai, T., et al. (2019). Constraint-induced or multi-modal personalized aphasia rehabilitation (COMPARE): A randomized controlled trial for stroke-related chronic aphasia. *International Journal of Stroke, 14*(9), 972–976. https://doi.org/10.1177/1747493019870401

Seeley, W., Menon, V., Schatzberg, A., Keller, J., Glover, G., Kenna, H., et al. (2007). Dissociable intrinsic connectivity networks for salience processing and executive control. *The Journal of Neuroscience, 27*(9), 2349–2356. https://doi.org/10.1523/JNEUROSCI.5587-06.2007

Simmons-Mackie, N., Raymer, A., & Cherney, L. (2016). Communication partner training in aphasia: An updated systematic review. *Archives of Physical Medicine and Rehabilitation., 97*(12), 2202–2221. https://doi.org/10.1016/j.apmr.2016.03.023

Yorkston, K., Beukelman, D., & Strand, H. (2010). *Management of motor speech disorders in children and adults* (3rd ed.). Pro-ed.

Emotions

11

Jens Bo Nielsen

Abstract

Emotional expressions, proposed by Darwin in 1896 as inherited motor patterns, have since been confirmed as universal across cultures, indicating a genetic basis. These expressions, like fear, anger, joy, and sadness, facilitate social communication and bonding. Physiological responses, behavioral reactions, and conscious experiences form the basis of emotional processing, with the amygdala playing a central role in integrating these aspects.

In neurorehabilitation, emotional expressions provide insights into motor control and response to stimuli. Lesions affecting emotional control areas can result in socially inappropriate responses, but training can improve emotional regulation. Emotional experiences influence decision-making processes, mediated by connections between the ventral-medial forebrain and prefrontal cortex. Emotional decision-making, often rapid and unconscious, is vital for adaptive behaviors.

Depression commonly accompanies brain injuries, impacting rehabilitation outcomes. Early detection and treatment of depression are essential for effective rehabilitation. Challenges arise from motivational deficits in depressed individuals, emphasizing the importance of addressing mental health alongside physical recovery in neurorehabilitation.

Keywords

Emotional expressions · Emotional processing · Amygdala · Decision-making · Depression

Box 11.1 Case Story

John presented with a severe traumatic brain injury (TBI) following a motor vehicle accident, leading to reduced consciousness and heightened muscle tension in response to sensory stimuli and sudden sounds. On the Glasgow Coma Scale (Box 12.3), John scored a 6, indicating significant impairment of consciousness. An MRI revealed extensive damage to the frontal and temporal lobes, including the prefrontal cortex, crucial for emotional regulation and executive functions. The observed muscle tension was linked to impaired emotional processing. Later, John demonstrated a gradual improvement in both consciousness and emotional regulation. Over time, his responses to sensory stimuli became less pronounced, and signs of increased awareness and responsiveness began to emerge. In addition to his TBI, John faced challenges such as muscle weakness and paresis on both sides of his body, along with difficulty speaking and

(continued)

J. B. Nielsen (✉)
Department of Neuroscience, University of Copenhagen, Copenhagen, Denmark
e-mail: jbnielsen@sund.ku.dk

J. B. Nielsen et al. (eds.), *Neuroplasticity-based Neurorehabilitation*,
https://doi.org/10.1007/978-3-031-81120-3_11

Box 11.1 (continued)

swallowing. While he regained mobility and speech through physical rehabilitation and speech therapy, his emotional expression remained impaired, contributing to a sense of social awkwardness. Cognitive-behavioral therapy, counseling, and emotional expression exercises became integral components of his recovery plan. Through these interventions, he learned strategies to reconnect with his emotions and improve expression. Over time, John showed significant progress in emotional expression, overcoming social challenges, and gradually re-engaging with social activities.

11.1 Our Emotions Influence Our Movements

Charles Darwin, in 1896, was the first to propose that emotional expressions are primarily inherited motor patterns with adaptive and survival significance (Darwin, 1896 (2009)). Subsequent research has supported Darwin's idea, revealing that many emotional facial expressions, such as fear, anger, joy, sadness, and surprise, are universally recognizable across various cultures even in a primitive and simple form (Fig. 11.1). This universality is evident in very young infants, even those who are blind or deaf from birth, indicating a strong genetic component. Correct interpretation of facial expressions is of vital importance in a social group, such as in primates, where misinterpretations may be punished immediately through violence or in the long-term through social isolation. The universality of emotional behaviors goes beyond that of facial expression. Motor behaviors such as laughing and yawning are also in all likelihood socio-emotional behaviors that help communication and establishment of connections between individuals in a group.

Emotional expressions and behaviors have their evolutionary roots in fight and flight reactions with their evident survival advantages for predators and prey. They also illustrate the three fundamental reactions involved in emotional processing: (1) A physiological (or autonomous) response generated from the hypothalamus, (2) a behavioral response generated from the brain stem, and (3) an emotional experience for which the cerebral cortex is responsible.

Both fight (anger) and flight (fear) are coupled to release of adrenaline, endorphins, and activation of the sympathetic nervous system, which ensures, among a range of reactions, that the heart beats faster and the muscles receive more

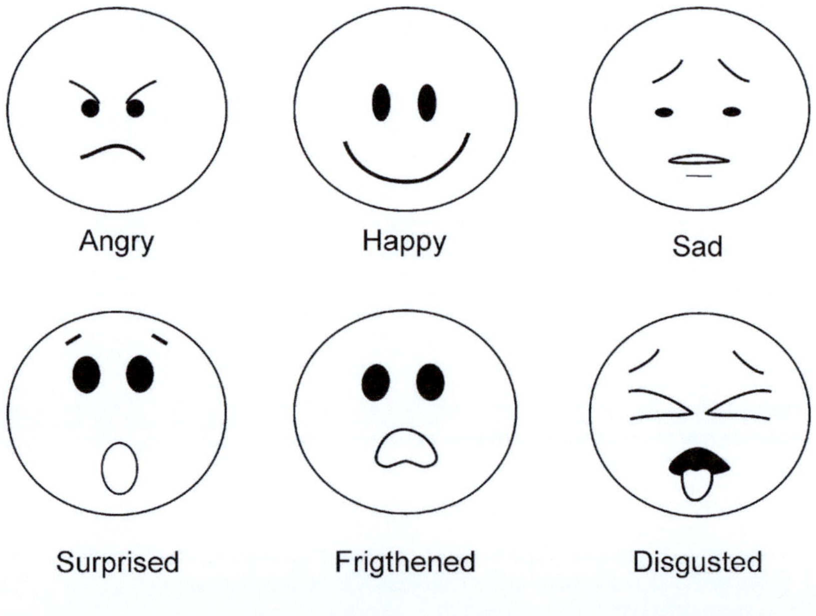

Fig. 11.1 Cartoon faces depicting different moods

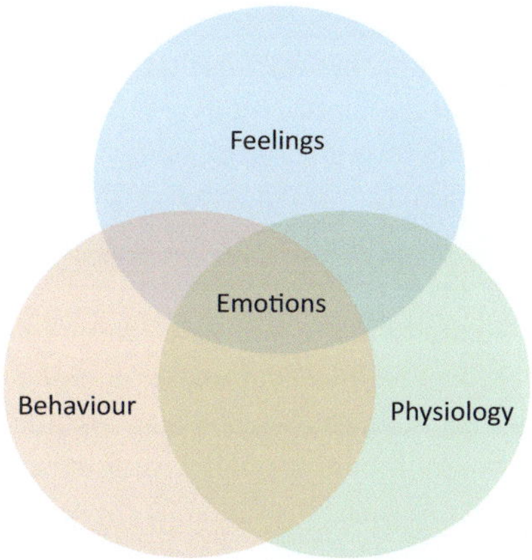

Fig. 11.2 Feelings (blue circle): Represents the subjective experience of emotion, encompassing thoughts, perceptions, and sensations associated with various emotional states. Behavior (red circle): Signifies observable actions or reactions linked to emotional states, including facial expressions, body language, and verbal responses. Physiology (green circle): Refers to the physiological changes occurring in the body during emotional arousal, such as heart rate, sweating, and hormonal fluctuations. Where the circles intersect, emotions emerge, reflecting the interplay between feelings, behavior, and physiology in shaping overall emotional experiences

blood. Ready to fight or to flee. The behavior—to fight or to flee—is triggered by nuclei in the brainstem reticular formation as described in Chap. 5. The emotion itself—or the feeling—of being angry or frightened is in many ways a secondary phenomenon to the physiological and behavioral reactions. It requires cortical processing and is often only fully realized when the fight (or flight) is over. Despite this, the feeling of being angry or afraid is often used as explanation or justification of the behavior and not the other way around. The two are mixed and under normal circumstances deliberate decisions to perform one or another behavior are heavily influenced by emotional influences from subcortical structures. Similarly, emotional reactions are typically regulated by cortical circuits, notably the prefrontal cortex, to prevent socially awkward behavior resulting from the outward expression of inner emotions. The physiological response (change of heart rate, change in blood supply, etc.), the behavior (fight or flight), and the feeling (anger or fear) are thus normally closely connected and influence each other (Fig. 11.2).

The emotional influence on movement may be revealed by comparing behavior in patients who have had specific lesions of either the descending corticospinal and/or corticobulbar pathways or the descending projections form the areas in the ventromedial forebrain around the hypothalamus, which are involved in controlling emotional reactions (Fig. 11.3). In case of lesion in one hemisphere only, some of the former patients may be unable to produce a symmetric smile when asked to do so voluntarily (when smiling to a photographer), but readily smiles with both sides of their face when told a (good) joke. In contrast, some of the latter patients may produce a symmetric smile in front of the photographers' lens, but fail to do so when told a joke later. These two types of smiles—the voluntary (fake) smile and the emotional (Duchenne) smile—are usually readily distinguished by most people and often used (consciously or subconsciously) to determine the sincerity and intentions of other people. Although many studies have pointed to contraction of small facial muscles around the eye as a signature of the emotional smile, there are probably many more subtle differences, which are picked up subconsciously through pattern recognition in the cortical visual areas achieved by years of practice and experience.

Similarly, many people can identify emotional changes in their friends or colleagues from their posture, the way they walk or drink their coffee. Small changes in speed of walking or posture may indicate the first signs of depression and the opposite changes may indicate a happy event. Courses in reading body language and body signs are common on the internet and are mostly designed to help people determine the true intent of other people (or rather their hidden emotions, i.e., telling fake, pretended movements from genuine emotional expressions). Given the significant role of social interaction in primates, especially humans, it is understandable that many individuals invest time in understanding social cues, even though they naturally excel at interpreting subtle emotional expressions from others.

Box 11.2 Anatomy

Emotional processing in the brain is often associated with the limbic system. The idea of a limbic system originates from Paul Broca, who used the term to describe several subcortical structures surrounding the hypothalamus on the border (Limbus in Latin) between the cortex and the brain stem. Among the structures that are or have been considered part of the limbic system are: hippocampus, amygdala, nucleus accumbens, hypothalamus, orbitofrontal cortex, and the parahippocampal cortex. However, it is now clear that the limbic system is not an isolated entity, that other structures are also involved in emotional processing and that the structures described as part of the limbic system have other roles (such as learning and memory) in addition to emotional processing. The limbic system is therefore rather seen as part of the larger neural network involved in visceral autonomic processing and focus has shifted to the functional role of the individual structures and areas. Chief among these is the amygdala.

The amygdala coordinates areas related to (1) the physiological expression of emotions (hypothalamus and brainstem nuclei), (2) those linked to behavioral reactions (reticular formation), and (3) those linked to unconscious (gyrus cingularis, parahippocampus) and conscious (prefrontal cortex) emotional processing (Fig. 11.4).

Electrical stimulation in the amygdala causes anxiety reactions in laboratory animals and lesions make the animals tame and disinterested in their surroundings. People with bilateral degeneration of the amygdala never learn to recognize the signs

(continued)

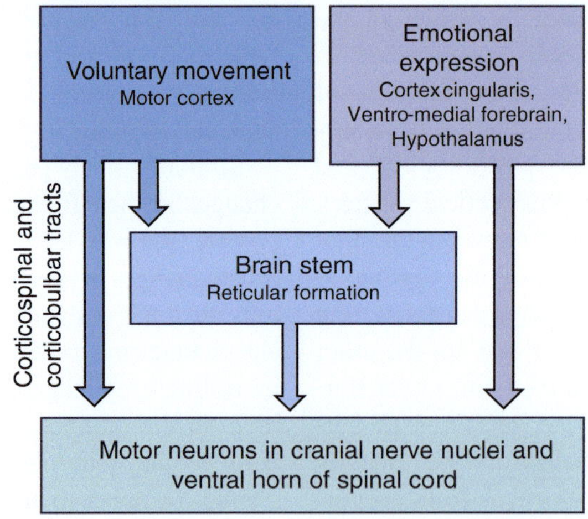

Fig. 11.3 Voluntary Movement Pathways (red Arrows): Represent neural pathways responsible for initiating and controlling voluntary movements. These pathways typically involve cortical regions, such as the primary motor cortex, supplementary motor area, and premotor cortex, which send descending signals to the spinal cord to execute planned movements. Emotional Reaction Pathways (yellow Arrows): Depict neural circuits involved in generating emotional responses. These pathways often include subcortical structures like the amygdala, hypothalamus, and brainstem nuclei, which integrate sensory input and coordinate autonomic and behavioral responses to emotional stimuli. Overlap of Pathways (Depicted in Purple): Where the pathways intersect, interactions between voluntary movements and emotional reactions occur. This overlap illustrates how emotions can influence voluntary actions and vice versa, highlighting the interconnectedness of these processes in regulating behavior and affect

Box 11.2 (continued)

that enable others to recognize, e.g., anxiety in a facial expression. On the other hand, they can easily recognize faces from, e.g., family members, even if they do not associate any emotional reaction with them. Consistently, it has also been shown that recognizing emotional facial expressions leads to activation of the amygdala. The amygdala receives information from all the sensory modalities, including the visual system (and especially the inferotemporal region where facial recognition is processed) and is connected to the hypothalamus, thus ensuring a somatic and autonomic physiological response. The amygdala is also involved in learned anxiety responses. The pairing of an otherwise neutral sound with an unpleasant experience can thus lead to the neutral sound giving rise to the physiological anxiety reaction due to plastic changes in the processing of the sound by the amygdala. The amygdala also appears to have a similar role in relation to pleasant stimulus and is thus probably of great importance, e.g., the pleasurable intake of certain foods to be quickly associated with positive emotions. Finally, the amygdala is also of great importance for memory of certain localities. If a particular place or person triggers a positive emotion, the amygdala is responsible for ensuring that the place or person is better remembered and that a laboratory animal (or a human) therefore visits that place (or person) more frequently.

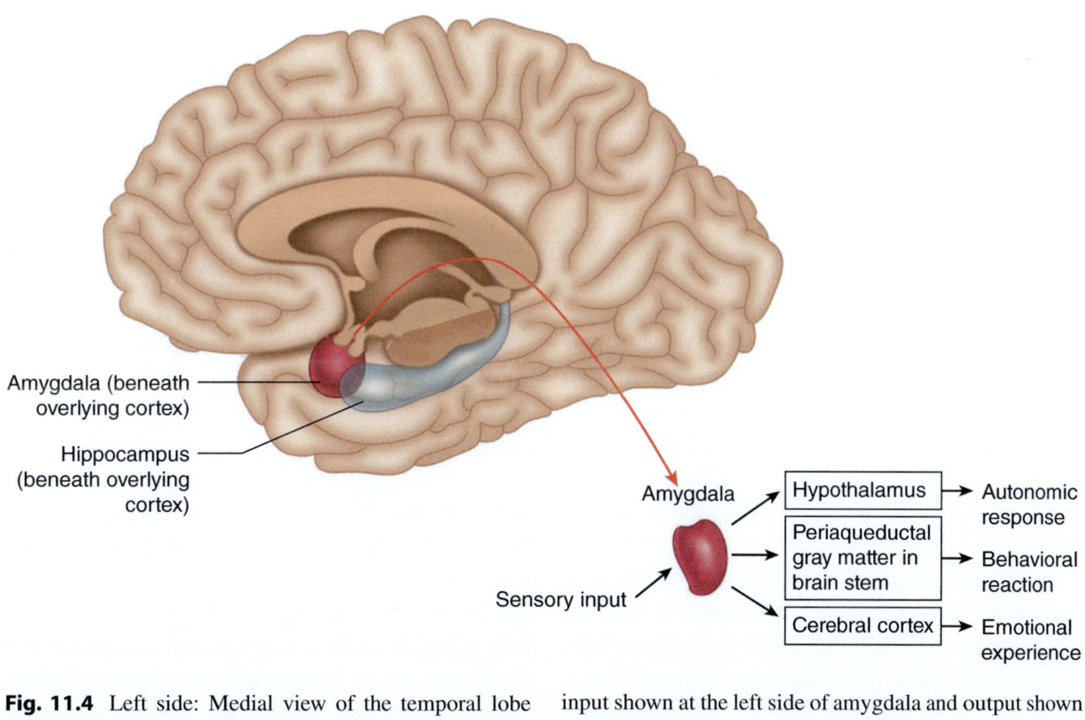

Fig. 11.4 Left side: Medial view of the temporal lobe showing the location of amygdala in relation to hippocampus. Right side: Amygdala is enlarged with sensory input shown at the left side of amygdala and output shown on the right side

11.2 Cause or Effect? The Experience of Emotion, the Behavior and the Physiological Reactions

As already mentioned, emotional experience, emotional behavior (the emotional expression), and physiological reactions are closely knit together and influence each other. During experiences of fear or anxiety, there is a notable involvement of cognitive thoughts regarding these emotions, alongside the sensation of physiological manifestations associated with fear and anxiety. Beta-blockers, which slow down the heart rate and diminish other physiological (autonomous) signs of activation of the sympathetic nervous system are efficient in diminishing the experience of fear and anxiety and are therefore frequently used in people with fear of flying or prior to examinations. Consistent with this, people with loss of peripheral sympathetic nerve fibers experience less anxiety than other people and also show less activation in the central areas of the brain involved in emotional processing (amygdala, cingular gyrus) (Critchley et al., 2001).

Behavior also influences emotional experience: It has been shown that people who engage in voluntary behaviors associated with happiness (e.g., voluntarily laughing or smiling) experience themselves becoming happier (Levenson et al., 1990). People who are asked to activate specific facial muscles designed to emulate different emotions, show autonomic (physiological) responses corresponding to the proper facial expression and report experience of the proper emotion without consciously realizing which emotion they had produced (Levenson et al., 1990).

Such findings make it obvious to consider how the interconnectedness of the three manifestations of expression can be used clinically to help people with mood disorders or movement disabilities. Certainly, engaging in fun and happy activities has its place in the treatment and care of people with depression, but it is not a substitute for anti-depressive treatment (and the other way around). Ensuring a generally happy and positive atmosphere and environment around a patient undergoing neurorehabilitation is similarly important, but also does not do the trick on its own.

11.3 Emotional Expressions Also Have Significance for Neurorehabilitation

The nuclei in the brain stem reticular formation that mediate emotional reactions project to the spinal motor neurons and interneurons and contribute to the excitability of the spinal circuitries (Chap. 5). A nervous or anxious patient usually tense up due to increased drive from the reticular nuclei and may be unable to fully relax during the neurological examination. This must be considered when evaluating the examination's outcome since the increased muscle activity may be misinterpreted as spasticity or other symptoms of pathological involuntary muscle activity. This is particularly a problem in patients with reduced consciousness or impaired communication as well as in children, in all of whom it can be difficult for the examiner to determine whether the patient cooperates sufficiently to relax. Increased muscle tension may therefore often be interpreted as spasticity in patients with reduced consciousness and communication due to brain lesion, when in fact it may be an emotional reaction to the situation or discomfort due to pain. The adequate treatment in such cases would be to remove the emotional *stimulus* (the pain) rather than the emotional *expression* (the muscle activity).

The subcortical and cortical areas and pathways involved in emotional expressions are mostly separate from those involved in voluntary movements (Fig. 11.3). As a result, patients with challenges performing voluntary movements may still show adequate emotional expressions as illustrated above in the fake and genuine (emotional) smile. This may be used as an advantage in relation to neurorehabilitation, since adequate activation of emotional reactions may facilitate and help to ease the performance of voluntary movements. Adding an emotional component to a training session and learning how to utilize that emotional component to its full extent, has the potential to increase the output from the spinal cord to the muscles and help to make voluntary movements stronger and more powerful.

People with lesions that involve the brainstem reticular formation and the areas that control them often suffer from inadequate control of emotional responses. In some cases, people laugh when they are sad and the other way around. This inadequacy can be socially disabling, but through training, it is possible to improve the voluntary control of the emotional expressions and gradually learn to either conceal the inadequate responses or ensure adequate responses to an increasing extent.

11.4 Emotional Influence on Decision Making

The connections from the ventral-medial forebrain to the prefrontal cortex are the basis for the conscious perception of emotion as feelings. The connections are also fundamental for executive functions including the ability to plan and make decisions that are socially acceptable and beneficial to the individual as part of a social group. This has been demonstrated by Antonio Damasio in his analysis of the now famous case of Phineas Cage. Phineas Cage had a brain lesion that severed the connections between the ventral-medial forebrain and the prefrontal cortex when using explosives to pave the way for the railroad across the US (Damasio et al., 1994). Within a short time, he changed personality dramatically. From being a well-organized and friendly family father and leader of a group of railroad workers, he started drinking heavily, getting into fights and soon lost both his job and family. Damasio interpreted this as an inability to make "good" decisions due to a lack of ability to apply emotional value to different decisions. The lack of initiative and social withdrawal observed in many lobotomy patients is also consistent with impaired integration of emotional processes in the executive function of the prefrontal cortex. Both human and animal studies indicate that quick and correct decision making may rely significantly on emotional (unconscious) processes. One often cited example is that of the American Quarterback who manages within a few seconds to choose a teammate to pass to before being tackled by opponents. With no time for conscious deliberation, these decisions rely on sensations from the unconscious brain centers, processing information more efficiently than conscious thought in the brief timeframe available. In well-controlled experiments, subjects, when presented with a "go" or "stop" signal shortly after initiating a movement, often make the correct choice even when unaware of the signal's nature (Leukel et al., 2012; Newell & Shanks, 2014). While they may report being unsure of the signal, their actions consistently align with the correct response, highlighting the power of unconscious decision-making processes (Leukel et al., 2012).

Box 11.3 Depression and Neurorehabilitation

One major challenge in neurorehabilitation is that depression (meeting symptoms required for a clinical diagnosis) is exceedingly common following brain injury with a reported prevalence around 30% following stroke, 20% following spinal cord injury, and 40% following traumatic brain injury. Although it is conceivable that brain injury may affect some of the molecular, cellular and/or network mechanisms that are responsible for development of major depression, it is more likely that this high prevalence is mainly explained by a psychological reaction to the sudden loss of physical and/or cognitive abilities. Humans vary in the way that they cope with life-changing events such as losing a near rela-

(continued)

Box 11.3 (continued)
tive or suffering a lesion to the nervous system. According to the current understanding of major depression, the likelihood of developing it during a lifetime depends on life events and individual genetic profiles. Chronic stress and negative experiences are preconditioning factors that increase the likelihood of a depressive state following brain injury or other events. It is important for health personnel and therapists to identify early signs of depression to ensure it is adequately treated as early in its development as possible. It is a challenge for a person with major depression to find sufficient motivation and energy to take active part in training and follow the guidelines of the therapists in daily life.

11.5 Final Remarks

In conclusion, emotional expressions and behaviors, deeply rooted in evolutionary fight and flight responses, involve a complex interplay of physiological, behavioral, and subjective components. Physiological arousal, triggered by the hypothalamus, prompts adaptive reactions like increased heart rate and muscle activity. Concurrently, behavioral responses, driven by brainstem circuits, manifest in observable actions such as fighting or fleeing. These immediate reactions intertwine with emotional experiences, primarily governed by cortical processing, which may fully materialize after the event. The relationship between these elements underscores their mutual influence, with feelings, behaviors, and physiological responses closely interacting to shape overall emotional experiences. Understanding this interconnectedness offers insights into conditions like mood disorders and movement disabilities, where profound understanding of emotional expressions may aid therapeutic interventions. Emotional expressions significantly impact decision-making processes, integrated into executive functions mediated by connections between the ventral-medial forebrain and the prefrontal cortex. The case of Phineas Gage exemplifies how disruptions in neural connections can profoundly alter personality and decision-making capacities, underscoring the pivotal role of emotions in guiding socially advantageous behaviors. Similarly, the case of John, who experienced substantial emotional and behavioral alterations after a severe traumatic brain injury (TBI), shows the interplay between neural dysfunction and emotional regulation. Advances in neuroscience and psychology continue to elucidate the mechanisms governing emotional processing and their profound implications for human behavior and well-being.

Review Questions

- What is the definition of emotions and why are these important in relation to neurorehabilitation?
- What is the function of the limbic system including amygdala?

References

Critchley, H. D., Mathias, C. J., & Dolan, R. J. (2001). Neuroanatomical basis for first- and second-order representations of bodily states. *Nature Neuroscience, 4*(2), 207–212. https://doi.org/10.1038/84048

Damasio, H., Grabowski, T., Frank, R., Galaburda, A. M., & Damasio, A. R. (1994). The return of Phineas Gage: Clues about the brain from the skull of a famous patient. *Science, 264*(5162), 1102–1105. https://doi.org/10.1126/science.8178168

Darwin, C. (1896 (2009)). *The expression of the emotions in man and animals*. Cornell University Library.

Leukel, C., Lundbye-Jensen, J., Christensen, M. S., Gollhofer, A., Nielsen, J. B., & Taube, W. (2012). Subconscious visual cues during movement execution allow correct online choice reactions. *PLoS One, 7*(9), e44496. https://doi.org/10.1371/journal.pone.0044496

Levenson, R. W., Ekman, P., & Friesen, W. V. (1990). Voluntary facial action generates emotion-specific autonomic nervous system activity. *Psychophysiology, 27*(4), 363–384. https://doi.org/10.1111/j.1469-8986.1990.tb02330.x

Newell, B. R., & Shanks, D. R. (2014). Unconscious influences on decision making: A critical review. *The Behavioral and Brain Sciences, 37*(1), 1–19. https://doi.org/10.1017/S0140525X12003214

Consciousness, Circadian Rhythms, and Sleep

12

Troels W. Kjær

Abstract

Consciousness is a state of brain function. It can be described in two or more dimensions. The two principal dimensions being level (wakefulness) and content (awareness). Healthy people are awake and aware during the day and during sleep they pass reversibly through different phases of reduced wakefulness and awareness. Many clinical conditions are associated with disorders of consciousness including traumatic brain injury, stroke, anoxia, infection, intoxication, and inflammation. The three main clinical states are coma, minimally conscious state, and vegetative state. Clinical examination is important when managing disorders of consciousness. Standardized testing schemes are used to identify the reason for the critical condition and to evaluate to which extent consciousness is affected. Instrumental tools such as brain scans and measures of brain electrical activity play an increasing role when working with disorders of consciousness both for diagnostic and prognostic purposes.

Sleep is characterized by well-defined physiological states that can be described by brain electrical activity combined with measures of muscle activity, eye movement, and heart activity among others. The presence and change between states are referred to as sleep architecture. While sleep architecture follows a general pattern in healthy subjects, that is not the case in disorders of consciousness. During coma, sleep architecture is absent, while elements of normal sleep architecture may appear in the minimal conscious state and the vegetative state.

Keywords

Consciousness · Disorders of consciousness · Arousal · Sleep · Wakefulness · Awareness

Box 12.1 Case Story

An 18-year-old man is brought to the emergency room by the rescue team. He was found unconscious, alone on the highway next to his bike. No bike helmet. He is bleeding from his mouth. He is transported on a spine board with a neck collar. The initial vital signs reported by the rescue team are stable, including pulse, blood pressure, and respiratory rate.

The ABCDEF scheme is applied (please see Box 12.2 for further explanation):

(A) Inspecting the mouth for foreign bodies that could obstruct breathing reveals that the bleeding seems to come from a tongue bite. Nothing else of notice. **(B)** An asymmetry of the thorax is noticed especially during inhalation. Suspicion of broken ribs right side of the thorax. Reduced

(continued)

T. W. Kjær (✉)
University of Aalborg, Aalborg, Denmark
e-mail: neurology@dadlnet.dk

J. B. Nielsen et al. (eds.), *Neuroplasticity-based Neurorehabilitation*,
https://doi.org/10.1007/978-3-031-81120-3_12

Box 12.1 (continued)
respiration sounds. (**C**) The patient appears pale with profuse sweating, and a heart rate of 120 bpm is recorded. The ECG shows normal results besides tachycardia. (**D**) Asymmetric pupils with slow reactions to light are noted, along with the absence of speech, vocalization, or response to pain. Muscle twitches are observed in the left arm, and the capillary blood glucose level is extremely low. (**E**) The patient's temperature is normal, but needle marks are found on the abdominal skin and after finger pricks. (**F**) The patient carries no identification papers.

Given the clinical presentation and findings, there is suspicion of a person with type 1 diabetes experiencing an insulin shock while riding his bike, possibly combined with a traumatic brain injury.

Some of the identified dysfunctions are compensated by clinical intervention, but focal neurological deficits persist. An acute MR-scan reveals intracerebral hemorrhage, and a standard Electroencephalography (EEG) indicates ongoing seizure activity.

The impairment of consciousness after normalization of the blood glucose, could be attributed to brain damage or status epilepticus; thus, both conditions are treated simultaneously. The patient is placed in an artificial coma to stabilize the critical cerebrovascular condition. Artificial coma is also known to dampen seizure activity. However, anti-seizure medication is also initiated to ensure proper management. Long-term EEG monitoring reveals cessation of seizure activity, but wake-up calls do not result in the regaining of awareness. Nonetheless, the seizure activity remains well controlled with the chosen anti-seizure medication. Polysomnography (a multiparameter study of sleep) shows the presence of sleep-wake cycles, and a thorough clinical examination suggests that the patient is in a minimally conscious state (MCS).

12.1 Definition of Consciousness

Human consciousness is inherently subjective, constituting a distinctive experience for each individual. While a person can comprehend his or her own perception of the color red, it is more difficult to fully grasp what it signifies in another person's conscious awareness. Consequently, arriving at a single, all-encompassing definition of consciousness proves challenging. Many people would concur that articulating one's conscious experience in a manner that enables another person to precisely comprehend what it feels like to be them is, indeed, an insurmountable task.

Despite the challenges in explaining consciousness, several attempts have been made to formulate practical definitions. Here are a couple of such definitions: Consciousness can be defined as that stream of thoughts which purposefully self-examines and takes others into account, over long time periods (Lemaire et al., 2022). Another descriptive definition is "Consciousness is the individual awareness of your unique thoughts, memories, feelings, sensations, and environments. Essentially, your consciousness is your awareness of yourself and the world around you." (Cherry, 2023). Both definitions emphasize the significance of a self-perspective, which is the core element that renders consciousness a personal experience. It could be likened to an inner subjective video capturing our individual awareness.

In the realm of consciousness, healthcare professionals and scientists, employ various tools and paradigms to investigate and describe this complex phenomenon. The examination encompasses behavioral observations, the study of specific brain regions' activities, and the correlation of physiological measures with conscious experiences. David Chalmers, a philosophy professor, refers to this aspect as the "easy problem." The easy problem pertains to understand the structure and functioning of dynamic systems related to consciousness. However, it falls short in explaining the fundamental reason behind the existence of an inner subjective experience, which lies at the heart of the consciousness problem. This enigma is known as the "hard problem" (Chalmers, 1995).

As of now, the hard problem remains unresolved, but there is hope that someday it may find an answer. The hard problem will be set aside in the rest of this chapter in order to focus on the easy problem of consciousness.

In traditional clinical perspectives, consciousness was often simplified into a binary concept, determining whether a person could interact or not. If a person responded appropriately, they were considered conscious, whereas if they did not, they were categorized as unconscious. This simplistic view still persists in the general public's understanding.

However, it has become evident that consciousness is far more complex than this binary model suggests. For instance, a person who is fast asleep but can be awakened through stimulation exists in a distinct state different from someone in a coma following a traumatic brain injury, who remains unresponsive due to the injury's severity.

When patients undergo anesthesia during surgery, the primary goal is to ensure they do not experience pain, remain still, maintain stable blood pressure, and have no recollection of the procedure afterward. This state induced by general anesthesia is a coma-like condition. It allows medical professionals to perform necessary operations safely. However, the situation would be quite different if the patient were merely asleep—in that case, they could wake up, move, and report pain. Thus, it is essential to recognize that sleep and anesthesia are distinct conscious states, even though a casual observer may see similarities between the two. The depth and effects of general anesthesia far exceed those of ordinary sleep, ensuring a controlled and pain-free surgical experience for the patient.

When dealing with consciousness in patients, it is necessary to go in more detail than just conscious/unconscious. There is a range of states reflecting wakefulness: awake, light sleep, REM sleep/deep sleep, pre-coma, coma, or even better a continuous scale. The best-known continuous scale depth of anesthesia is the bispectral index or BIS-spectrum (Avidan et al., 2008). The BIS-spectrum ranges from 0 to 100. This scale changed the understanding of the depth of consciousness. Anesthesiologists started to talk about a one-dimensional continuous scale of consciousness level in the 1990's (Hoffman et al., 1996).

In the second half of the twentieth century, it gradually became clear that describing consciousness by one dimension alone is inadequate. For instance, deep sleep and REM sleep are very different both subjectively and objectively but are still considered the same level of consciousness. Another clear difference is that deep sleep is a state without dreams mostly appearing in the beginning of the night. REM, however, occurs in short periods mostly toward the end of the night and is associated with vivid dreaming and functional decoupling of the motor system. Some people experience that when waking up from REM they are paralyzed for some seconds. On this background it is clear that one dimension of consciousness is simply not enough to fully describe these phenomena. Another issue is that people in vegetative state are awake but with little or no awareness. To resolve these discrepancies, a new understanding reflecting both the level and the content of consciousness was developed. Several researchers have worked with describing these two dimensions (Laureys, 2009). Consciousness is now clinically defined as a combination of level of consciousness and content of consciousness. Level of consciousness is also referred to as wakefulness and content of consciousness as awareness (Fig. 12.1).

Sometimes even the two dimensions of consciousness (level and content) are insufficient. Martial et al. has suggested a third dimension of consciousness, namely, connectedness to understand near-death experience (Martial et al., 2020). Connectedness is a reflection within the brain. When someone has a near-death experience, the brain is characterized by disconnectedness. The authors therefore argue that a novel framework distinguishing awareness, wakefulness, and connectedness is necessary to understand near-death experience.

Other researchers have focused on the interaction between the observer and the patient. For

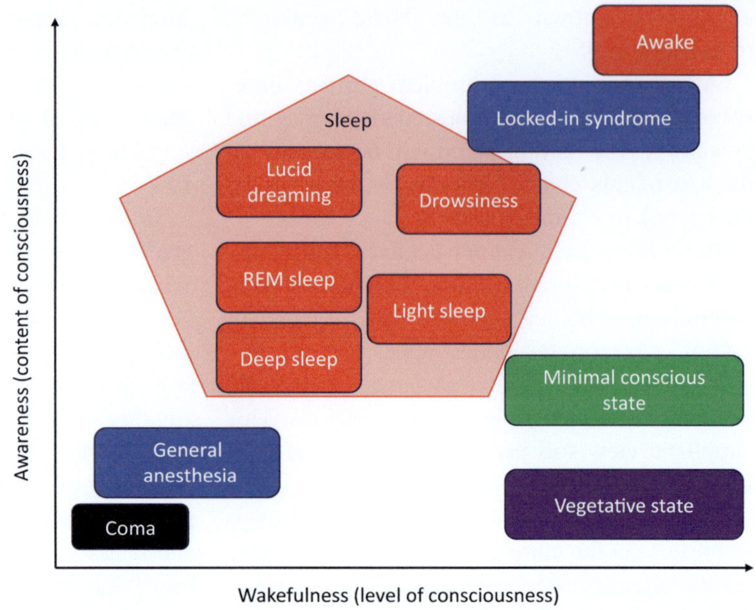

Fig. 12.1 Currently accepted definition of normal consciousness and impairment consciousness. The red states are normal consciousness when awake and asleep. The black, green, and purple states are the three main states of disorders of consciousness. The locked-in syndrome is a special case with normal level and content of consciousness, but inability to communicate

that purpose, responsiveness is important. That could be a reaction to pain, speech, or light. This is also considered as a third, but different dimension of consciousness. This chapter will focus on consciousness as a three-dimensional phenomenon of level, content, and responsiveness.

12.2 Clinical Assessment of Consciousness

When faced with a critically ill patient requiring urgent attention, it is essential to employ a systematic approach to assess various critical parameters, including consciousness, to identify and manage life-threatening conditions. Oftentimes, patients experiencing impaired consciousness are unable to effectively communicate their feelings such as fear, pain, thirst, or other concerns. The widely utilized method for this evaluation is known as ABCDEF, where each letter represents a specific aspect of bodily or social function that requires focused attention and prioritization (Box 12.2).

Often, it is unclear why a person is unconscious. It could be due to several causes including infection, trauma, or intoxication. Irrespective of cause, the ABCDEF approach is generally useful for diagnosis and monitoring of the critically ill

Box 12.2 ABCDEF Scheme

A: **Airway**. Evaluate voice and breath sounds. Inspect for foreign bodies.

B: **Breathing**. Evaluate respiratory rate, should be 12–20/min. Inspect movement of chest wall. Listen to the lungs with stethoscope and perform chest percussion. Measure oxygen saturation in the capillaries, should be 97–100%.

C: **Circulation**. Look at skin color and sweating. Measure blood pressure, systolic should preferable be 100–140 mmHg. Listen to heart sound with a stethoscope. Count pulse should be 50–100 bpm. Perform capillary refill test. Should fill in maximum 2 s. Do electrocardiography monitoring.

D: **Disability**. Evaluate consciousness with Glasgow Coma Scale (GCS) Score or Full Outline of UnResponsiveness (FOUR) score. Measure blood glucose.

E: **Exposure**. Examine skin for bleeding, skin reactions, needle marks. Measure body temperature.

F: **Family**. Identify the persons social situation.

patient. This chapter will focus on consciousness the "D" in the ABCDEF scheme.

Many scoring systems of consciousness with various focus and level details exist. Two systems are especially well known. They are the Glasgow Coma Scale (GCS) and the Full Outline of UnResponsiveness (FOUR). GCS has been used for several decades as the gold standard to objectively describe the degree of impairment of consciousness. It is composed of three parameters and the score is a number between 3 and 15 (best) (Box 12.3).

GCS has some shortcomings. It is not optimal for patients in respirator since a tube for ventilation affects the verbal response. Another problem is that it does not evaluate spontaneous breathing patterns and brainstem reflexes. These could have high value for estimating the level of consciousness (Wijdicks et al., 2005).

For these and other reasons, the FOUR score is increasingly used. The scale is a sum of four parameters and the score is a number between 0 and 16 (best) (Box 12.4).

Skilled observers in the intensive care unit have demonstrated the reproducibility of the FOUR score. This scoring system proves to be more accurate in reflecting the severity of coma compared to the GCS, resulting in a more reliable prognosis estimation. Moreover, the evaluation of brain stem reflexes through this scoring system enables the monitoring of signs of incarceration, particularly when the brain stem herniates across structures within the skull. Additionally, the systematic assessment of respiratory patterns provides a reliable estimate of the

Box 12.3 The Glasgow Coma Scale

The best eye response is

1. No eye opening
2. Eye opening to pain
3. Eye opening to sound
4. Eyes open spontaneously

The best verbal response is

1. No verbal response
2. Incomprehensible sounds
3. Inappropriate words
4. Confused
5. Orientated

The best motor response is

1. No motor response.
2. Abnormal extension to pain
3. Abnormal flexion to pain
4. Withdrawal from pain
5. Localizing pain
6. Obeys commands

Box 12.4 The FOUR Score

Eye Response

0. Eyelids remain closed with pain
1. Eyelids closed but open to pain
2. Eyelids closed but open to loud voice
3. Eyelids open but not tracking
4. Eyelids open or opened, tracking, or blinking to command

Motor Response

0. No response to pain or generalized myoclonus status
1. Extension response to pain
2. Flexion response to pain
3. Localizing to pain
4. Thumbs-up, fist, or peace sign

Brainstem Reflexes

0. Absent pupil, corneal, and cough reflex
1. Pupil and corneal reflexes absent
2. Pupil or corneal reflexes absent
3. One pupil wide and fixed
4. Pupil and corneal reflexes present

Respiration

0. Breathes at ventilator rate or apnea
1. Breathes above ventilator rate
2. Not intubated, irregular breathing
3. Not intubated, Cheyne–Stokes breathing pattern
4. Not intubated, regular breathing pattern

respiratory drive required for long-term survival.

12.3 The Clinical Presentations of Disorders of Consciousness

Based on the full clinical picture and paraclinical testing, several different states of impaired consciousness can be identified. Habitual consciousness has two main components: normal wakefulness and normal awareness. There are three main states of disorder of consciousness (DoC). They are coma, minimally conscious state, and vegetative state or unresponsive wakefulness. Each of these states has different locations in the two dimensions of wakefulness and awareness (Fig. 12.1).

Disorders of consciousness can appear based on a range of different etiologies and in patients with or without comorbidities. Various clinical conditions are associated with disorders of consciousness including traumatic brain injury, stroke, brain tumors, anoxia, infection, intoxication, and inflammation.

The neurological deficits vary from patient to patient. Additionally, the duration or chronicity plays a significant role in determining the prognosis. This wide variability in both causative factors and clinical presentations poses a considerable challenge when trying to establish standardized treatment guidelines. Each case demands careful consideration and personalized approaches to address the unique complexities of disorders of consciousness effectively.

12.3.1 Vegetative State (VS)

The vegetative state (VS) syndrome is characterized by wakefulness without awareness and responsiveness—also known as unresponsive wakefulness syndrome (UWS). It is a rare, but chronic, devastating neurological disorder based on severe dysfunction of the brain. Recent functional neuroimaging results have shown that some segments of the cortex are functioning in these patients. External stimulation. e.g., painful stimuli, will still activate the primary sensory cortex. But when this part of cortex is functionally disconnected from higher order associative sensory areas, the stimulation will not reach awareness. Studies have revealed that such disconnection plays a central role in the vegetative state syndrome (Laureys, 2005).

While there is significant disruption of the cerebral hemispheres, there is often sufficient sparing of the brain stem and diencephalon to allow sleep-wake-cycles and some autonomic and somatic reflexes. A patient in the vegetative state can maintain blood pressure, cardiac functions, and respiration, but demonstrate little or no cognitive functions.

When a vegetative state that lasts more than 1 month is considered a persistent vegetative state. In rare cases, e.g., after traumatic brain injury the persistent vegetative may improve to a minimally conscious state or even higher level of consciousness.

12.3.2 Minimally Conscious State

The minimally conscious state (MCS) is characterized by wakefulness with responsiveness and reproducible but not consistent evidence of awareness of self or surroundings. Thus, the minimally conscious state, unlike the vegetative state, is characterized by some evidence of awareness of self and/or the environment.

The minimally conscious state often fluctuates. Some patients regain limited consciousness. The shorter the duration of the minimally conscious state, the better a chance of recovery. The prognosis is better if the cause of the minimally conscious state is traumatic brain injury than if it is due to global anoxia. The minimally conscious state may be the first state after damage to the brain or it may be following coma or a vegetative state.

12.3.3 Coma

Coma is a state of both reduced level and content of consciousness. When a patient is in coma, he or she is unresponsive to the environment, e.g., there is no response to pain stimulation. The critical reflexes such as pupillary, gag, and corneal reflexes are absent. Coma may be induced with pharmaceutical compounds to stabilize patients in an emergency. It may also be due to traumatic brain injury, bleeding, anoxia, intoxication, infection, among others.

Coma can arise due to damage to various parts of the brain, including the cerebral cortex and the brain stem, leading to both depressed awareness and wakefulness. Specifically, the reticular activating system (RAS) in the brain stem is responsible for maintaining awareness in disorders of consciousness and regulating sleep cycles.

Regularly initial focal brain damage in coma is succeeded by diffuse affection of the brain due to increased intracranial pressure. Swelling, bleeding, or loss of blood supply to the brain can lead to increased intracranial pressure. This further impairs brain function by squeezing the brain stem and causing a coma.

The prognosis of coma patients depends on the underlying cause, extent of brain damage, and timely medical intervention. Coma may be a terminal condition, or it may be gradually reversible, either to complete recovery or to the persistent vegetative state or the minimally conscious state.

12.4 Diagnosis of the Acutely Ill Patients with Impairment of Consciousness

When health care providers only had access to clinical evaluation it was difficult to tell the various disorders of consciousness apart. Nowadays a range of paraclinical testing also called instrumental tools play an increasing role in intensive care units (Allyn et al., 2022).

The instrumental tools in use for assessing disorders of consciousness include electroencephalography (EEG) (Sect. 12.6), polysomnography (PSG) (Sect. 12.6.3), functional magnetic resonance imaging (fMRI) (brain activity detected by changes in blood flow and oxygenation levels), diffusion tensor imaging (DTI) (structural connections between different brain regions measured by the diffusion of water molecules), positron emission tomography (PET) (brain metabolism or receptor binding detected by positron-emitting radioactive tracers), single photon emission tomography (SPECT) (specific neurochemical processes detected by a radioactive tracer), and combined techniques (e.g., transcranial magnetic stimulation and EEG; TMS-EEG). All these methods can detect diagnostic aspects of brain function not demonstrable with behavioral assessment (Magnani et al., 2022). Furthermore, these paradigms seem to be of increasing prognostic value. It is important to keep in mind that these tools give an indication but are never diagnostic in themselves. Furthermore, different hospitals may prioritize in different ways, due to absence of certain tools, shortage of expertise, and insufficient economic resources. It is therefore considered state of the art to combine clinical examination and paraclinical testing when making a diagnosis of disorder of consciousness.

12.5 Treatment of the Acutely Ill Patients with Disorder of Consciousness

It is important to recognize most of the critical conditions in the patients within a few minutes. The gold standard is the ABCDEF scheme explained above. Once dysfunctions are identified, compensatory treatment is initiated, including respiratory support, circulatory stabilization, antibiotic, and inflammatory medication among many others. While this treatment focuses on compensating the identified dysfunctions it is also essential to perform supportive care.

Supportive care includes prevention of infections, thromboembolic disease, and pressure ulcers. It also focuses on the necessity to provide good nutrition and perform physical therapy to avoid contractures. Therapy using music and light may be useful for some patients with disorder of consciousness.

There is no specific treatment for the vegetative state. Decisions about whether to discontinue life-sustaining care is a large problem in these cases. For instance, maintaining life support for patients in a prolonged vegetative state is associated with several ethical and resource utilization issues.

Most patients in a minimally conscious state do not respond to specific treatments. However, for some patients, treatment with apomorphine, zolpidem, or amantadine has been found to lead to improvement in neurologic responsiveness during treatment. The evidence, however, is limited.

When patients with disorder of consciousness open their eyes, it is a common misunderstanding that the patient has recovered consciousness and has awakened. This is normally not the case, but rather a wish among family and caregivers, who experience a very stressful situation and look for any sign of hope. The family and caregivers also have a high prevalence of depression and posttraumatic stress disorder (Jaffa et al., 2023). Rather eye opening is a sign of structural and functional reorganization of cerebral networks (Lemaire et al., 2022).

Patients acutely ill may also experience a less severe but noticeable decrease in consciousness and experience delirium. Delirium is a clinical condition characterized by fluctuations in awareness. It is associated with altered processing of external stimuli and cognition. The cause is typically medical conditions like infection, metabolic disturbance, or other acute medical illnesses. It can also be triggered by trauma or surgery. Treatment of delirium includes perceptual shielding, pharmacological intervention, and electrical stimulation. Delirium often is reversible in a short time range of hours to days, as opposed to the much slower pace of normalization of disorders of consciousness.

12.6 The Role of EEG in Assessment of Consciousness and Sleep

Electroencephalography (EEG) is a neurophysiological method to measure the electrical activity of the brain, also known as brain waves. The brain waves especially reflect the postsynaptic activity of cortical pyramidal neurons, but due to cortical-subcortical circuits large parts of the brain affect the appearance of the EEG.

Electrodes are placed on the skull, either as several individual electrodes or in a cap system. Both methods have advantages and disadvantages. The cap cannot be used if there are recent skull defects or drains. Also prolonged use may be associated with pressure ulcer. But it is easy to use and electrodes do not get swapped. With individual electrodes, it is possible to make small adjustments of position to keep the skin intact and a reduced number of electrodes may be used. A central issue when using individual electrodes is that they may fall off or get swapped.

The EEG is characterized by some basic rhythms and may also present pathological discharges. The basic rhythms of the EEG are referred to as frequency bands, named, delta (<4 Hz), theta ([4;8 [Hz), alpha ([8;13 [Hz), beta ([13;30 [Hz), and gamma (≥30 Hz) (Fig. 12.2). There are several different setups for EEG recording, but only the standard EEG, long-term EEG monitoring, and the polysomnography (PSG) will be described here.

EEG is also the modality of choice for most brain computer interfaces. If a person can control brain waves in a given region like the motor cortices, by performing imaginary movement of the right and left hand and one foot, EEG-recordings from the active regions can be fed into a computer for interpretation (see Chap. 16). In that way EEG can tell us whether an otherwise non-communicating patient has cognitive functions and corresponding EEG activity. Based on these, EEG measures a system of simple communication from patient to surrounding. Perception of information by the patient is often auditory or visual—since especially the former is preserved in several patients.

12.6.1 Standard EEG

Typically, 21 electrodes are placed on the skull according to the 10–20 system, where four fixpoints on the skull define two axes, spanning a two-dimensional grid of electrode positions. The

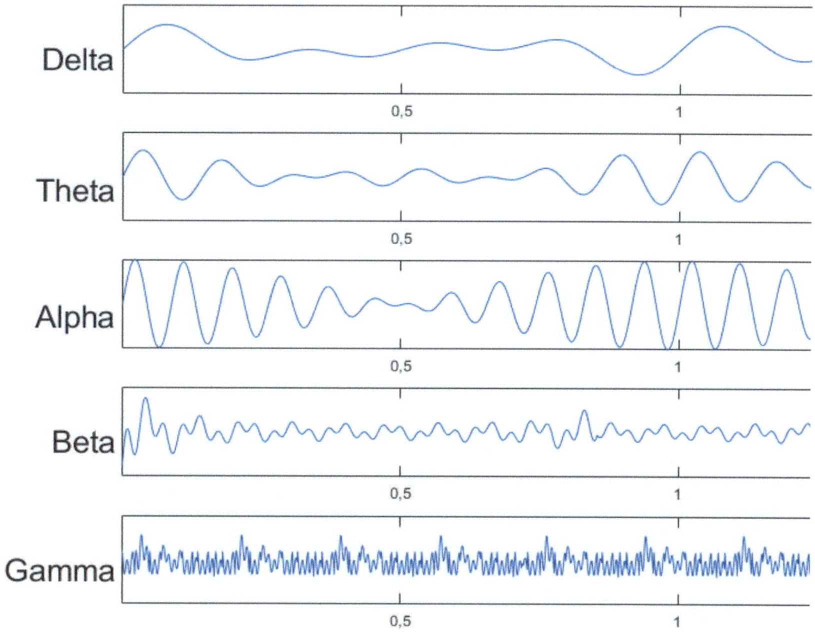

Fig. 12.2 The five frequency bands of EEG. The unit of the *x*-axis is seconds. Alpha in posterior leads is typical for an awake resting healthy person with eyes closed. Reduced level of consciousness is often associated with theta occurrence and coma with delta occurrence. Beta and gamma are seen during certain cognitive tasks. However, many other EEG findings exist. Courtesy of Christian Musaeus

anterior point is the nasion between the eyebrows and the posterior point is the inion at the protrusion on the back of the head. The lateral points are the mandibular caput just in front of the ears. All distances between the electrodes are 10% or 20% of these axes, hence the name 10–20 (Fig. 12.3). Recordings typically last 20–30 min. Patients may be sitting or lying. Spontaneous activity is the goal of a standard EEG, but provoked activity (stroboscopic light, hyperventilation, and sleep) may also be recorded.

A standard EEG is useful for getting information about the state of arousal/sleep, focal pathology and interictal epileptiform discharges. Sometimes other pathologies may be detected, e.g., seizure patterns and periodic discharges. Intermittent standard-EEG is often performed in patients with disorders of consciousness to make sure that they are not in non-convulsive status epilepticus or when it is needed to estimate arousal during muscle relaxation.

12.6.2 Long-Term EEG Monitoring

Long-term EEG monitoring is used to follow the continuous cerebral activity of patients. In the intensive care unit, it is typically used when non-convulsive status epilepticus is suspected or to estimate arousal or drug effects. Recordings typically last a few days to weeks.

Usually, the full set of 21 electrodes is used, but sometimes reduced electrode numbers are sufficient. Ultra long-term EEG monitoring with a limited number of electrodes from subcutaneously implanted EEG devices may be used over months to years.

Long-term EEG monitoring is associated with certain difficulties, like care when handling the patients, electrodes falling off, or rarely electrodes inducing pressure ulcers.

12.6.3 Polysomnography

Polysomnography (PSG) is the gold standard for sleep recording. It involves recording of EEG with a reduced number of electrodes, typically nine. Simultaneous recording of other modalities includes eyes (EOG), muscle (EMG), heart (ECG), sound, oxygen saturation, airflow, thoracic and abdominal movement using individual sensors or electrodes. PSG is rarely used in the acute phase of disorders of consciousness but

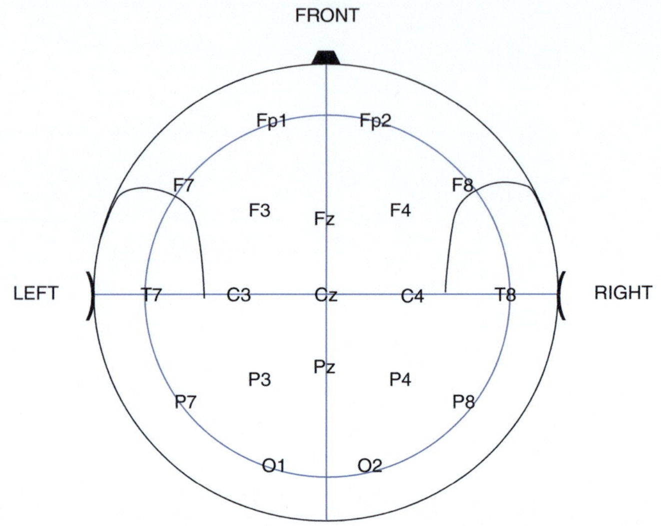

Fig. 12.3 The 10–20 system for standard placement of EEG-electrodes. The capital letters refer to prefrontal, frontal, central, temporal, parietal, and occipital regions. The letter "z" is midline, odd numbers are left of the midline, even numbers are right of the midline. Larger numbers are further from the midline. Here are 19 active electrodes, plus one reference, and one ground. Different EEG schools use different locations of reference and ground. The Fpz and Oz active electrodes are not illustrated in this figure since they are rarely used in clinical practice. Created by the author

plays an important role in the workup of associated sleep disorders.

Polysomnography can detect factors associated with dysfunction of specific neuroanatomical areas. Recognizing which impairments affect each patient is essential for accurate diagnosis, prognosis, and the selection of an appropriate treatment. When a patient exhibits reduced awareness and wakefulness, the hope for the future among their loved ones is compromised, often leading to a prevailing sense of despair. However, when there is an improvement in sleep architecture, it serves as a small ray of hope.

Polysomnography thus is an instrumental tool when estimating the sleep-wake cycles in patients with obvious disorders of consciousness. But also, when patients fluctuate in and out of coma, i.e., patients in hepatic coma, sleep assessment also plays an important role. When a patient in an apparent non-coma period starts to complain of irregular sleep or reduced sleep quality, the health care provider suspects an increase in hepatic encephalopathy associated with reduction of wakefulness and development of pre-coma or coma. When the patient is in coma and is no longer able to communicate sleep experience subjectively, PSG may serve as an objective measure of sleep status.

12.7 Circadian Rhythm

Biological rhythms play a crucial role in regulating numerous aspects of the human body's function. It is common to divide these rhythms based on periodicity into three types. If the period is shorter than 24 h, it is considered ultradian, when approximately 24 h, it is circadian, and when longer than 24 h, it is labeled infradian. These cyclic changes influence behaviors, body temperature, blood pressure, hormone levels, brain activity, and numerous other parameters.

Circadian rhythms, with a periodicity of around 24 h, are synchronized with changes in light and temperature. They encompass the sleep/wake cycle, reaction time, alertness levels, temperature variations, gastro-intestinal functions, and endocrine activities.

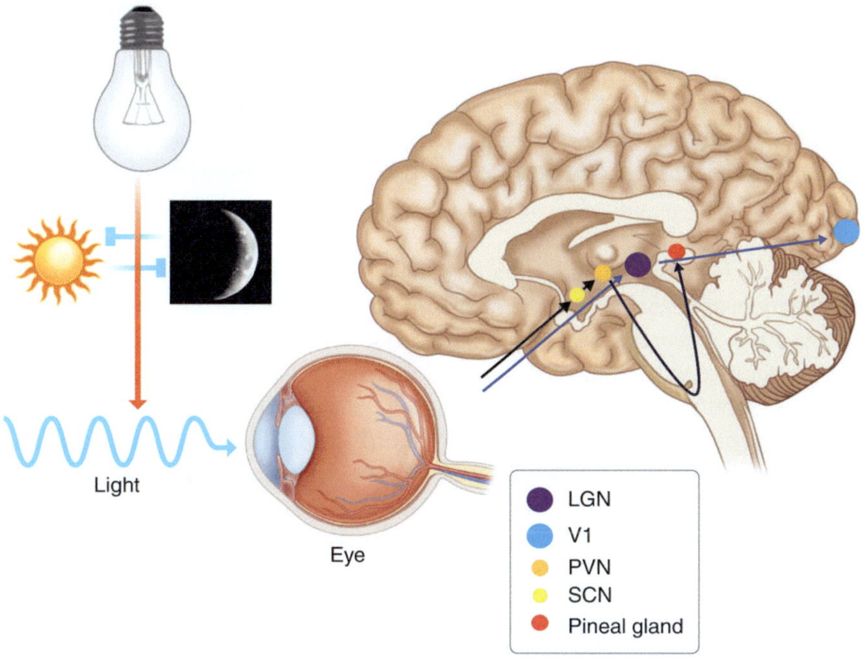

Fig. 12.4 The pathway between the suprachiasmatic nucleus (SCN) and the pineal gland is a key circuit regulating circadian rhythms, specifically controlling melatonin secretion. The SCN receives light information from the retina and sends projections to the paraventricular nucleus (PVN). The PVN projects to the intermediolateral cell column of the spinal cord, which then activates sympathetic neurons in the superior cervical ganglion. The superior cervical ganglion sends noradrenergic signals to the pineal gland, stimulating melatonin synthesis at night. Light inhibits this pathway, suppressing melatonin secretion and aligning the circadian rhythm with the external light-dark cycle

On the other hand, ultradian rhythms have shorter periods and are mainly regulated by internal factors like hormone levels. Examples of ultradian rhythms include pulse rate, blinking, appetite, arousals, and urination patterns.

Infradian rhythms, with longer periods, are typically influenced by hormonal changes and variations in light exposure. Examples of infradian rhythms include menstrual cycles and seasonal fluctuations in sleep patterns and mood.

The circadian system, consisting of a network of tissue clocks, is regulated within the suprachiasmatic nucleus (SCN) in the anterior hypothalamus (Fig. 12.4). This cluster of cells in the hypothalamus is often referred to as the "master clock." Rhythmic transcriptional pathways are regulated by molecular clock machinery, where clock genes encode proteins that induce circadian rhythms. The circadian pacemaker is directly aligned with the 24-h solar cycle through light synchronization (Khan et al., 2018). The SCN receives external cues, primarily light exposure, and processes this information to synchronize the body's internal clock with the natural day–night cycle. Through intricate interactions of genes and proteins, the SCN generates a rhythmic pattern that impacts the entire body.

Light is the primary external cue that helps synchronize the circadian rhythm. Photoreceptors in the retina of the eye respond to changes in light levels and send signals to the SCN, signaling the time of day. Exposure to natural light during the day and limited exposure to artificial light at night help maintain proper entrainment of the circadian rhythm.

In addition to light, social cues, known as "zeitgebers," also play a significant role in entraining the circadian rhythm. Mealtimes, social interactions, and daily routines can influence the body's internal clock, helping it stay aligned with the external environment.

The circadian rhythm directly influences the sleep-wake cycle. When the circadian rhythm is disrupted, such as in shift work or jet lag, it can lead to sleep disorders like insomnia or excessive sleepiness. Understanding the circadian rhythm's role in sleep regulation has paved the way for chronotherapy, a treatment approach that aligns sleep schedules with the individual's circadian preferences.

While the significance of circadian rhythms for healthy life and disease in general is well understood, much less is known when it comes to patients with disorders of consciousness. The circadian rhythm is a fundamental aspect of human physiology, governing a wide range of bodily processes and maintaining a fine balance between internal and external cues. Patients with disorders of consciousness lack many of the external cues normally entraining the circadian rhythm. It is therefore essential that health care professionals understand circadian rhythms and provide the possibility for the patient to detect daytime and nighttime to enhance sleep, restore cognitive function, and overall well-being.

12.8 Sleep

Sleep is widely acknowledged as crucial for both the brain and the body, it is a fundamental aspect of human life, essential for overall health and well-being. While it may appear as a passive state of unconsciousness, sleep is a highly complex and dynamic process, influenced by various physiological and psychological factors. The complexities of sleep and the different sleep stages will be explored below. The role of sleep in disorders of consciousness and its consequences for successful neurorehabilitation will also be touched upon.

Sleep is a naturally recurring state of reduced consciousness and physical activity, characterized by altered EEG patterns and decreased responsiveness to the environment. It is essential for cognitive functions, emotional regulation, memory consolidation, and overall physical restoration. Although the exact purpose of sleep remains a subject of ongoing research, several theories suggest that it plays a role in neural plasticity and restoration of bodily functions.

Sleep is regulated by the physiology of the sleep/wake cycle based on the circadian rhythm, and homeostatic phenomena like the sleep pressure, that builds up during wakefulness and decreases during sleep.

Many anatomically distinct areas and networks of the brain are essential to obtain sleep. The suprachiasmatic nucleus described above is in the hypothalamus and contains the master clock that receives information about light levels. The brain stem plays an important role in the transition between sleep and wake. Some cells in the brain stem are sleep promoting via inhibitory neurotransmitters, released to the hypothalamus. The basal forebrain is involved in keeping us awake. The brain stem also plays a key role in uncoupling movement for the dreams in REM sleep. The pineal gland acts on signals from the suprachiasmatic nucleus to increase production of the hormone melatonin, promoting sleep when lights are turned down (Fig. 12.4).

Sleep is not a uniform entity but rather consists of distinct stages that cycle throughout the night. These stages are broadly classified into two categories: Non-Rapid Eye Movement (NREM) sleep and Rapid Eye Movement (REM) sleep (Box 12.5).

Box 12.5 Sleep Stages

Non-Rapid Eye Movement (NREM) Sleep. The three stages of NREM sleep are referred to as N1, N2, and N3:

- N1: This is the transition phase between wakefulness and sleep often referred to as dosing. It is characterized by slow eye movements and theta brainwave activity. It is a light sleep stage, and individuals can be easily awakened during this phase. While vivid dreaming is associated with REM sleep, some people also experience more dull dream-like phenomena during N1.
- N2: In this stage, brainwave activity becomes more synchronized with occasional bursts of rapid brain activity known as sleep spindles and K-complexes. It is a deeper stage of sleep than N1, and the state in which healthy adults spend most of the night.

(continued)

Box 12.5 (continued)

- N3: Also referred to as slow-wave sleep (SWS) or delta sleep, this stage is characterized by the presence of slow, high-amplitude delta brainwaves. It is the deepest stage of NREM sleep and plays a crucial role in physical restoration and growth. It has been suggested that a specialized system, the glymphatic system, is responsible for the clearance of the potentially harmful metabolic waste of the central nervous system. Dysfunction of the glymphatic system has also been suggested to be associated with neurodegeneration like Alzheimer's disease. This system is especially active during N3 sleep (Astara et al., 2023).

Rapid Eye Movement (REM) Sleep:

- REM sleep is the stage during which most vivid dreaming occurs. It is characterized by rapid eye movements, increased brain activity resembling wakefulness, and temporary paralysis of voluntary muscles other than eye muscles to prevent acting out dreams. REM sleep is vital for cognitive processing, memory consolidation, and emotional regulation.

The sleep architecture reflects the appearance of the various sleep stages, awakenings, and arousals. Often it is possible to identify 4–5 sleep cycles. The sleep cycle typically follows this pattern: N1—N2—N3—N2—REM sleep. While this cycle repeats multiple times it is never identical from cycle to cycle, but varies during the night. Typically, N3 sleep periods become shorter during the night and REM sleep periods become longer during the night.

Insufficient sleep has profound effects on cognitive function. Cognitive processes such as attention, memory, and problem-solving are compromised when an individual consistently experiences inadequate sleep.

Sleep plays a key role for memory consolidation. Recently formed memories undergo spontaneous reactivation during sleep especially REM sleep. The spontaneous reactivation leads to enhanced neural plasticity and thus strengthening of the memories (see also Chap. 6). This reactivation process may be activated by delivering cues during sleep. Such intervention is called targeted memory reactivation and may play a role not only in memory consolidation in healthy subjects but also in rehabilitation (Antony & Schechtman, 2023). The cognitive impairment can impact daily activities, work performance, and overall quality of life.

Sleep deprivation is linked to mood disturbances, including increased irritability, anxiety, and susceptibility to stress. Chronic sleep deficiency can contribute to the development of mood disorders such as depression and exacerbate existing mental health conditions.

Prolonged sleep deprivation is associated with a heightened risk of various physical health issues, including cardiovascular diseases, obesity, diabetes, and impaired immune function. The body's ability to regulate glucose metabolism and maintain cardiovascular health is compromised without sufficient sleep.

Recent research and diagnostic guidelines have focused on the use of sleep-wake patterns and EEG in patients with disorders of consciousness (Raciti et al., 2023). The role of EEG and sleep characteristics of disorders of consciousness is controversial, but some phenomena are gaining increasing interest. Epileptiform activity such as spikes in the EEG is associated with worse outcome in disorders of consciousness. The absence of sleep spindles, K-complexes, and REM sleep is a biomarker of poor prognosis especially in patients with unresponsive wakefulness syndrome.

A predominant concept is that the regulation of sleep involves distinct processes, namely, circadian rhythmicity, and sleep homeostasis, which were traditionally considered functionally and mechanistically separate. New literature suggests that these phenomena overlap (Franken & Dijk, 2024).

It has been observed that changes in genes central to circadian rhythmicity not only impact the timing of sleep but also influence potential indicators of sleep homeostasis, such as delta activity in the EEG. It has also been demonstrated that perturbations of sleep affect the rhythmicity in the expression of core clock genes in tissues outside the master clock. Changes in the expression of many genes in response to sleep loss outlast the effects on the EEG and time spent asleep. These and other findings support the newer concept that circadian and sleep-wake-driven processes are to some degree dependent.

Although sleep and disorders of consciousness may appear similar in terms of apparent unconsciousness, they have distinct underlying mechanisms. Sleep is a natural and reversible process that serves vital functions, whereas disorders of consciousness are abnormal and potentially life-threatening conditions resulting from brain dysfunction. Nonetheless, understanding the brain's intricacies in sleep and disorders of consciousness can help researchers to get a better understanding of the human brain and its complexities, and health care providers to develop more effective tools of diagnosis and treatment of disorders of consciousness.

Review Questions

- How is consciousness defined and assessed?
- What characterizes different sleep stages?
- Why is circadian rhythm important in relation to neurorehabilitation?

References

Allyn, J., Devineau, M., Oliver, M., et al. (2022). A descriptive study of routine laboratory testing in intensive care unit in nearly 140,000 patient stays. *Scientific Reports, 12*, 21526.

Antony, J. W., & Schechtman, E. (2023). Reap while you sleep: Consolidation of memories differs by how they were sown. *Hippocampus, 33*, 922–935.

Astara, K., Pournara, C., de Natale, E. R., et al. (2023). A novel conceptual framework for the functionality of the glymphatic system. *Journal of Neurophysiology, 129*, 1228–1236.

Avidan, M. S., Zhang, L., Burnside, B. A., et al. (2008). Anesthesia awareness and the bispectral index. *The New England Journal of Medicine, 358*, 1097–1108.

Chalmers, D. (1995). Facing up to the problem of consciousness. *Journal of Consciousness Studies, 2*, 200–219.

Cherry, K. (2023). *Consciousness in psychology*. https://www.verywellmind.com/what-is-consciousness-2795922. Updated 2023-05-19. Downloaded 2023-12-29.

Franken, P., & Dijk, D. J. (2024). Sleep and circadian rhythmicity as entangled processes serving homeostasis. *Nature Reviews. Neuroscience, 25*, 43–59.

Hoffman, W. E., Zsigmond, E., & Albrecht, R. F. (1996). The bispectral index during induction of anesthesia with midazolam and propofol. *Journal of Neurosurgical Anesthesiology, 8*, 15–20.

Jaffa, M. N., Kirsch, H. L., & Creutzfeldt, C. J. (2023). Curing Coma Campaign Collaborators. Common data elements for disorders of consciousness: Recommendations from the working group on goals-of-care and family/surrogate decision-maker data. *Neurocritical Care, 39*, 600–610.

Khan, S., Nabi, G., Yao, L., et al. (2018). Health risks associated with genetic alterations in internal clock system by external factors. *International Journal of Biological Sciences, 14*, 791–798.

Laureys, S. (2005). The neural correlate of (un)awareness: Lessons from the vegetative state. *Trends in Cognitive Sciences, 9*, 556–559.

Laureys, S. (2009). Coma. In L. R. Squire (Ed.), *Encyclopedia of neuroscience* (pp. 1133–1142) https://www.sciencedirect.com/referencework/9780080450469/encyclopedia-of-neuroscience. Downloaded 2023-12-29

Lemaire, J. J., Pontier, B., Chaix, R., et al. (2022). Neural correlates of consciousness and related disorders: From phenotypic descriptors of behavioral and relative consciousness to cortico-subcortical circuitry. *Neuro-Chirurgie, 68*, 212–222.

Magnani, F. G., Barbadoro, F., Cacciatore, M., et al. (2022). The importance of instrumental assessment in disorders of consciousness: A comparison between American, European, and UK International recommendations. *Critical Care, 26*, 245.

Martial, C., Cassol, H., Laureys, S., et al. (2020). Near-death experience as a probe to explore (disconnected) consciousness. *Trends in Cognitive Sciences, 24*, 173–183.

Raciti, L., Raciti, G., Militi, D., et al. (2023). Sleep in disorders of consciousness: A brief overview on a still under investigated issue. *Brain Sciences, 13*, 275.

Wijdicks, E. F., Bamlet, W. R., Maramattom, B. V., et al. (2005). Validation of a new coma scale: The FOUR score. *Annals of Neurology, 58*, 585–593.

Part II

Neuroplasticity in Neurorehabilitation

Neuroplasticity: What Is It?

13

Jens Bo Nielsen, Jakob Lorentzen, and Rasmus Feld Frisk

Abstract

Neuroplasticity, the nervous system's ability to undergo structural and functional changes, is fundamental to the brain's adaptability. William James and Santiago Ramon y Cajal were early proponents of this concept, highlighting its role in habit formation and personality development. Research has since revealed complex mechanisms underlying neuroplasticity at molecular, cellular, and network levels. Long-term potentiation (LTP) and long-term depression (LTD) exemplify how synaptic efficiency is enhanced or diminished, demonstrating the bidirectional nature of synaptic plasticity.

Neuronal activity triggers structural modifications, such as spine formation and synaptic strengthening, influenced by recent and past experiences. Representational changes in cortical maps, as seen in somatosensory and motor cortex adaptations following sensory deprivation or amputation, further illustrate neuroplasticity. Cross-modal plasticity highlights the brain's ability to repurpose regions for alternative functions, showcasing its flexibility.

Following brain injury, functional recovery is driven by regeneration of damaged tissue and reorganization of neural connections. While the central nervous system faces challenges due to inhibitory factors and scar formation, studies on neurogenesis in the hippocampus and olfactory bulb offer therapeutic insights. Reorganization involves surviving pathways compensating for lost functions, emphasizing the brain's adaptability. Early intervention post-injury is crucial for guiding plastic changes toward recovery.

Understanding neuroplasticity mechanisms has significant implications for neurorehabilitation and regenerative medicine, potentially leading to effective interventions for brain injuries and neurodegenerative disorders, ultimately improving patient outcomes and quality of life.

Keywords

Neuroplasticity · Long-term potentiation · Synaptic plasticity · Cortical maps · Regeneration · Reorganization

Box 13.1 Case Story

Heidi, a 12-year-old girl, volunteers to participate as an able-bodied control person in a scientific study of neural mechanisms responsible for controlling hand movements. She scores high in all tests of motor abilities including fine manipulative control of finger movements using both hands. As part of the study, a structural magnetic

(continued)

J. B. Nielsen (✉) · J. Lorentzen · R. F. Frisk
Department of Neuroscience, University of Copenhagen, Copenhagen, Denmark
e-mail: jbnielsen@sund.ku.dk; jlorentzen@sund.ku.dk; frisk@sund.ku.dk

J. B. Nielsen et al. (eds.), *Neuroplasticity-based Neurorehabilitation*,
https://doi.org/10.1007/978-3-031-81120-3_13

Box 13.1 (continued)
resonance image of her brain is obtained. It reveals that she lacks the main part of the right cerebral hemisphere, including all the motor and sensory areas of the frontal and parietal lobes. Subsequent tests show that transcranial magnetic stimulation over the left primary motor cortex elicits contraction of finger muscles on both the left and the right side. Somatosensory evoked potentials elicited by stimulation of both the left and right hand are shown to have a hot spot over the somatosensory cortex of the left hemisphere. Careful motor and sensory testing reveal no deficits in motor performance or sensory perception. The girl also shows above normal IQ and scores high on all cognitive tests. It is speculated that the loss of parts of the right hemisphere is explained by a lesion early during development of the brain at a time where the surviving left hemisphere has been sufficiently plastic to take over function from the lost parts of the right hemisphere.

13.1 Neuroplasticity Is the Ability of the Nervous System to Change—Structurally and Functionally

The word plasticity is derived from the Greek word "plastikos," which in verb form (plassein) means to shape or form. It designates the ability of a solid to deform when it is affected by an external force. It is also used as a description of the brain's ability to change and adapt. The American psychologist William James (1842–1910) was probably the first to use the term plasticity in this sense when writing that "organic tissue, especially nerve tissue, seems endowed with an extraordinary degree of plasticity" and that the "phenomena of habits in living beings are due to the plasticity of the organic tissues of which their body is composed" (James, 1890 (rev. 1950)). This was echoed by the founder of modern neuroanatomy and Nobel prize winner Santiago Ramon Y Cajal (1852–1934) who wrote about the ability of young persons to develop their own unique personality that "...a young person must – in order to cope with the frothing flow of new impressions – bring to action regions of the brain that hitherto lay dormant" and that "When the plastic adaptation is completed, the organization of the brain is enriched and refined; one knows more, and one's judgment is correspondingly improved" (Ramon y Cajal, 1917 (1989)).

Research since the days of William James and Santiago Ramon Y Cayal has aimed to achieve a mechanistic understanding of this plasticity. Not surprisingly, there is no single mechanism involved. The ability of the nervous system to change and adapt—and indeed recover function following lesion sometimes, though rarely, to the same extent as the girl described in the case story in the beginning of this chapter—involves multiple interrelated changes and adaptations at molecular, cellular, and network level. Neuroplasticity is a broad concept encompassing any changes in the nervous system over time. It ranges from the downregulation of dopaminergic receptors in the brains of Parkinson's disease patients taking L-DOPA to our ability to learn and shift perspectives. The relationship between these changes at both the behavioral/functional and mechanistic/physiological levels is often unclear. Frequently, documented cellular changes lack apparent significance at the functional/behavioral level, and clear improvements in function may lack a solid mechanistic explanation.

However, for neurorehabilitation to advance, it is crucial to bridge the gap between these two ends of the spectrum. Progress in neurorehabilitation relies on bringing together the diverse aspects of neuroplasticity to create effective and impactful interventions. In the following, an overview of neuroplasticity at different levels of the nervous system is given.

13.2 Cellular Plasticity

In the middle of the nineteenth century, when William James wrote about plasticity, it had not yet been clarified that the neural tissue consists of networks of interconnected neurons and that it is changes in these neurons and their connections that are the basis of neural plasticity. This understanding only started to emerge when Santiago Ramon Y Cajal provided decisive evidence that the nervous system consists of myriads of individual neurons. Around the same time Charles Sherrington (1857–1952) noticed a delay in the transmission of signals between neurons and introduced the idea (and indeed the name) of "the synapse," but it was not until the discovery of chemical transmitters by Otto Loewi (1873–1961) and Henry Dale (1875–1968) in the 1920s and 1930s that the synapse started to achieve the central role that it has today in our understanding of not only communication between neurons, but also how this communication may change and adapt over time as a fundamental mechanism of plasticity.

The theoretical framework for the role of the synapse in plasticity, learning, and memory was developed by the Canadian psychologist, Donald Hebb (1904–1985) and made public in his 1949 book (Hebb, 1949). Based on purely theoretical considerations, he suggested that synapses are formed or increase their size when one neuron assists another in its firing and that growth and metabolic processes will be initiated when neuron A excites and makes neuron B active, so that the efficiency of neuron A in activating neuron B will be increased. It is this idea which has been trivialized in "Hebbs law": What fires together, wires together. Experimental evidence to support this theory had to await the development of new electrophysiological techniques in the 1960s and 1970s. Chief among these is the discovery of long-term potentiation (LTP). It was made originally by Terje Lømo (1935) in Oslo. He observed that the responses of hippocampal neurons to stimulation of their input from other neurons were potentiated following a train of stimuli at high rate. He observed that the responses would remain larger for hours following a single train at 30 Hz lasting only 30 s. Terje Lømo was joined by Tim Bliss (1940) and the two of them subsequently made the first detailed study of the phenomenon, which was named Long-term Potentiation (LTP). Tim Bliss continued a long series of experiments into the mechanisms underlying LTP for which he was awarded the Lundbeck Brain prize in 2016 together with Richard Morris (1948) and Graham Collingridge (1955), who have made significant contributions to the understanding of the behavioral correlates and molecular mechanisms of LTP, respectively. LTP is now well established as a model for learning and memory and is thought to reflect the physiological processes related to activity-dependent modifications of neural networks throughout the nervous system (see also Chap. 6).

The heightened effect of associating two stimuli stems from prior nerve pathway activation and increased intracellular calcium. This explains Hebb's principle: "what fires together, wires together." The molecular mechanisms involved in this effect are described in Chap. 6.

Through the use of fiber optics and advanced laser microscopes, it has become possible to visualize the individual synaptic connections. Consequently, it is possible to observe how these connections alter after being influenced, for instance, by the electrical stimulation of a nerve fiber linked to the dendrites of a specific neuron (Fujii et al., 2008). Within a brief timeframe, new spines emerge from the dendrites of the stimulated nerve cell, which receives the signal from the activated nerve fiber. Additionally, dormant synaptic connections become metabolically active, reactivating and facilitating the transfer of information between neurons. As a result, there is a continuous process of modulation in the connectivity among individual neurons, contingent upon the specific preceding activities in those connections, ranging from recent occurrences (milliseconds) to events in the more distant past (hours to days). This means that the efficiency of synapses is continually adjusted based on prior activities (experiences) within the network, and the strength of transmission across the network's connections is consequently altered in accordance with the prevailing activity pattern. Notably, these changes do not solely involve variations in the release of neurotransmitters from terminals but also include structural modifications, such as the generation of new neurotransmitters in the presynaptic neuron, the production of receptors in the postsynaptic neuron, and the formation of novel synapses, entailing the production of all essential cell components in both the presynaptic and postsynaptic neurons.

13.3 Representational Changes: Changes in Cortical Maps

Undoubtedly, alterations in synaptic strength and, potentially, the establishment of new synapses are key mechanisms underlying the plastic changes in representational maps found in all sensory modalities as well as in the motor system (see also Sects. 5.5.5 and 7.6). The pioneering research of Michael Merzenich (1942) and his team, initially conducted in monkeys, unveiled these plastic changes. They observed that neurons in the somatosensory cortex, initially responsive only to the touch of a specific finger, would quickly adapt to responding to touch from adjacent fingers following the amputation of a finger or following nerve lesion. Subsequent studies have confirmed similar adaptations in individuals with peripheral nerve damage or following amputation of an arm or leg (Chen et al., 2002). Similar plastic alterations have also been reported for the representation of muscles in the primary motor cortex as described in Chaps. 5 and 7. An example is also given in Fig. 13.1.

Multiple studies have indicated that during development, cells in the cerebral cortex receive input from various parts of the body, but many of these inputs are functionally suppressed through various inhibitory mechanisms. Through early childhood experiences and the utilization of different body parts, these inputs are selectively organized. For example, only input from a specific finger activates a particular cell in the somatosensory cerebral cortex, while input from other fingers, hand, and arm is inhibited. However, this does not imply that these suppressed inputs vanish entirely. Instead, they remain dormant and can be "reawakened" under certain conditions. Notably, GABAergic inhibition, orchestrated by local cortical interneurons, plays a pivotal role in this immediate functional reorganization. Over subsequent weeks, more structural changes occur, with inactive synaptic components gradually downregulated, and active components further upregulated through the molecular changes described earlier.

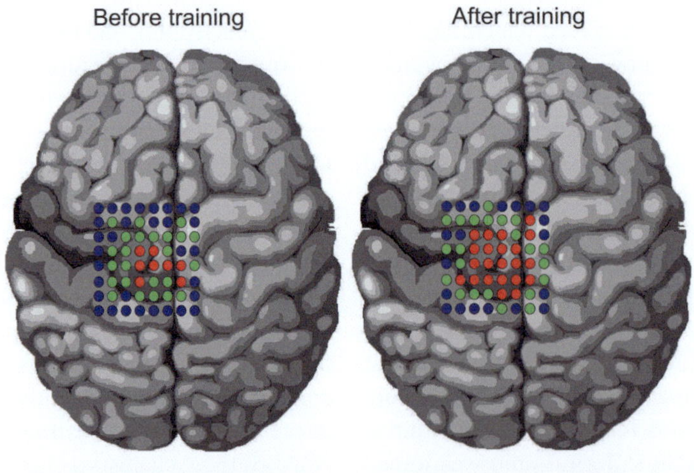

Fig. 13.1 Map of representation of the Tibialis anterior muscle in the motor cortex before and after visuo-motor training using the right foot. Transcranial magnetic stimulation (TMS) was used to elicit motor evoked potentials (MEPs) in the Tibialis anterior muscle. Stimulations were applied in a 8×8 grid around the hotspot for eliciting the MEP. A stimulation intensity of 1.1 × MEP threshold at the hotspot was used. Each circle represents a stimulation site. The color indicates the size of the MEP: Red: >100 μV; Green: 50–100 μV; Blue: <50 μV. It is observed that MEPs were larger after training

13.4 Cross-modal Plasticity

Cross-modal plasticity refers to the phenomenon where the brain exhibits adaptive changes in response to sensory deprivation or altered sensory input. In a seminal study by Mark Hallett (1943) and colleagues in 1996, it was observed that individuals blind from birth displayed activity in their visual cerebral cortex while reading Braille (Sadato et al., 1996). This contrasted with sighted individuals and those who became blind later in life, who only showed activity in the somatosensory and motor cortex associated with Braille reading.

Initially, it was believed that such significant neural changes were limited to early development, suggesting a critical period beyond which plastic changes were improbable. However, subsequent research has challenged this notion. For instance, individuals blindfolded for just 5 days demonstrated activation in the visual cerebral cortex when using their hands for tactile exploration (Merabet & Pascual-Leone, 2010). Moreover, blind individuals exhibited the ability to use the visual cerebral cortex to perceive electrical stimulations on the tongue (Ptito et al., 2005).

These adaptive changes underscore the brain's remarkable flexibility, as it possesses numerous connections that may become functionally significant under specific conditions. Rather than simply growing connections from skin receptors to the visual cerebral cortex, it appears that many nerve cells in the visual cortex receive inputs from diverse sources. Each nerve cell, on average, receives around 10,000 different inputs, highlighting the complexity of neural processing.

Contrary to the simplistic view that primary visual cortex nerve cells solely receive input from the retina, they actually receive inputs from various areas within the visual cortex, as well as from other brain regions, particularly those processing somatosensory information. Many sensory areas of the brain are not dedicated to a single modality but are multimodal, receiving inputs from multiple senses.

An illustrative example is found in nerve cells processing taste impressions on the tongue. These cells respond not only to taste but also integrate inputs from smell, vision, pressure on the tongue, palate, and sound. This multimodal integration enhances our overall sensory experience, as evidenced by imagining the altered experience of eating a tasteless, colorless, and soggy chip. Thus, cross-modal plasticity highlights the intricate interplay of sensory modalities in shaping our perception of the surrounding environment.

The contemporary understanding of the brain emphasizes its interconnected nature, refuting the notion that specific brain areas operate in isolation. Instead of perceiving the brain as a collection of independent functional modules, it is more accurate to view it as an extensive network where specialized regions serve distinct functions. These functionally identified areas can be likened to nodes within this intricate network, challenging the previous belief in isolated functional modules.

Recent evidence challenges conventional views, revealing that language function, for instance, is not confined to specific regions like Broca's and Wernicke's areas (see Chap. 10). Rather, it involves networks spanning both the left and right hemispheres of the brain. Similarly, motor control extends beyond traditionally defined motor areas, incorporating vital processing in visual and somatosensory regions.

Advanced imaging techniques, such as diffusion tensor imaging, coupled with computer models, provide a comprehensive overview of the brain's expansive and complex network (Johansen-Berg, 2013).

Surprisingly, despite the complexity of the nervous system, calculations suggest that the distance between individual nerve cells is relatively short. There are approximately six interposed links between any given nerve cell and another in the nervous system. This proximity implies that information does not need to traverse extensive distances to move from one part of the nervous system to another.

This understanding holds significant implications, suggesting that the brain can compensate for dysfunction in one part of the network. If a portion of the network is damaged and ceases to function, other regions may adapt and take over the lost function. In contrast, if specific brain areas were solely responsible for particular functions, any damage to those areas would result in the permanent loss of those functions.

13.5 Plasticity Following Lesion: What Is the Basis for Recovery of Function?

The process of functional recovery after a brain lesion can be conceptually simplified into two main mechanisms: either the damaged neural tissue undergoes re-establishment of its function, or there is a re-organization of neural connections, allowing other brain regions to compensate and take over the function previously performed by the affected area.

13.5.1 Regeneration and Repair of Damaged Tissue

The nervous system of invertebrates shows a remarkable capacity for regeneration and recovery of function following lesion. Cutting some worms in halves will result in two fully functioning worms due to regeneration from both the tail and the head end. Studies on frogs and fish have also shown a very remarkable capacity for regeneration. Peripheral nerves in vertebrates are also able to regrow and re-establish functional connectivity following lesions. Human axons in peripheral nerves may grow up to 3 cm per month and make functional connections with both muscle fibers and appropriate sensory organs at distances of tens of centimeters if sufficient time is allowed.

This is in stark contrast to axons within the central nervous system of vertebrates including humans. The longest recorded distance that a central axon has grown within the central nervous system following a lesion is about 5–8 mm. Damage to a central axon has severe consequences not only for the two parts of the neuron distal and proximal to the lesion, but also for its surroundings. Deprivation of energy supply from the cell soma triggers an active and irreversible degenerative process in the part of the axon distal to the lesion involving accumulation of intracellular calcium, activation of proteases, and cytoskeletal disassembly. This Wallerian degeneration (after Augustus Waller (1816–1870) who was the first to describe it) deprives target neurons or target tissue from their normal innervation including trophic factors and the consequence is often that the target neurons or target tissue atrophy and may even die. The proximal part of the axon is also affected by the lesion and both the axon and the neuron itself may degenerate and die (retrograde degeneration)—presumably due to lack of neurotrophic factors supplied from the target neurons and/or target tissue. Transsynaptic degenerative effects may thus propagate through a circuit in both anterograde and retrograde direction and have secondary consequences at sites remote from the primary lesion.

It has then come as a surprise that central neurons and their axons may regenerate quite well if provided with the appropriate environment. Grafts of peripheral nerves have thus been shown to create a medium that central axons proximal to a spinal cord lesion may grow in to and thereby bridge several centimeter wide lesion to reach the distal stump of the spinal cord. Mature central axons also readily grow into grafts of the immature nervous system and neural stem cells and may grow over very long distances. Numerous studies have now identified a range of neurite outgrowth promoting factors in these tissues, such as neurotrophins and cell adhesion molecules (which are components of the Schwann cell basal lamina). These attract and promote the growth of central and peripheral axons but are not present to any large extent in the mature central nervous system. In addition, studies have shown that the mature nervous system in contrast is rich in growth inhibiting factors, some of which are derived from myelin. Since there are many of these neurite-growth inhibiting factors, blocking or abolishing any of them has failed to facilitate axonal regeneration, but trials to interfere with a shared pathway for their production are under way. In addition to these growth inhibiting factors that are intrinsic to the nervous system, a lesion to the nervous system also activates astrocytes that generate scar tissue to limit the size of the injury. The scar tissue not only establishes a mechanical barrier for axonal growth but also liberates several growth inhibiting factors such as Chondroitin sulfate proteoglycans (CSPG). Pharmacological suppression of scar tissue (prednisolon) or CSPG has been shown to promote axonal regeneration and in animals to facilitate functional recovery following lesion.

13.5.2 Neurogenesis: Does It Play a Role?

If injury and degeneration lead to death of neurons, these will need to be replaced unless other neurons and networks can take over their function. For a long time, it was believed that the mature human nervous system lacked the potential to generate new neurons (neurogenesis). Since the 1960s, strong evidence has been accumulated to show that new neurons continue to be born in (at least) two areas of the brain: the dentate gyrus of the hippocampus and in the olfactory bulb. In both areas, the neurons mature and become integrated into the neural circuitry, where they play important functional roles for memory and olfaction, respectively (see Box 13.2). There is still no consensus about the possibility of neurogenesis occurring in other areas of the nervous system and there is no evidence that neurogenesis plays a role in repairing lesions or in the functional recovery following brain injury. However, the discovery of neurogenesis and hence active neural stem cells in the adult brain has led to significant interest in harvesting stem cells with the goal of transplantation and/or production of sufficiently large number of neurons to replace those lost through lesion. Transplantation of olfactory glial stem cells, olfactory ensheathing cells (OEC), has shown great potential for promoting regeneration and functional recovery in animal models of spinal cord injury. OECs have the advantage that they can be harvested from the olfactory epithelium of the patient and thereby circumvent any issues regarding tissue incompatibility. However, clinical trials have so far not produced convincing results in humans.

Box 13.2 Evidence of Human Neurogenesis Is Provided by Nuclear Bomb Testing

When cells divide, they incorporate carbon from the environment and some of that carbon comes from the atmosphere. Between 1955 and 1963, there was a significant surge in the atmospheric Carbon-14 content caused by nuclear bomb testing. However, since then, it has reverted to its stable pre-testing level. As a result, it is now feasible to ascertain whether cells or neurons were formed during an individual's adulthood by comparing the concentration of Carbon-14 in them with the individual's age.

A post-mortem examination of the brains of 120 individuals unveiled that only neurons in the hippocampus exhibited Carbon-14 levels that aligned with their generation during the individual's adulthood. It was also possible to determine that around 700 neurons were born every day in the individual. This means that almost one-third of the cells in the hippocampus may be replaced by new neurons during a lifetime.

13.5.3 Re-organization Following Injury: Can Other Surviving Pathways or Areas Take Over Function?

The idea that undamaged areas or surviving pathways may take over function from damaged areas and pathways is not new but was proposed already in the eighteenth century and demonstrated experimentally by Marie Jean Pierre Flourens (1794–1867) in a series of lesion experiments in rabbits and pigeons. He observed that functions, which disappeared following small lesions of the brain, would re-appear after some time. Flourens interpreted his findings as evidence that functions cannot be localized in the brain. This was proved wrong soon afterwards by a series of observations in human subjects, most importantly Pierre Paul Brocas (1824–1880) observation of loss of language function following lesion of what is now called Brocas language area in the frontal part of the left hemisphere (Broca, 1861). Flourens' findings have therefore been ignored for a long time but have recently been "re-discovered" and re-interpreted as one of the first descriptions of plasticity and re-organization of function in the brain. It has also been largely forgotten that Broca reported a case of re-appearance of language function in a child following lesion in the left hemisphere and suggested that the right hemisphere had the ability to take over language function at least in children (Broca, 1861). As discussed further in the next chapter, the brain of children up to the age of around 10 years may show an extraordinary ability for re-organization. However, there is abundant evidence that re-organization also occurs in the adult brain although to a much more limited extent than appears to be possible in children (see Box 13.3).

It is well documented that injuries to the corticospinal tract or the motor cortex are accompanied by re-organization of the somatotopic

Box 13.3 Age-Dependent Neuroplasticity

Understanding age-dependent neuroplasticity is essential for tailoring neurorehabilitation interventions to the specific needs and capabilities of individuals across different age groups. Rehabilitation programs should consider factors such as developmental stage, cognitive reserve, and age-related changes in brain structure and function.

Early childhood is characterized by rapid and extensive neuroplasticity as the brain undergoes critical periods of development (see Chap. 14). During these sensitive periods, the brain is highly adaptable and responsive to environmental input, allowing for the establishment of neural circuits underlying sensory, motor, cognitive, and socio-emotional functions. Early identification and intervention for developmental disorders or neurological injuries can maximize neuroplasticity and functional outcomes.

While neuroplasticity in adulthood is more limited compared to childhood, the adult brain retains the capacity for structural and functional reorganization in response to learning, environmental changes, and rehabilitation interventions. As one example, structural changes have been documented in the hippocampi of taxi drivers in London regardless of their age. Navigation through the maze of streets in London is considered one of the most challenging memory tasks, and the continued learning and memory processes required to be able to find the most efficient way from point A to point B apparently leads to pronounced growth of parts of the hippocampi judged from MRI scans.

Neuroplasticity in adulthood primarily involves synaptic plasticity, such as long-term potentiation (LTP) and long-term depression (LTD), which underlie learning and memory processes.

Factors such as cognitive engagement, physical activity, and social interaction can promote neuroplasticity and cognitive resilience in adulthood. While the extent of neuroplasticity may decline with age, older adults can still benefit from such interventions and maintain cognitive function. Adaptive plasticity mechanisms, such as compensatory recruitment of alternative brain regions or neural circuits, may also contribute to functional preservation and cognitive reserve in older adults.

Aging is associated with structural and functional changes in the brain, including

(continued)

Box 13.3 (continued)

synaptic loss, reduced neurogenesis, and alterations in neurotransmitter systems. However, research suggests that the aging brain remains capable of specific forms of neuroplasticity such as synaptic plasticity and functional reorganization.

Normal aging brings about morphological and biophysical changes in neurons, including reduced dendritic branching and dysregulated calcium homeostasis, along with alterations in synaptic density in crucial regions like the hippocampus and prefrontal cortex (PFC). These regions are not only vital for learning, memory, and executive functions, but undergo age-related shifts in gene expression and protein synthesis. Such changes potentially influence cognitive abilities. Older adults often engage additional brain structures during cognitive and motor tasks, observed via BOLD fMRI, possibly compensating for these changes. Motor tasks require more cognitive resources for older individuals. This is particularly the case after brain injuries. Performance disparities between age groups are most pronounced in complex tasks like dual tasks, where cognitive demands intensify. This heightened cognitive demand for motor tasks in older adults, coupled with diminished resources, may contribute to issues like falls, especially when navigating challenging environments. Studies have linked motor function performance with gray matter volume, white matter integrity, and biochemical alterations in neurotransmitter systems like dopamine, serotonin, acetylcholine, and noradrenaline in the aging brain. These correlations underscore the relation between neural structure, function, and biochemistry in the context of aging and motor performance.

organization of the motor cortex (Chen et al., 2002). This is most strikingly illustrated by complete lesions of the spinal cord, where the cortical areas representing muscles distal to the lesion are quickly re-organized to represent muscles proximal to the lesion. In such cases, the re-organization naturally has no functional consequence for the control of the muscles distal to the lesion, which remain paralyzed. However, in relation to partial lesions following spinal cord injury or stroke, it has been demonstrated that the re-organization in the representational map is closely related to functional improvements. Importantly, therapeutic strategies may facilitate and direct changes in the representational maps closely associated with the functional improvements. Animal experiments have documented that the changes in representational maps and the functional recovery observed following lesions to the corticospinal tract are related to sprouting of collaterals from surviving corticospinal tract fibers, which re-innervate synaptic sites/spines on motor neurons and interneurons in the spinal cord made vacant by the loss of injured fibers. In parallel with this, synaptic connections in the local cortical circuitry are also re-organized through downregulation of inhibitory connections to surviving neighboring corticospinal neurons, sprouting and establishment of new synaptic connections and other regulatory mechanisms. Such "spontaneous" re-organization following lesion is not necessarily of functional benefit but may lead to establishment of connections that prevent a more beneficial re-organization later. This has been used as one argument in favor of intervention early after lesion to drive the plastic changes in a functionally beneficial direction (Nudo, 2003).

This is also evidence that other areas outside the primary motor cortex may take over function following stroke. Convincing evidence has been presented that the premotor cortex may take over functional control of muscle activity from the primary motor cortex following stroke.

Significantly larger bilateral activity is observed in the premotor cortex of stroke survivors during relatively simple movements than in intact control subjects and inactivation of the premotor cortex by repetitive TMS may interfere with the movement in the stroke survivors but not in the intact individuals (Grefkes & Ward, 2014). This observation is not too surprising since the premotor cortex contributes significantly to the corticospinal tract and cortical and spinal re-organization allowing surviving corticospinal neurons in the premotor cortex to take over function from lesioned corticospinal neurons from the primary motor cortex, and is well in line with observations in animals. Although the functional significance of ipsilateral corticospinal connections (the ventral corticospinal tract) is still under some debate, there is good evidence to suggest upregulation of these connections following lesions involving the contralateral motor cortex. Also in this case, early intervention following lesion appears of importance to guide the plastic changes in a functionally beneficial direction.

Similar re-organization following lesions have been documented for the various sensory modalities and areas, and should be seen as a universal, spontaneous response to an injury. However, whether the re-organization is functionally beneficial, or the opposite depends on whether it is driven by appropriate activity. Similar to what is observed during development (see next chapter), the re-organization following lesion is activity-driven and may be directed and shaped through environmental stimuli. The period following a lesion is in its essence an opening of a critical period, where appropriate motor and/or sensory stimuli are necessary to ensure correct (re-)establishment of neural connections. In clinical practice, there are many other factors that have to be taken into account, which may prevent or argue against early intervention following lesion, but when it comes to harvesting the plastic potential created by this opening of a critical period following lesion, there is no doubt that early is always better.

Box 13.4 Why Is There Limited Regenerative Capacity in the Mature Vertebrate Central Nervous System?

The mature vertebrate central nervous system exhibits a remarkable contrast to other animals, as it lacks the ability for regenerative processes and neurogenesis. In contrast, in various animals, the developing nervous system of vertebrates and the peripheral nervous system, demonstrate significant regenerative capabilities. The question arises: what sets the adult vertebrate central nervous system apart in this regard?

Although speculative, it is reasonable to suggest that this lack of regenerative capacity may be linked to the need for maintaining stable fundamental connectivity, ensuring long-term memory functions, and fostering superior intellectual capacity in vertebrates. During critical periods of development, neural circuitries are pruned and re-organized in response to environmental influences. Consequently, some degree of stability might be necessary to retain these experiences ingrained in the neural circuitry.

Moreover, one may ponder whether a consistent sense of self, experienced every morning upon waking up, would persist if our nervous system retained the same level of plasticity found in the immature nervous system. The loss of regenerative capacity and vulnerability to lesions could potentially be the price paid to attain consciousness.

In essence, the absence of regenerative abilities in the mature vertebrate central nervous system might be intertwined with the imperative of maintaining stable neural connections to support cognition and memory functions effectively. Although conjectural, it is plausible that this trade-off of regenerative potential contributes to our conscious experiences and sense of self.

Review Questions

- What is neuroplasticity?
- What are the molecular and cellular basis of neuroplasticity?
- Why is neuroplasticity important for learning?

References

Broca, P. (1861). Sur le principe des localisations cérébrales. *Bulletin de la Société d'Anthropologie, 2*, 190–204.

Chen, R., Cohen, L. G., & Hallett, M. (2002). Nervous system reorganization following injury. *Neuroscience, 111*(4), 761–773. https://doi.org/10.1016/s0306-4522(02)00025-8

Fujii, R., Ichikawa, M., & Ozaki, M. (2008). Imaging of molecular dynamics regulated by electrical activities in neural circuits and in synapses. *Neurosignals, 16*(4), 260–277. https://doi.org/10.1159/000123037

Grefkes, C., & Ward, N. S. (2014). Cortical reorganization after stroke: How much and how functional? *The Neuroscientist, 20*(1), 56–70. https://doi.org/10.1177/1073858413491147

Hebb, D. O. (1949). *The organization of behavior*. John Wiley and Sons Inc..

James, W. (1890 (rev. 1950)). *The principles of psychology*. Dover publications.

Johansen-Berg, H. (2013). Human connectomics—What will the future demand? *NeuroImage, 80*, 541–544. https://doi.org/10.1016/j.neuroimage.2013.05.082

Merabet, L. B., & Pascual-Leone, A. (2010). Neural reorganization following sensory loss: The opportunity of change. *Nature Reviews. Neuroscience, 11*(1), 44–52. https://doi.org/10.1038/nrn2758

Nudo, R. J. (2003). Functional and structural plasticity in motor cortex: implications for stroke recovery. *Physical Medicine and Rehabilitation Clinics of North America, 14*(Suppl. 1), S57–S76. https://doi.org/10.1016/s1047-9651(02)00054-2

Ptito, M., Moesgaard, S. M., Gjedde, A., & Kupers, R. (2005). Cross-modal plasticity revealed by electrotactile stimulation of the tongue in the congenitally blind. *Brain, 128*(Pt 3), 606–614. https://doi.org/10.1093/brain/awh380

Ramon y Cajal, S. (1917 (1989)). *Recollections of my life*. : MIT Press.

Sadato, N., Pascual-Leone, A., Grafman, J., Ibanez, V., Deiber, M. P., Dold, G., & Hallett, M. (1996). Activation of the primary visual cortex by Braille reading in blind subjects. *Nature, 380*(6574), 526–528. https://doi.org/10.1038/380526a0

14 Neurodevelopment and Neuroplasticity

Jens Bo Nielsen and Andrea Guzzetta

Abstract

This chapter will describe the development of the nervous system from the first neurons occurring around 17 days after conception until the end of puberty. The interaction between signaling factors in the environment, cell receptors, and transcription factors in the regulation of cell proliferation, cell differentiation, cell survival, and in the establishment of connections between neurons prior to birth will be described. It will be emphasized how functional connectivity in the nervous system develops through pruning mechanisms where only neurons and neuronal pathways which establish functionally effective connections with each other survive. This competitive regulation of connectivity ("survival-of-the-fittest connection") is the basis of the ability of the immature brain to generate functional neural networks despite significant lesions early during development. The significance of environmental stimuli for optimal neurodevelopment during critical periods after birth and for efficient early interventions aiming to facilitate neurodevelopment will be discussed. The continued cognitive and motor development of children will be presented. The neuroplastic potential of the nervous system at different ages will be evaluated, and the challenges and possibilities that lesions at each of the developmental stages poses will be discussed.

Keywords

Neural development · Activity-dependent re-organization · Age-related neuroplasticity · Interaction between genes and environment

J. B. Nielsen (✉)
Department of Neuroscience, University of Copenhagen, Copenhagen, Denmark

Elsass Fonden, Charlottenlund, Denmark
e-mail: jbnielsen@sund.ku.dk

A. Guzzetta
University of Pisa, Fondazione Stella Maris, Pisa, Italy
e-mail: andrea.guzzetta@fsm.unipi.it

Box 14.1 Case Story

Jamie, a one-year-old boy, lives with his parents in a suburban neighborhood. Genetic testing, soon after birth revealed that he had hereditary spastic paraparesis (HSP), a condition causing progressive muscle stiffness and weakness in the lower limbs.

As Jamie grew older, it became apparent that he was failing to meet important motor milestones typical for his age, such as sitting up unaided and crawling.

Concerned, Jamie's parents sought guidance from healthcare professionals and began interventions such as physical therapy and assistive devices. Despite these efforts, Jamie continued to struggle with motor skills development, highlighting the challenges posed by his condition.

(continued)

J. B. Nielsen et al. (eds.), *Neuroplasticity-based Neurorehabilitation*,
https://doi.org/10.1007/978-3-031-81120-3_14

Box 14.1 (continued)

As Jamie approached his first birthday, his parents noticed small improvements in his mobility and motor skills, thanks to early interventions and ongoing support from medical specialists. They remained hopeful for Jamie's future, committed to providing him with the love, support, and resources he needed to thrive despite the challenges he faced.

14.1 Introduction

Development of the nervous system begins around day 17 after conception with specialization of groups of cells in the fetus into neurons. Within the next 8.5 months around 100,000,000,000 neurons are created (sometimes at a rate of 4200/s) and the full macroscopic outline of the nervous system is established at birth. However, the total number of connections in the brain continues to increase until around 18–24 months after birth and re-organization of these connections (neuroplasticity) in relation to learning and memory continues for the rest of our lives. The accelerated maturation of the nervous system during prenatal and early infancy stages gives rise to unique conditions that hold significance for nervous system injuries and our ability to enhance functional development and promote reorganization of neural function. This chapter will describe these unique conditions.

14.2 Prenatal Neurodevelopment

The nervous system develops around day 17 in the form of a cell layer known as the neural plate (Fig. 14.1). The neural plate soon folds to form the neural tube. The distal part of the neural tube gives rise to the spinal cord and the rostral region becomes the brain. Some cells migrate actively towards the sides and establish connections with the peripheral sensory organs of the skin, joints, and muscles. Failure of closure in the upper portion results in impaired brain development, leading to anencephaly, while incomplete closure in the lower part gives rise to spina bifida. Pregnant women often take folic acid supplements to prevent these types of birth defects associated with a deficiency of folic acid.

The subsequent development of the nervous system involves parallel proliferation, migration, and differentiation of neurons to populate the different areas and structures of the nervous system and then establish connections between them and with the surrounding tissues. Induction from the surrounding environment, along with the predetermined presence of receptors on the surface of the neurons, plays a critical role in this process.

The specialization of regions along the neuraxis is determined by gradients of secretion of different factors from the surrounding tissue. In addition to this, HOX genes play an important role (Fig. 14.2). The HOX genes are a family of genes that encode transcription factors responsible for the sequential activation of an entire cascade of genes important for the development of various body parts—not just the nervous system, but everything from arms and legs to eyes. If the wrong HOX genes are activated in the wrong place, it will result in malformations such as cleft palate, major malformations in the brain, or in the development of the extremities.

The simple division of the nervous system into motor and sensory functions, which is most evident in the spinal cord, is also determined by the interaction of secreted proteins from the surroundings and receptors and transcription factors in the local neurons (Fig. 14.3).

The neurotransmitters that the neurons use are determined by the transcriptional program that gives each neuronal type its characteristics (i.e., the factors described above). However, the electrical activity and various humoral factors may also lead to changes in neurotransmitter production.

During development, over 50% of neurons undergo cell death before the nervous system reaches full maturation. This process is driven by competition among neurons for a limited supply of neurotrophic factors. Each neuron possesses an inherent genetic cell death program called

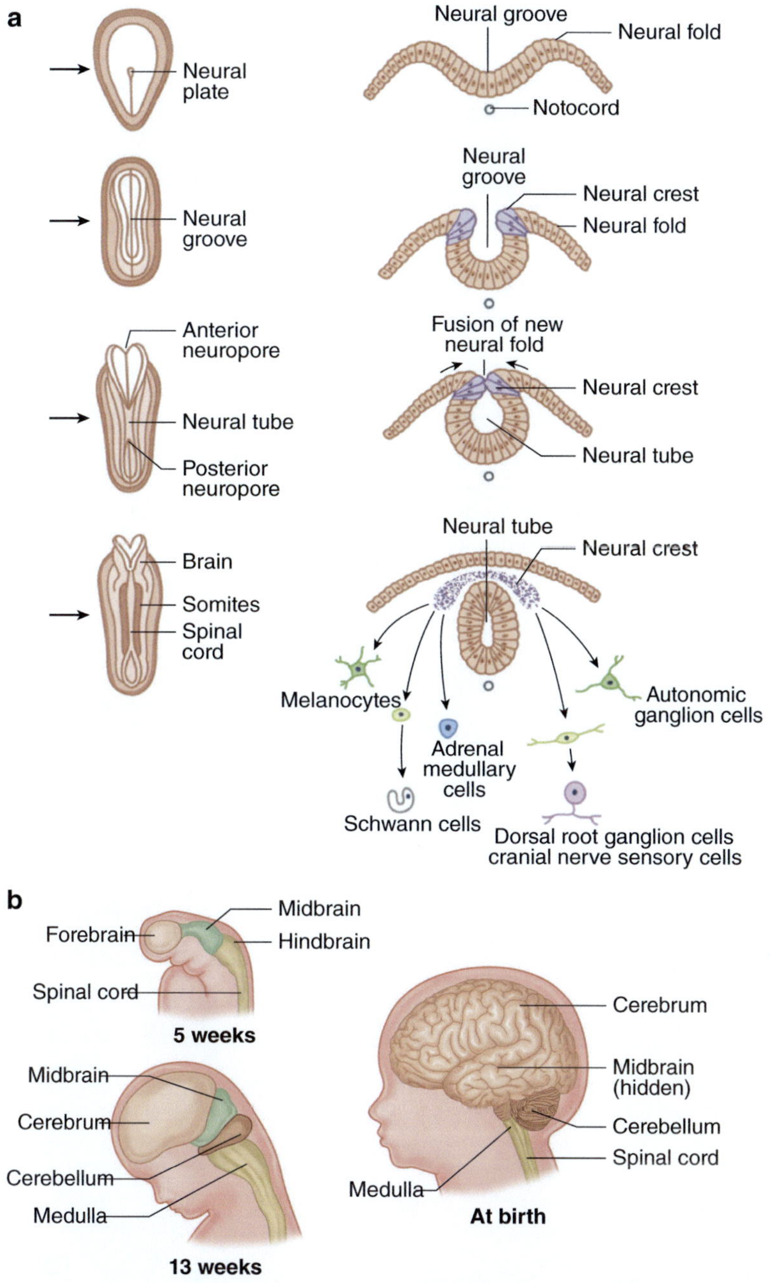

Fig. 14.1 Development of the human nervous system. (**a**) Schematic representation depicting the early stages of human nervous system development. On the left side of the figure, the neural groove is illustrated, showing the initial invagination of the neural plate. The neural tube formation process is depicted, where the neural folds converge and fuse to form the closed neural tube. Differentiation of the neural tube into various cell types, including neurons and glial cells, is represented, indicating the early stages of nervous system development. (**b**) Gross Anatomy of the Developing Brain. On the right side of the figure, the gross anatomy of the human brain at different developmental stages is depicted. At 5 weeks of gestation, the brain is shown in its early embryonic form, with basic structures beginning to take shape. At 13 weeks of gestation, significant development has occurred, with distinct regions of the brain, including the forebrain, midbrain, and hindbrain, becoming more defined. At birth, the gross anatomy of the brain is illustrated in its mature form, with well-defined structures such as the cerebrum, cerebellum, and brainstem clearly visible. Each developmental stage is labeled accordingly to indicate the progression of brain development from early embryonic stages to birth

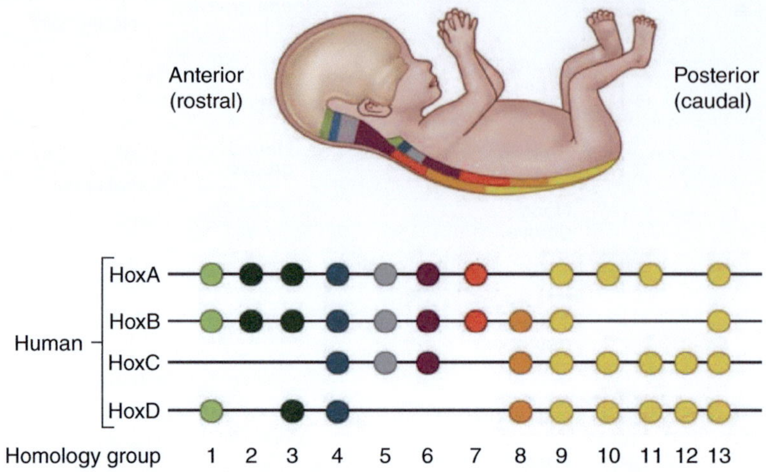

Fig. 14.2 This figure illustrates the spatial distribution of human Hox genes (HoxA to HoxD) along the midbrain and spinal cord, organized into homology groups 1–13. Homology groups 1–13 are color-coded to denote their respective positions along the midbrain and spinal cord. The midbrain and spinal cord are depicted as anatomical landmarks, providing a reference for the localization of Hox genes. Hox genes are positioned along the midbrain and spinal cord according to their homology groups, indicating their relative spatial organization

Fig. 14.3 This figure schematically depicts the process by which gradients of BMP protein (upper) and Sonic Hedgehog protein (lower) induce the differentiation of sensory neurons (blue) and motor neurons (green) in a segment of the spinal cord. Sensory neurons differentiate in response to high levels of BMP and low levels of Sonic Hedgehog signaling. Motor neurons differentiate in response to low levels of BMP and high levels of Sonic Hedgehog signaling

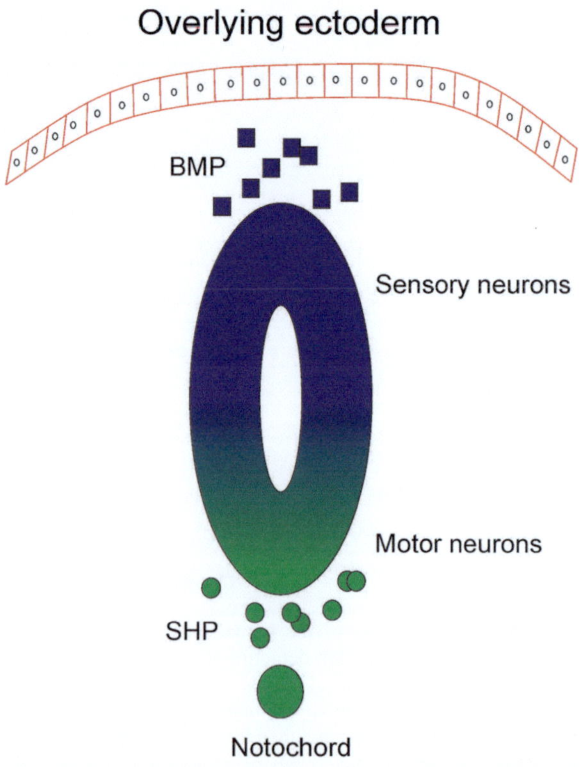

apoptosis, which is triggered in the absence of external trophic factors like nerve growth factor (NGF), brain-derived neurotrophic factor (BDNF), and others, released by the target tissue. Only neurons that establish functional connections with the target tissue and receive adequate neurotrophic factor support will survive, while less successful neurons will undergo apoptosis. Neurotrophins, such as NGF and BDNF, bind to and activate kinases (Trk receptors), which prevent the activation of the cell death program.

The axonal outgrowth occurs through distinct steps, resembling a series of road signs on a pathway toward the target. The response of the axon to these signals depends on the specific type of nerve cell and the receptors present in its membrane. The final establishment of functional connections involves activity-dependent reorganization of corticospinal connectivity during a critical period shortly after birth, where only the most functional connections survive. It is during this pruning process that corticospinal connections from the opposite hemisphere become dominant. In cats, this critical period lasts around 4 weeks from 2–3 months of age after birth (Martin et al., 2007). If a cat is prevented from using one paw during this period, the connections to the motor neurons for that paw do not develop normally, resulting in reduced usage of the paw in adulthood (Martin et al., 2007).

Similarly, in humans, connections with motor neurons and interneurons in the spinal cord are established before birth, and there appears to be a corresponding period of connection reorganization around 3–4 months of age (Hadders-Algra, 2021).

Various mechanisms are involved in the establishment of synaptic connections once axons have reached their target vicinity. Axons interact to ensure selectivity, and they possess the ability to convert their targets to appropriate types and eliminate inappropriate contacts. It is believed that a relatively small number of different recognition molecules, as few as a few hundreds, are sufficient to establish the intricate circuitry of the human brain. Spontaneous or experience-driven electrical activity, particularly during later stages of development, plays a vital role in establishing and maintaining many synaptic connections.

Once structural contact between pre- and postsynaptic neurons is established, signaling between the two neurons influences gene expression and leads to the production of synaptic material, including receptors and neurotransmitters. This ensures the establishment of functional connectivity between the two neurons. However, during development, most connections that are established in both the central and peripheral nervous systems are later eliminated due to competitive activity-dependent mechanisms. As a result, it is not uncommon for the number of connections a neuron receives to decrease dramatically during development. This is counterbalanced by an increase in the strength of the surviving synaptic connections.

14.3 Critical Periods During the Development of the Nervous System

Since the early 1960s, it has been understood that the development of the nervous system is not a pre-programmed process independent of the environment (Bence & Levelt, 2005). In addition to cell-to-cell interactions and their influence on each other's development, the environment also plays a crucial role in shaping nervous system development. This has been extensively studied in the visual system of felines (Bence & Levelt, 2005).

Newborn kittens are functionally blind, and visual function develops only after birth through neural activity triggered by light stimulation on the retina during a critical period of just two weeks. If a kitten is deprived of visual input from one eye during this period, the nerve cells in the visual cortex do not develop the necessary characteristics to respond to light from that eye, resulting in lifelong functional blindness. Before the critical period, nerve cells are formed in the visual cortex as part of a genetic program, but if they do not receive meaningful activity from the eye, they undergo pruning or elimination. Studies have also demonstrated that kittens exposed exclusively to vertical stripes during the critical period do not develop the ability to perceive horizontal surfaces and lines, such as the edge of a table.

Similar critical periods have been identified for sensory and motor systems in cats, rats, and other laboratory animals (Hensch, 2005). It is widely assumed that similar periods exist during human development, although they are likely more protracted and not as "critical." While there are sensitive periods when children's development is particularly influenced by external factors, the absence of such influences during these periods is unlikely to have catastrophic consequences for specific characteristics. Instead, external influences significantly enhance the development of the respective attributes. Therefore, terms like "sensitive period" or "window of opportunity" are used to describe these periods in human development.

14.4 Response to Lesion of the Developing Brain—Is Early Better?

As already discussed in Chap. 13, the developing immature nervous system differs from the adult mature central nervous system in its ability to regenerate following lesion. This is a consequence of the presence of neural stem cells (radial glia cells), which may divide and replace damaged neurons, the presence of environmental signals (neurotrophic factors, adhesion molecules, etc.) that may induce and guide growth of axons and the absence of environmental factors that inhibit and suppress regeneration (such as myelin). Early during development specific areas of the nervous system have also not yet been dedicated to specific functions. This appears to happen only after critical periods of development where environmental stimuli are crucial for inducing specific functional properties in specific areas of the nervous system through activity-dependent processes. Evidence that function may be allocated to other areas in the brain following lesion comes from observations in children and adults with Cerebral Palsy as well as chance observations of lesions on MR scans from apparently well-functioning individuals. Significant flexibility in allocation of function early during development is also evident from the observations that individuals who are blind from birth show activation of the visual cortex following touch of their fingers, whereas this is not the case for individuals who have become blind as adults (Basu et al., 2010). This may be related to the fact that cortical neurons initially send projections towards the spinal cord, but during normal development only those from the motor cortex survive due to establishment of successful functional connections through activity-dependent interaction with target neurons. In the absence of competition from motor cortex neurons, neurons in other areas of the brain may be successful in establishing functional connections with target neurons in the spinal cord and make functional control of muscle activity possible. A similar mechanism appears to play a role in the competition between corticospinal projections from the two hemispheres during development (Martin et al., 2007). During normal development, both hemispheres send projections to both sides of the spinal cord, but through functional competition in a critical period following birth (in cats 2–4 weeks, in rats, the first week, and in humans possibly around 0–6 months), the majority of ipsilateral projections disappear again and the left hemisphere ends up controlling the right side of the spinal cord and vice versa. Following early lesions of one motor cortex, ipsilateral projections from the non-lesioned hemisphere can survive and may be responsible for some functional abilities in individuals with early brain lesions. The clinical observation that it is possible to remove one hemisphere in cases of severe epilepsy or other unilateral severe brain dysfunctions prior to the age of 10–12 years with only limited functional deficits consequently is also evidence of the capacity of the remaining parts of the nervous system to re-organize and take over function from the removed hemisphere. Needless to say, this degree of re-organizational capacity is not present in the adult brain.

Comparison of the behavioral effects of lesions in animals have also to some extent supported that lesions early during development are associated with a better outcome than lesions in adult animals. The idea that greater and quicker recovery of function is seen the younger the organism, is usually referred to as Kennards principle in recognition of the work performed in the 1930's by Margaret Kennard. However, later studies have revealed a much more complicated picture (Elliott, 2020). Comparison of lesions to young and old brains is complicated by the influence of the site and extent of the lesion. A lesion of a given size may affect more areas of a young small brain than an old big brain. In the immature brain, the lesion may also affect neural stem cells and environmental signaling mechanisms essential for the normal development of the nervous system. Early lesions may therefore fundamentally influence the development of the nervous system beyond that (in space and time) of the initial lesion and have a much larger and more significant effect on the nervous system than a lesion of similar size in an adult brain. The functional outcome of a lesion during development therefore must be seen as a balance between the larger plasticity and the larger vulnerability of the immature brain. The outcome of a lesion will depend on whether plasticity (good recovery) or vulnerability (bad recovery) dominates, and this balance will be determined by a combination of the exact time of the lesion during development, the site of the lesion, and the extent of the lesion. This interaction remains incompletely understood but significantly contributes to the remarkable variability observed in the relationship between functional capacity (clinical outcome) and anatomical lesions identified through brain scans in human infants. In addition to this, environmental factors and the possibility of providing efficient early interventions greatly influence the functional outcome and the future functional development of the child. Understanding the vulnerabilities and plasticity resulting from lesions at specific sites and times during nervous system development can improve care for children with early brain lesions, enhancing their developmental outcomes.

14.5 Sensori-Motor and Cognitive Development

14.5.1 The First Movements

All parents will know that fetal movements occur frequently in the third trimester of pregnancy and may be felt easily by both parents. The possibility of observing the fetus directly in the womb arose with the invention of the ultrasound technique in the early 1970s. With this technique, it has since been possible to describe several specific movement patterns throughout fetal life. The earliest movements, in the form of sideways movements, are observed already in the seventh to eighth week of pregnancy. A little later, in the fetal stage, from the 9th to 11th week, hiccups, yawning and breathing movements are also observed. Later, eye movements (14th week) and even asymmetrical patterns are also seen, where the right arm is more active than the left (15th week). The movements in question are probably generated by simple nerve cell networks in the spinal cord or nerve cells in the brain stem and should probably be seen as precursors to the simple movement patterns seen in the newborn child. They are generally referred to as "spontaneous movements," in that they are endogenously generated and not the result of external triggers (reflexes) nor of intentional processes. Also, some of those movements involve the entire body, including head neck, trunk, and the four limbs, and for that reason they are called "general movements," as opposed to more localized ones, involving only single body parts (Hadders-Algra & Prechtl, 1992). General movements (GMs) persist beyond birth, and gradually diminish between the fourth and sixth month of post-term age. Notably, the influence of increased gravity post-birth does not substantially alter the primary attributes of GMs, including complexity, variability, and fluency. This consistent pattern is evident in recordings both inside the uterus (fetal recordings) and outside it (neonatal recordings), emphasizing the pre/post-natal continuum defining the developmental profile of GMs. Throughout their existence, they retain their intrinsic quality of being endogenously generated, although, as time progresses, they undergo a subtle transformation, becoming increasingly modulated by experience.

14.5.2 Motor and Cognitive Development After Birth

The immature state of the human brain at birth has two functional implications of equal importance. One is that there are limits to how big the head of an infant may be at the time of birth. Bigger brains have undoubtedly had an evolutionary advantage, but the cost has been that women give birth with pain and with a considerably higher risk for both their own life and that of the child as compared to other animals. The evolutionary solution for allowing still bigger brains without too high a risk for the death of both mother and child has been to delay some of the development until after birth. The consequence of this and the other functional implication of an immature brain is that the newborn infant is virtually helpless as compared to other animals and relies heavily on its parents for feeding, protection, and transportation. As it turns out, this has the advantage of creating a close child–parent bond which lasts throughout childhood and adolescence—for many more years than in any other animal—and allows the child to learn both motor, cognitive, and social skills before being able to severe those bonds and lead an independent life. The immature state of the brain at birth and its high level of plasticity throughout childhood and adolescence allows the human infant, child, and youth to maintain a high degree of adaptability and acquire new cognitive and motor skills through experience-dependent learning processes rather than to have to rely on innate hard-wired solutions. From the time of birth, the newborn infant essentially probes with every movement how its body interacts with the surroundings. Every movement—big or small, complex, or simple—is a small experiment, where the neural circuits in the sensori-motor areas of the brain of the infant investigate the sensory consequences of interaction with the environment. As described already in Chaps. 5, 7, and 8, a predictive model, which becomes increasingly precise at predicting the sensory consequences of movement, is established and updated with every movement the infant is doing by comparing the expected (calculated) sensory feedback and the actual sensory feedback from the movement. It is a slow process which takes years to perfect even for some of the most basic motor skills. Studies have shown that although human infants begin to walk upright around the age of 1 year, their gait pattern is still more unstable, more variable, and costs more energy than in adults up to the age of 11–12 years (Petersen et al., 2010). The ability to reach and grasp an object quickly and precisely is also optimized through practice and only becomes as precise and efficient as in adults around the age of 14–15 years (Forssberg et al., 1991). The development of speech and language also illustrates the importance of the immaturity of the human brain at birth and the ability of the human brain to flexibly adapt to its specific surroundings through learning from the time of birth and onwards: It is now known with certainty that all human infants are born with the ability to learn any human language. Which language they end up speaking only depends on which language they are exposed to. They learn by mimicking their parents. They produce sounds which they gradually optimize by comparing them to those that their parents make. This is probably one of the clearest examples of how a sensori-motor learning process is closely coupled to development of cognitive abilities and vice versa. Interestingly, a critical period has been determined in the development of human language. If an infant is not exposed to certain sounds or differences in sounds (such as the sound of ‘r’ and ‘l’) in Indo-European languages before the age of 10 months, it may be difficult and maybe even impossible to learn that sound or difference in sound later in life (as many Japanese people experience). There are also sounds in the Mandarin language which speakers of Indo-European languages are not exposed to and therefore, have profound difficulties learning later in life. However, if they are exposed to those sounds—even in a video recording—for some minutes each day before the age of 10 months, they have no difficulties detecting and pronouncing those sounds later in life (Liu et al., 2022).

14.5.3 Developmental Stages: Motor and Cognitive Milestone

Given the immature state of the infant brain and that development depends on experience-dependent plasticity and learning, it is understandable that there is a very considerable variation in the motor and cognitive abilities of infants and children of different ages. This is illustrated in Fig. 14.4 which not only shows the age where most infants achieve different gross motor skills such as lifting their head, rolling over, sitting, standing, and walking but also the considerable variability (the horizontal bars) between infants. This variability is a clinical challenge since it makes it difficult to determine whether an individual child develops normally or not. The concept of "typical development" encompasses a wide spectrum, leading to potential delays in identifying deviations warranting intervention.

Cognitive and language milestones are more difficult to define and show even greater variability, but some of the approximate ages for achievement of some cognitive and language skills are given in Figs. 14.5 and 14.6.

Despite the variability in all milestones, failure to achieve one or more of them is often what raises the first suspicion of a neurodevelopmental disorder in an infant or child. To aid in the diagnosis and the monitoring of children with neurodevelopmental disorders, several different tests exist, some of which have been validated and are used relatively routinely worldwide (see Box 14.2).

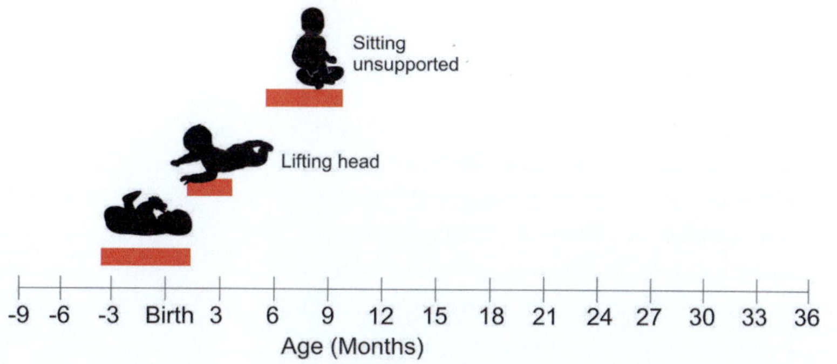

Fig. 14.4 Development of basic motor skills in human infants. Typical development is characterized by large variability between individual infants indicated by the red bars in the figure. Many of the skills are also overlapping and development of new skills is not necessarily serial

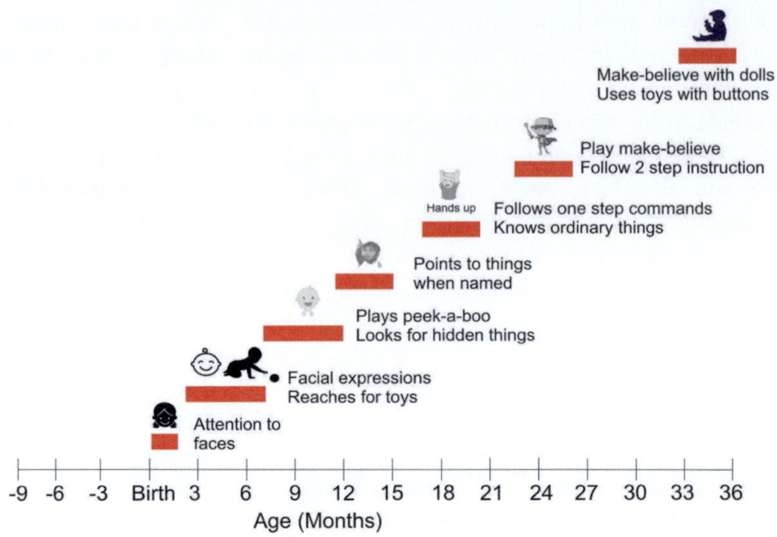

Fig. 14.5 Development of cognitive abilities. Only some selected abilities have been illustrated. As for motor skills, cognitive abilities develop at vastly different rates in individual infants as indicated by the red bars

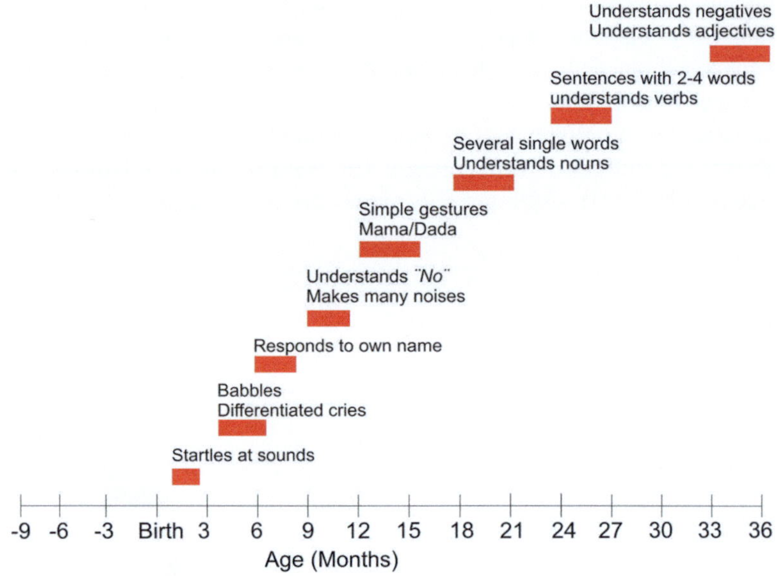

Fig. 14.6 Development of communication abilities. Red bars indicate the large variability in the age at which individual infants achieve the ability

Box 14.2 Neurodevelopmental Test

General Movement Assessment **(GMA) (Einspieler & Prechtl,** 2005)—General Movement Assessment is an assessment of an infant's spontaneous movements when lying on its back calm and alert. If performed by a trained therapist, it may be used to determine abnormal or absent general movements from birth until about 4–5 months post-term, which is highly predictive of neurodevelopmental disorder. The observation may be done from a video recording and takes 10–15 min. The possibility of using artificial intelligence to identify general movements from video recordings shows great promise.

Test of Infant Motor Performance **(TIMP) (Madayi et al.,** 2021)—Test of

(continued)

Box 14.2 (continued)
Infant Motor Performance was developed for use in neonatal intensive care units (NICU) and has been validated for infants 34 months post-conception until 4 months post-birth. It involves observation of the infant in the NICU and includes 42 items, such as head orientation, movements of the limbs, antigravity control, and reaction to auditory, visual, and postural stimuli.

Alberta Infant Motor Scale **(AIMS) (Eliks & Gajewska,** 2022)—Alberta Infant Motor Scale was developed based on observations of the development of 2200 infants in Alberta, Canada. It has been validated for infants from term until 18 months post-term and scores 58 in four situations: prone (21 items), supine (9 items), sitting (12 items), and standing (16 items).

Bayley scales of infant development (Del Rosario et al., 2021)—The Bayley scales were developed by the psychologist Nancy Bayley to assess the development of infants 1–42 months of age. The scales have been developed further and exist in different versions. The Bayley III is at present the most widely used of them. It has three subtests, which provide scoring of the child's achievements as compared to typically developing infants of the same age in the cognitive (attention, imagination, pretend play), language (naming of objects, follow directions), and motor domains (grasping, sitting, climbing stairs). The tests take around 45–60 min to perform.

Review Questions

- What are the main characteristics of neurodevelopment disorders?
- What are critical and sensitive periods and why are these important?
- What test can be applied to identify neurodevelopmental disorder?

References

Basu, A., Graziadio, S., Smith, M., Clowry, G. J., Cioni, G., & Eyre, J. A. (2010). Developmental plasticity connects visual cortex to motoneurons after stroke. *Annals of Neurology, 67*(1), 132–136. https://doi.org/10.1002/ana.21827

Bence, M., & Levelt, C. N. (2005). Structural plasticity in the developing visual system. *Progress in Brain Research, 147,* 125–139. https://doi.org/10.1016/S0079-6123(04)47010-1

Del Rosario, C., Slevin, M., Molloy, E. J., Quigley, J., & Nixon, E. (2021). How to use the Bayley scales of infant and toddler development. *Archives of Disease in Childhood. Education and Practice Edition, 106*(2), 108–112. https://doi.org/10.1136/archdischild-2020-319063

Einspieler, C., & Prechtl, H. F. (2005). Prechtl's assessment of general movements: A diagnostic tool for the functional assessment of the young nervous system. *Mental Retardation and Developmental Disabilities Research Reviews, 11*(1), 61–67. https://doi.org/10.1002/mrdd.20051

Eliks, M., & Gajewska, E. (2022). The Alberta infant motor scale: A tool for the assessment of motor aspects of neurodevelopment in infancy and early childhood. *Frontiers in Neurology, 13*, 927502. https://doi.org/10.3389/fneur.2022.927502

Elliott, D. (2020). The legacy of the Kennard principle. *Journal of Undergraduate Neuroscience Education, 19*(1), R11–R14.

Forssberg, H., Eliasson, A. C., Kinoshita, H., Johansson, R. S., & Westling, G. (1991). Development of human precision grip. I: Basic coordination of force. *Experimental Brain Research, 85*(2), 451–457. https://doi.org/10.1007/BF00229422

Hadders-Algra, M. (2021). Early diagnostics and early intervention in neurodevelopmental disorders-age-dependent challenges and opportunities. *Journal of Clinical Medicine, 10*(4). https://doi.org/10.3390/jcm10040861

Hadders-Algra, M., & Prechtl, H. F. (1992). Developmental course of general movements in early infancy. I. Descriptive analysis of change in form. *Early Human Development, 28*(3), 201–213. https://doi.org/10.1016/0378-3782(92)90167-f

Hensch, T. K. (2005). Critical period plasticity in local cortical circuits. *Nature Reviews. Neuroscience, 6*(11), 877–888. https://doi.org/10.1038/nrn1787

Liu, L., Gotz, A., Lorette, P., & Tyler, M. D. (2022). How tone, intonation and emotion shape the development of infants' fundamental frequency perception. *Frontiers in Psychology, 13,* 906848. https://doi.org/10.3389/fpsyg.2022.906848

Madayi, A., Shi, L., Zhu, Y., Daniel, L. M., Noordin, A. A., Sherwood, S. A. M., et al. (2021). The Test of Infant Motor Performance (TIMP) in very low birth weight infants and outcome at two years of age. *Journal of Perinatology, 41*(10), 2432–2441. https://doi.org/10.1038/s41372-021-01067-w

Martin, J. H., Friel, K. M., Salimi, I., & Chakrabarty, S. (2007). Activity- and use-dependent plasticity of the developing corticospinal system. *Neuroscience and Biobehavioral Reviews, 31*(8), 1125–1135. https://doi.org/10.1016/j.neubiorev.2007.04.017

Petersen, T. H., Kliim-Due, M., Farmer, S. F., & Nielsen, J. B. (2010). Childhood development of common drive to a human leg muscle during ankle dorsiflexion and gait. *The Journal of Physiology, 588*(Pt 22), 4387–4400. https://doi.org/10.1113/jphysiol.2010.195735

Neuroplasticity as a Basis for Neurorehabilitation

15

Jens Bo Nielsen, Ivana Bardino Novosel, Jakob Lorentzen, Rasmus Feld Frisk, and Lisbeth Højkjær Larsen

Abstract

Central to neurorehabilitation is the understanding that repetitive, task-specific training can drive plastic changes in the brain. This involves intensive practice of motor and cognitive tasks, promoting synaptic strengthening and the formation of new neural pathways.

Incorporating neurobiological insights, neurorehabilitation also emphasizes the role of timing and environment. Early intervention post-injury can harness periods of heightened plasticity, optimizing recovery outcomes. Furthermore, enriched environments, which provide a variety of stimuli, are known to enhance synaptic plasticity, aiding rehabilitation. Training as part of daily life is crucial, as it ensures consistent, real-world practice of skills, reinforcing neural pathways in relevant contexts.

High doses of training in natural surroundings are particularly effective, as they integrate rehabilitative exercises into familiar, functional settings, enhancing motivation and contextual learning.

Keywords

Neuroplasticity · Deliberate training · Motivation · Goal setting · Enriched environments · Daily life integration

J. B. Nielsen (✉)
Department of Neuroscience, University of Copenhagen, Copenhagen, Denmark

Elsass Foundation, Charlottenlund, Denmark
e-mail: jbnielsen@sund.ku.dk

I. B. Novosel · J. Lorentzen · L. H. Larsen
Department of Neuroscience, University of Copenhagen, Copenhagen, Denmark

Department of Pediatrics, University Hospital Rigshospitalet, Copenhagen, Denmark
e-mail: ivana.novosel@sund.ku.dk; jlorentzen@sund.ku.dk; lihl@sund.ku.dk

R. F. Frisk
Department of Neuroscience, University of Copenhagen, Copenhagen, Denmark
e-mail: frisk@sund.ku.dk

Box 15.1 Case Story

Henry, a 65-year-old man with no previous medical history, is presented to a primary stroke unit due to an ischemic stroke affecting the left hemisphere. Neurological examination shows right-sided weakness with poor voluntary muscle activation, especially in distal muscles. As a result, his mobility is very limited to basic transfer from supine position to sitting on the edge of the bed with support from one person. At the time of admission, he was unable to get from sitting to standing as he has trouble with weight-bearing on his affected leg and impaired postural control, leading to reduced balance. Cognitively, Henry is well preserved with a good insight into his situation; however, he experiences fatigue after a short time of concentration.

(continued)

J. B. Nielsen et al. (eds.), *Neuroplasticity-based Neurorehabilitation*,
https://doi.org/10.1007/978-3-031-81120-3_15

Box 15.1 (continued)

Henry is treated acutely with thrombectomy removing the cerebral blood clot, which helps to restore blood flow to the affected brain area. Henry shows good spontaneous remission with a greater ability of voluntary muscle activation and transfer skills in the days following surgery. Subsequently, physical therapy is initiated to restore an independent and efficient gait function.

The therapists at the neurorehabilitation unit designed a task-specific program for him, breaking down the gait function into sub-tasks and -goals gradually introduced with progressive difficulty to encourage and motivate Henry throughout the rehabilitation. They let him start with easier tasks and progressively increase the difficulty as Henry improves his transfer and walking skills.

The therapists supervise Henry´s training, with a focus on facilitating his engage ment and active participation by incorporating visual, auditory, and proprioceptive feedback that can support and facilitate his gait ability.

Following discharge from the neurorehabilitation unit, Henry and his therapists discussed the goals for Henry´s rehabilitation program and decided to focus on structured home-based training to emphasize repetitive and intense practice of gait-related exercises. This is routinely evaluated to ensure that Henry is practising at his optimal challenge point. A team of therapists also visits Henry's home and helps him to arrange it to be suitable for self-managed home-based training. Over the following 2 years, Henry steadily becomes more and more proficient at walking and eventually manages to go shopping in the local mall using a cane.

This chapter describes how a fundamental grasp of neurobiology and neuroplasticity can inform practical approaches and interventions in neurorehabilitation. The chapter does not seek to introduce a new concept in neurorehabilitation with strict guidelines and regulations on how to conduct practical neurorehabilitation. Instead, it aims to empower therapists to create personalized neurorehabilitation programs that are most likely to succeed in promoting the functional recovery of the individual, based on the current understanding of neurobiology and neuroplasticity as discussed in earlier chapters. The principles outlined below should be considered as a set of ideas that can inspire ways for clinicians to assist the individual optimally at various stages of rehabilitation and in different practical situations. It is up to clinicians, neurorehabilitation units, and departments to determine when each of these principles is applicable to an individual undergoing a neurorehabilitation program. Various sets of principles, ideas, or recommendations, originating from fundamental neuroscience, neuroplasticity, and/or motor learning, have been proposed for this objective in various review papers (Kleim, 2011; Maier et al., 2019; Nielsen et al., 2015; Warraich & Kleim, 2010). While the reviews exhibit minor variations, they complement one another by emphasizing different facets of neurorehabilitation and drawing on diverse aspects of knowledge in neurobiology, neuroplasticity, and motor learning. In the subsequent discussion, arguments, and ideas from all these reviews have been consolidated and organized in relation to key topics in neurorehabilitation to explore the implications in a practical setting (Fig. 15.1).

Arguably, the most significant practical implication arising from the understanding of neuroplasticity and motor learning is that barring the initial post-injury phase, the therapist's role must transition into that of a personal coach. The therapist should primarily guide, motivate, and supervise the patient. Meaningful functional improvements result from hours of daily practice integrated into the patient's daily life, rather than relying solely on the limited weekly or monthly hours a therapist can provide. This is not to diminish the importance of therapy sessions; they remain crucial for supporting the patient, identifying missing components that can help to optimize function and improvement toward specific goals, providing feedback, and sustaining moti-

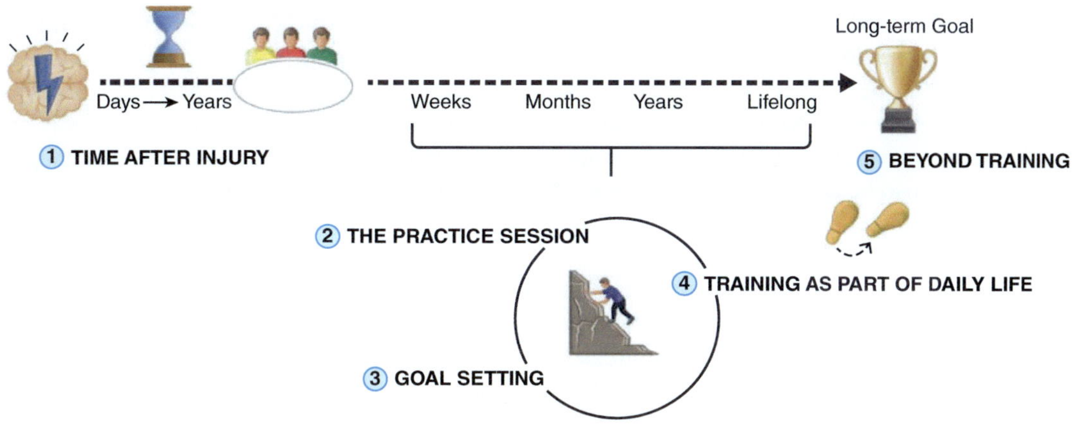

Fig. 15.1 An overview of key topics in neurorehabilitation: 1) Time After Injury, 2) The Practice Session, 3) Goal Setting, 4) Training as Part of Daily Life, and 5) Beyond Training

vation and progression. However, emphasis should shift toward the patient's actions when the therapist is not present, whether the patient resides in a neurorehabilitation center or at home.

While it may seem harsh to suggest that neurorehabilitation becomes the responsibility of the patients themselves, it is unfortunately necessary if maximum functional recovery is to be achieved. Therapists and healthcare providers can offer support and guidance, but the burden lies on the patient to put in the training efforts over an extended period. In neurorehabilitation, training refers to a structured process that helps individuals learn and enhance their performance of skilled tasks. It involves engaging in deliberate practice with specific goals until the skill is automated.

Ultimately, it falls upon the therapist to instruct the patient on the most effective training methods and, in a broader context, how to lead a post-injury life conducive to efficient recovery of function. Consequently, the therapist has a role not only in relation to the training itself but also in addressing other factors that influence recovery during daily life, such as sleep, exercise, and nutrition. The ensuing sections will explore (1) when training should commence, (2) how to plan and enhance training, (3) the significance of establishing goals in neurorehabilitation and assessing progress, (4) the significance of training in daily life, and finally, and (5) how other factors can be optimized to facilitate recovery (see Fig 15.1).

15.1 Time After Injury

15.1.1 Training Should Start As Soon As It Is Possible and Safe

From a purely neuroplasticity point of view, there is every reason to start training as early as is practically possible. The neural tissue reacts to injury by initiating a cascade of signaling factors that aim to promote (self-)repair of damaged neurons and promote functional communication in the involved neurons and networks. This surge of signaling factors makes for a period after lesion where the neural networks are very amenable to change, similar to sensitive periods during development (Chap. 14). There is no clear understanding of how long such a sensitive period—if it exists—lasts in humans, since all the knowledge arises from animal experiments, where it is a matter of days or at most a few weeks after injury.

However, in practice, there are usually many reasons why focused training aimed at recovery of function must be delayed. One is whether the patient is in a state, physically, cognitively, and mentally, where focused training is possible and relevant. The patient may be unconscious or unable to participate cognitively in the training, so it makes little sense to initiate focused training. Passive training aiming at the prevention of contractures or mobilization aimed at "training" (automatic) postural reactions and functions of the autonomic nervous system (blood pressure regulation) may be relevant in such cases, but pursuit of motor learning goals will have to await active participation from the patient. Patients may also be depressed or in other ways in a mental state in the early period following a life-changing event such as brain or spinal cord injury where their motivation for participation in a training program is limited. It may therefore make little sense to use valuable resources to start training until the patient is better able to respond and take an active part in the training. Importantly, some studies have suggested that training may be directly counter-indicated early following stroke and traumatic brain or spinal cord injuries. The conditions warrant careful multidisciplinary considerations to minimize the risk of exacerbations (see Part III for knowledge of specific neurological disorders). During the early period after an injury, surviving neurons near the site may be especially vulnerable to reduced nutrition. Edema and other factors that limit the supply of nutrition can be exacerbated by mobilization and physical activity. Repair mechanisms that aim to remove injured tissue may also potentially be affected by early mobilization and physical activity. There are therefore reasons to be concerned and clinical findings also indicate that very early mobilization (i.e., within an initial 24 h) should be avoided.

15.1.2 It Is Never Too Late to Pursue Motor Learning or Performance Enhancement

While starting training as early following injury as possible is likely of importance, there is no reason to argue—again from a strict neuroplasticity point of view—that it is ever too late to start training. Admittedly, there may be missed opportunities in the early stages following an injury, where rehabilitation efforts can have significant and quick effects on functional recovery. Nevertheless, this does not imply that training later is futile. The available evidence indicates that the nervous system remains plastic throughout life, with the potential for recovery of function and learning new ways to perform tasks, regardless of the time elapsed since the injury.

In practice, the decision comes down to cost-benefit considerations. In a healthcare system where numerous individuals require assistance, is it justifiable to continue allocating resources when the improvements in an individual's function are minimal, requiring increasing efforts for ever-smaller effects? Similarly, for the individual, is it sensible to devote a substantial portion of their life to achieve marginal gains in function, or does a point come when the inclination to accept the attained level of functional recovery becomes overwhelming?

Such decisions are up to the individual or the decision takers in the respective healthcare systems. There are no endless resources available—either as individuals or as societies, and such decisions probably will always need to be taken despite a lingering potential for further recovery of function.

15.2 The Practice Session

15.2.1 It Is the Patient, Who Has to Perform—Not the Therapist

One of the key principles emphasized in motor learning- and neuroplasticity-based neurorehabilitation is the crucial role of active patient participation for effective functional recovery. It is the patient who must perform—not the therapist. Considering what is known about motor learning—and learning in general—this seems like stating the obvious. As described in Chap. 7 improved motor performance and acquisition of new skills rest on error signals generated from the comparison of the intended movement and the performed movement. The error signals update a predictive model of the interaction of the body with the environment and passive movements or manipulations without the active participation of the patient (who has an intention and a plan for the movement) therefore will not and cannot generate learning and induce the required plastic changes in the nervous system (Perez et al., 2004). Despite this, passive manipulations or passive limb movements as well as technical aids that take over function from the patient are a fundamental part of many neurorehabilitation programs. Early following brain injury, the patient may not be able to cooperate and take an active part in a training program. Should one then simply do nothing? Likewise, is an ankle orthosis, which prevents training and recovery of function of the ankle muscles, but helps the patient to walk, good or bad? Unfortunately, answers that apply to all patients and circumstances for such questions are not available. Strong evidence suggests that passive mobilization of a patient reduces the risk of stroke or trauma-associated pneumonia. Furthermore, it is well established that learning is impossible without active participation. While ankle orthosis may enable intense unsupported treadmill training with many steps, the ankle strategy is compensatory. Individual therapists are strongly encouraged to utilize their fundamental understanding of neurobiology, neuroplasticity, and motor learning to judge how to best help the individual patient, while being diligently aware of the intended goal of the chosen intervention. It should be mentioned that it is naturally a prerequisite that the patient is motivated to train and that the therapist should only be involved at the patient´s explicit request. The fundamental principle of active engagement in training must therefore in practice be balanced by other factors. The case of Constraint-Induced Movement Therapy illustrates this point (see Box 15.2).

Box 15.2 CIMT

Constraint-induced movement therapy (CIMT) is the epitome of a therapy based on active patient involvement. The therapy originates from observations of learned non-use in macaque monkeys by Edward Taub (Taub et al., 2006). Deprived of sensation from one arm, the monkeys would "forget" to use the arm and mainly use the arm with intact sensory feedback. This would lead to the deterioration of the motor function of the arm without sensation, but the deterioration could be counteracted if the monkey was forced to use the arm by restricting use of the arm with intact sensory feedback. Taub suggested that neurological injuries in humans could lead to similarly learned non-use and that constraining the use of the non-affected arm in persons with hemiplegia could be an efficient way to promote functional recovery. Since then, CIMT has been evaluated in a large number of clinical trials, which have been reviewed in a number of systematic reviews and subjected to meta-analysis (Corbetta et al., 2015). Although there is general agreement that the fundamental idea of getting the patient to use the affected hand as much as possible during daily living is scientifically sound and should theoretically be superior to more conventional therapies, there are challenges in practice, which have made the actual improvements in functional recovery less convincing. The main problem is—unsurprisingly—patient compliance. In a situation where a patient has just recently experienced a life-changing event in the form of a brain injury requires significant mental resources and strong motivation and commitment to accept further restriction of functional abilities. CIMT only makes sense in patients who are mainly affected on one side of the body and for many—if not all—of them, it will greatly influence their function and abilities in daily life if the use of their unaffected side is also restricted. In this relation, it is especially challenging that studies suggest that CIMT must be applied for more than 4 h per day to produce significant functional effects. This is a very long time for the patient to accept. CIMT is therefore a therapy, which makes good sense in theory, but in practice, it is probably only a very small number of carefully selected patients who can benefit from the intervention and are able to accept it at the intensity and the duration that is required.

15.2.2 What Is the Optimal "Dose" of Rehabilitation?

The question of how much training is necessary to regain function is on the mind of every person who has acquired a brain injury. How long will it take before I can walk again? How much time do I need to train per day or per week? Is it better to train 1 h every day than 2 h every 2nd day? Unfortunately, there are no definite answers to questions such as these. The answers depend on the severity of the injury and the functional deficit, the type of skill, the type of training, the time after injury, the engagement and motivation of the patient, the prior training state of the patient, the genetics of the patient, what the patient is doing in between training sets, the goal sought to achieve, and a long range of other factors some of which will be highlighted in the present chapter. With so many different factors at play, it is impossible to provide guidelines regarding the dosage of rehabilitation applicable to every patient undergoing neurorehabilitation. The large number of factors is also part of the reason why there are only a few controlled clinical trials that have attempted to provide evidence of how much training should be provided and how it should be organized. Intensity is a term often used in practice and research when describing training dose. It might be helpful to consider dose as an interplay between frequency, repetition, task difficulty, duration of training sessions, and length of training period—reserving the term intensity for endurance training. From the understanding of neuroplasticity and motor learning, there are, however, some general principles that may be of help when seeking to improve function most effectively.

1. Motor learning and hence recovery of motor function takes a long time, and neurorehabilitation is usually considered in months and years rather than days and weeks. Although initial progress may be relatively quick and lead to steep improvements in function in the associative phase of learning within days or weeks (cf. Chap. 7), the subsequent autonomous phase proceeds much more slowly and improvements rely on continuous practice over months and years. At this time, it becomes a question of how much effort and resources the patient, the therapist, and society want to put into relatively small functional gains. However, as demonstrated by elite musicians and athletes, improvements in function may still be obtained following 3 h of daily practice for 10 years. Certainly, it is not the goal of neurorehabilitation for the patient to reach perfection in performance similar to elite athletes and musicians, but such estimates still give an idea of how much effort and time needs to be put into achieving functional benefits or goals. It is few patients who will have the mindset and the necessary resources and time to train for several hours every day for several years, but the experience from elite performers suggest that this is what it takes to reach the full theoretical potential for functional recovery. In practice, more modest goals will need to be applied, but it is important that the patient realizes from the start that there is no miracle cure and that recovery/relearning will take a very long time. Slow progress may be disappointing, and the patient may lose motivation and stop training. It is therefore important for the therapists to communicate clearly from the outset that slow progress is to be expected following an initial quick improvement phase and that continuous practice over months and years has a very high likelihood of being beneficial.
2. There are limits to how often and for how long at a time an individual patient may concentrate on practice and deliberately try to recover function. This is both a question of motivation, attention, and fatigue. In addition, there are physical constraints if the practice involves training of relatively weak muscles at relatively high **dose** since muscle fatigue and delayed-onset muscle soreness (DOMS) may develop. Practice sessions may therefore have to be scheduled to allow for muscles to recover and to involve progressively higher **dose** according to muscle capacity. In addition to a basic understanding of neuroplasticity and motor learning, the

therapist therefore needs to have a good understanding of the personality and cognitive abilities of the patient as well as the basic principles of exercise and muscle physiology to plan the neurorehabilitation program most efficiently for the individual patient. It is personality, cognitive, exercise physiology, and muscle physiology factors that limit how often and for how long at a time practice can be performed in the individual patient. In contrast, the nervous system does not appear to have similar limitations in establishing new connections and adapting network activity to promote functional recovery. It is therefore not neuroplasticity or motor learning capacity, which sets the limit for how often or for how long practice sessions can take place. It is only the other psychological, cognitive, and physiological factors, which need to be considered in the individual patient. From a strict neuroplasticity point of view, it is "full steam ahead."

3. Motor learning shows high specificity. Generally, one becomes good at what is practiced, and there is only relatively little transfer between skills, although they may resemble each other. Time is therefore best spent for the patient to do what they want to be good at. This will usually mean relatively common everyday tasks that are best practiced in natural surroundings as part of everyday life rather than in a neurorehabilitation unit. Transitioning patients to real-world environments, where they encounter the complex challenges of everyday life, must be done as quickly as possible. When out of the protected and supervised environment of a neurorehabilitation unit it becomes important to differentiate between learning compensatory movements and achieving genuine recovery. While compensatory movements may help task completion, true recovery requires reintegrating basic motor skills into everyday activities, promoting adaptability and functional independence beyond the confines of impairments. Patients must be informed about these conflicting strategies and their implications for interventions along the journey toward independence.
4. It is often stated that a high number of repetitions is necessary for motor learning to proceed and to recover function. While it is true that animal studies have shown that functional recovery following both brain and spinal cord lesion requires training over a long time (months) involving a high number of repetitions of either upper limb reaching or walking, the idea that "all it takes is a high number of repetitions" needs to be moderated. In the early (associative) stage of pursuing a novel motor learning goal, improved performance may be achieved quickly with few repetitions. The patient must find the optimal strategy to solve the task and accomplish the skill. This is best accomplished by letting the patient try out different strategies and deliberately practice different possible solutions. It is only much later in acquisition, the autonomous (adaptive) phase, where motor learning proceeds much more slowly, that a high number of repetitions is required. This is most efficiently achieved by integrating the practice into everyday life. The high number of repetitions required may translate into several hours of practice per week, if not per day.
5. Adding the above points together it is clear that the dose of training offered by public centralized neurorehabilitation units is insufficient. The level of functional recovery achieved is probably far from its potential with the ideal allocation of human resources and time. Lang et al. highlighted this in a comprehensive observational study, revealing that neurorehabilitation providers offer only a fraction of the practice repetitions demonstrated to be effective in studies on neuroplasticity in animal models and human motor learning.

Studies also support that increasing the amount of scheduled therapy time can lead to better outcomes. For example, Lohse et al.'s 2014 study found consistent benefits for stroke patients receiving increased therapy time compared to those receiving usual care therapy. A more recent systematic review indicated that at least 240% more therapy time was necessary for clinically significant benefits, translating to 120 min a day compared to the mean usual time of 25 min (Schneider et al., 2016). It is worth mentioning that the review relied on the surrogate measure of scheduled therapy time rather than active practice time, which is generally not reported. Research indicates that patients are only active for 40% of their therapy time (Lang et al., 2009) as they might require breaks, interruptions may occur, and equipment may malfunction, among other factors. Therefore, in the pursuit of enhancing active practice time, it is essential to plan interventions carefully.

15.2.3 Deliberate Practice and Optimal Challenge Point

The concept of deliberate practice, introduced by K. Anders Ericsson and his colleagues in the 1990s, has garnered substantial interest. Deliberate practice intersects with the notions of active participation on one hand and feedback, goal setting, and motivation on the other (these will be further discussed below). Deliberate practice extends beyond active participation by not only stipulating that patient, not therapists, should conduct the training but also emphasizing the cognitive engagement of patients in setting training goals. Deliberate practice entails training outside one's comfort zone, with focused attention on performance, clear feedback, and progression monitoring. Ericsson et al. derived this concept from their study of how musicians most effectively acquire and enhance their skills. While they highlighted the necessity of intensive and prolonged practice as already mentioned, they underscored that repetitions do not lead to improved performance without a mental focus on identifying and deliberately strengthening weaknesses. In other words: Doing what one is already good at may be fun and create a sense of control, but it will not contribute to improving performance or expanding skills. This ties into the necessity of ensuring progression in training and thereby also the necessity of adequately judge when the patient has reached a level of performance where the increase of challenge and progression in training is necessary. Identifying and addressing what a patient cannot do is crucial, aligning with the theoretical framework of motor learning introduced by Fitts and Posner (discussed in Chap. 7) and expanded upon by Guadagnoll and Lee (2004).

Guadagnoli et al. stressed the significance of considering task difficulty relative to an individual's skill level and the conditions of task performance. As a task becomes more challenging, there is an optimal level where interpretable information increases, enhancing learning. However, surpassing an individual's processing capacity can overwhelm with information, diminishing the learning benefit. This relationship between learning, performance, and the optimal challenge point is vital in developing rehabilitation programs for those with motor and cognitive impairments.

As can be seen from Fig. 15.2, the point of optimal task difficulty for maximizing learning does not align with the point of peak practice performance. This implies that although practice enhances performance, it is not flawless. Clinicians must remember the optimized challenge point and stages of learning when aiming to induce neuroplastic change for motor skill (re-) learning.

15.2.4 Practice Protocols

Time is valuable for a person who has had a brain injury. It is important to gain as much as possible from each practice session whether this is in the start of the neurorehabilitation program at a centralized neurorehabilitation unit or at home following discharge. Active participation and deliberate practice are necessary for success, but how should the practice session be organized most efficiently? In this relation, there is an ongoing discussion in the motor learning literature regarding block and random training. Block training with repeated practice of a certain skill or subskill appears in most studies to lead to quicker improvements in performance than random practice where different skills or subskills are practiced interspersed in a random fashion. However, random practice seems more robust to interference and leads to better retention of performance in the long term.

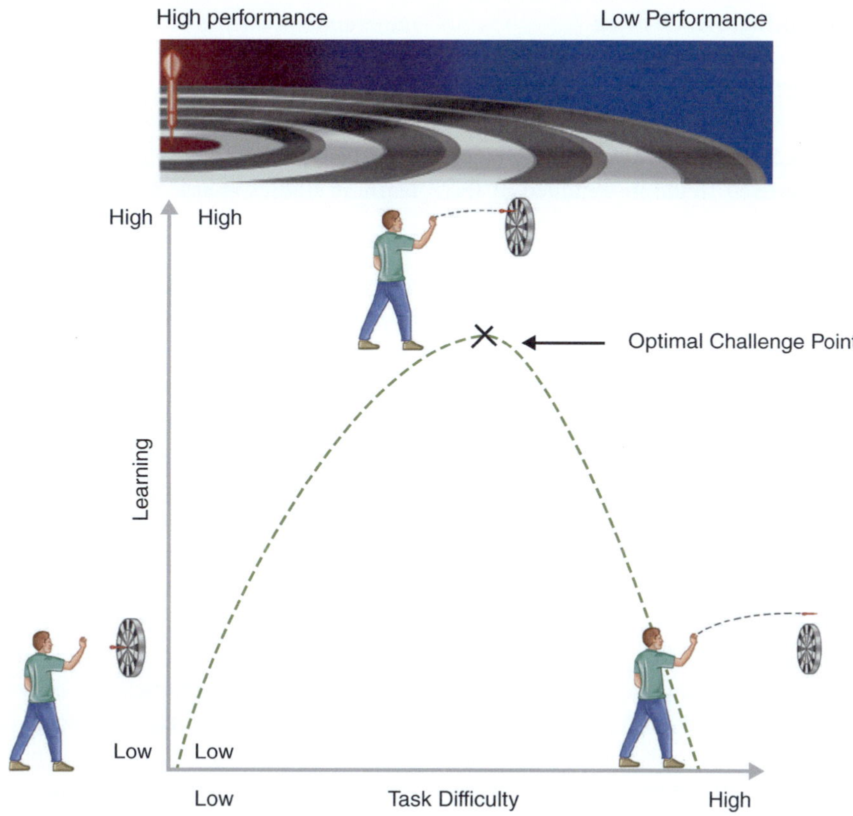

Fig. 15.2 A graph illustrating the relationship between learning and task difficulty, showing a learning curve that peaks at the "Optimal Challenge Point" where both task difficulties and performance are challenged and balanced. The y-axis represents learning, increasing from low to high, while the x-axis represents task difficulty, increasing from low to high. A person is depicting throwing darts in three different scenarios: at the bottom left with low difficulty resulting in high performance but low learning, at the bottom right with high difficulty resulting in both low performance and low learning and finally, in the middle where task difficulty is balanced between high and low with a trade-off in performance but with high learning = the optimal challenge point

There is no good evidence to support whether one or the other approach is superior to the other in relation to neurorehabilitation and no general guidelines can be provided. However, based on experience from motor learning and sports science, it may be assumed that focus on specific skills or subskills that are trained repeatedly in a block-like fashion may be beneficial initially to ensure that the person acquires basic skills. This may involve repeated training of reaching and grasping of objects or repeated training of balancing tasks or basic gait on a treadmill or over-ground with or without body-weight support. The drawback of this type of training approach is that the person may find the repeated performance of the same task boring and quickly lose interest and the necessary attention and focus on the task. This type of training therefore requires that the person is intrinsically highly motivated and/or that the therapists can provide the necessary support, guidance, and motivation to help the person maintain focus.

Later, when basic skills have been achieved to some extent, it may make sense to add practice of more skills and/or subskills and adopt a more randomized training design. Again, there is no evidence to point to a certain level of function that should be reached before practice of new skills and a more randomized approach is introduced. This will depend on the individual person and the experience of the therapist.

15.2.5 Consolidation, Offline Learning, and Risk of Interference

As described in Chap. 7, improved performance relies on the improved function obtained at the end of a practice session. What has been learned during the practice session will need to be consolidated in the form of structural changes in neural connectivity before permanent improvements in performance are achieved. In this consolidation period, what has been learned is fragile and may be lost if the consolidation process is interrupted or disturbed. This is the case if other tasks or skills activating the same neural network are learned during the consolidation period or if the neural network is disturbed in some other way (in the case of the motor cortex by applying transcranial magnetic stimulation or similar artificial disruptive activation). In relation to neurorehabilitation, there is not sufficient knowledge to determine the extent to which such interference may be a problem or not. However, as already mentioned interference is mainly a problem in relation to block training where specific tasks are learned through repeated performance in isolation, whereas randomized performance of different tasks and skills appears to be less vulnerable. A way to minimize this problem could therefore be to avoid repetitive training of the same task in a block fashion.

More importantly, the consolidation period following a practice session may also be used to facilitate the permanent storage of what has been learned during the session in line with reinforcement learning observed in experimental animal and human studies (see Chap. 7). There is now good evidence that sleep is associated with increased consolidation and that sleep immediately after practice may protect against interference. Importantly, sleep may also result in "offline learning" where the performance of the trained task improves beyond that achieved through the practice session itself (Chap. 7). Exercise has similarly been shown to facilitate consolidation when performed within some hours following practice (Thomas et al., 2016). There is insufficient evidence to determine to what extent interventions such as sleep and exercise during the consolidation period can be used in clinical practice to facilitate functional recovery, but it should be considered whenever practically possible based on the available evidence from motor learning studies in able-bodied subjects.

15.2.6 Enhancing Intrinsic Feedback and Providing Extrinsic Feedback

Improved function, as already mentioned and described in Chaps. 7 and 8, rely on the optimization of predictive motor programs based on comparison of the expected and the actual sensory consequences of the movement. Does it matter whether the focus is on how to move body parts or the intended goal while trying to improve function? Whether the focus is on adjustments of movement patterns (knowledge of performance) or clear functional accomplishments (knowledge of results). The understanding of how feedback influences motor performance and learning is essential for the development of optimal training methods and some answers may be drawn from knowledge of basic neurobiology.

As already emphasized feedback relies on an individual's own sensory-perceptual information about the movement being performed, also called intrinsic feedback. This poses a fundamental challenge for efficient functional recovery in a neurologic population since proprioceptive information may have been lost or strongly reduced due to injury or degeneration. Muscle weakness and impaired coordination of muscle activity may also challenge the predictability of the sensory feedback and lead to an unfavorable signal-to-noise ratio. As illustrated by the case of Ian Waterman and other "deafferented" people (see Chap. 2), it is possible to compensate for the loss of proprioceptive information and learn to perform a variety of skills with the use of other senses, in particular vision and vestibular information, but this comes at a cost, which is probably best expressed in Ian Waterman's reference to his situation as "a daily marathon" (Cole, 1995). Without the automatic updating of the predictive model for movements, which is ensured by proprioceptive feedback elicited by movement, conscious attention must be paid to visual and other sensory information, and the task or skill must be accomplished using a cognitive plan rather than an automatic (subconscious) program. Importantly, in the case of complete loss of proprioception, this does not change with practice. Without proprioceptive feedback to confirm the predicted sensory feedback, the person is stuck in the cognitive or associative phase of motor learning and never reaches the autonomous stage where conscious attention and visual control can be relaxed. Most neurological patients do not have complete loss of proprioception, but most, if not all of them, will have some degree of impairment in sensory feedback mechanisms and will consequently have challenges updating their predictive models for motor control and improving function as quickly and easily as neurologically intact people. It is the task of the neurorehabilitation provider to help the person to circumvent this challenge by finding ways to either enhance the proprioceptive information or compensate the loss of proprioceptive information through other sensory modalities.

Human studies have provided evidence that stimulation of sensory afferents that are timed appropriately to coincide with either the movement produced by the person or with transcranial magnetic stimulation (paired associative stimulation), may efficiently promote learning in neurologically intact individuals and there is also some indication that such procedures may be of use clinically (Christiansen & Perez, 2018). However, it seems premature to introduce this approach in routine practice.

Patients may also be helped by enhancing the sensory feedback from the tools and objects that they interact with. Training using objects that respond with somatosensory (vibration), auditory, or visual signals when touched or grasped may also greatly enhance the ability of the patient to interact with the objects and promote functional improvement.

Another way of guiding and improving performance is feedback provided by an external source such as a therapist, coach, or a mechanical device/monitoring system. This is called extrinsic feedback, also known as augmented feedback, and engages the brain's reward systems, enhances attention, corrects errors, and motivates behavior. It relates strongly to reinforcement learning and operant conditioning in experimental motor learning studies (Chap. 7). In neurorehabilitation, extrinsic feedback is usually delivered intuitively through verbal corrections or praise. Therapists need to understand that they are providing information leading to motor adaptation. Its purpose is to improve learning, and the accuracy of the feedback is crucial. Accurate extrinsic feedback, even when it is subliminal, enhances learning, whereas inaccurate feedback hinders it. Therefore, whenever possible, it is essential to prioritize purposeful, individually tailored tasks and environments that employ cues to promote task-intrinsic feedback.

Extrinsic feedback can also be data-driven. Biofeedback is a technology that enhances performance by augmenting physiological signals in real time. Other technologies, such as virtual reality systems, can monitor progress and perform kinematic analysis, providing objective extrinsic feedback. In Chap. 16, the role of technology in neurorehabilitation will be discussed in more detail.

An extension of this, which may not have been realized to its full extent, is that auditory and visual feedback signals may also act as stimuli for operant conditioning of the patients. Operant conditioning shares similarities but is not identical with reinforcement learning (or reward-based learning). Operant conditioning is the basis of "click training" in dogs, dolphins, and other animals. Operant conditioning was first discovered by Edward Thorndike (1874–1949) who observed that his cat would learn how to open his garden shed more quickly if he placed a fish outside the shed. This observation was developed further by Thorndike's pupil Burrhus Frederic Skinner (1904–1990), who invented the simple training cage where rats learn to press a lever to obtain food (the Skinner box). If the release of food when the lever is pressed, is paired with a sound, the rat learns to associate the sound to food and therefore does not need to receive the food immediately. The sound itself becomes sufficient as a promise of food. This simple learning paradigm, where a specific behavior (movement, task, or skill) is "rewarded" by a sound (a click), has been shown to be a very efficient way to teach animals of any species, including humans, to learn even very sophisticated skills. Although there is no reason why operant conditioning would not work in a neurorehabilitation context, it is not a procedure that most neurorehabilitation providers would feel comfortable in using since it may imply that the patient is similar to a "trained dog." Most importantly, in neurorehabilitation, language can be used efficiently to provide much more detailed and sophisticated feedback than a simple clicker sound.

Contrary to most animals, humans do not need immediate feedback in order to improve performance and humans can make use of their cognitive and social abilities to a much larger extent than any other species to learn new skills. While a rat in a Skinner box never learns to press the lever by observing a rat pressing the lever in the neighboring cage, an imaginary human in a similar situation would quickly pick up the idea. While chimpanzees may outcompete human children at playing computer games when left to their own individual resources, a group of children always outcompete a group of chimpanzees because the children are better at learning from each other. This human ability can be harvested to help neurological patients gain function by providing adequate verbal feedback. However, it is still essential that the feedback is correct, simple, and meaningful to be translated into improvements in function by the patient. While it is important to be supportive and provide encouragement, it will not help the patient if the therapist does not provide sufficiently correct and simple feedback. In practice, this often means that the therapist preferable should focus on clear functional accomplishments (i.e., knowledge of result) that the patient can aim for rather than adjustments of movement patterns or parameters (i.e., knowledge of performance) that are difficult to quantify and describe correctly with sufficient simplicity. The ability to lift a cup and bring it to the mouth to get something to drink is a simple measure of success. The exact way the cup is grasped or the trajectory of the movement toward the mouth is far more complex to describe and may require some kind of instrumented measurement to provide sufficiently correct measures that can be used by the patient to improve function.

Understanding the effect of feedback on learning outcomes, particularly in therapeutic settings, remains an area of ongoing investigation. While the relationship is not fully understood, evidence suggests therapists can optimize learning by enhancing intrinsic feedback and providing extrinsic feedback more intentionally. Objective feedback from equipment during training has been shown to enhance motor learning and performance, with knowledge of performance feedback appearing more immediately effective than knowledge of the result. If possible immediate, objective, and accurate information about movement should be prioritized, for example, task-oriented practice and biofeedback, over therapist communication. High-incentive feedback and rewards, such as those employed in virtual reality games, have shown promise in increasing patient compliance and engagement.

Finally, it is important to be aware that feedback has no effect without a purpose for a given movement or a specific objective to achieve. The purpose might be straightforward, such as trying to drink from a cup without spilling or taking a step without falling, or it may have a more long-term perspective, such as returning to work. Regardless, feedback must be aligned with the purpose or goal to be effective.

15.3 Goal Setting and Progress Assessment

A clear goal for practice is essential for the effectiveness of feedback and motivation. Having something to aim for is critical for maintaining commitment in daily practice. When the goal is meaningful and valuable, the human prefrontal cortex plays a key role in sustaining the motivation needed to pursue the goal. The prefrontal cortex is heavily involved in regulating behavior and evaluating the benefits and costs of different actions. Thus, if the cost of action is higher than the interest in pursuing the goal, motivation diminishes. Recognizing the importance of setting individualized goals for each patient is vital to ensure active engagement in rehabilitation. Indeed, knowledge of neuroplastic changes underpins the importance of active engagement in facilitating improvements.

Long-term goals are important for overall commitment and direction of practice, but short-term or partial goals may be as important to ensure compliance and keep patients continuously engaged. Achievements of partial goals may support the experience of success and generate a sense of accomplishment and reward which supports motivation. Conversely, failure to reach the goals may motivate to further practice or adjustments. Frequent assessment of goals with embedded feedback is an important tool to ensure engagement. Additionally, progress assessment is crucial for the therapist to determine whether the chosen intervention is relevant and sufficient or needs to be adjusted according to obstacles.

It is important to recognize that goals are often more meaningful for patients if they are set at an activity and participation level rather than at an impairment-level (see ICF model Fig 1.1). While goals are easier to quantify at the impairment level, it is primarily helpful for therapists to measure body structure and functional changes and less important for the patient. However, the achievement of goals at an activity and participation level may be scored (or quantified) using the Goal Attainment Scaling (GAS) (Turner-Stokes, 2009). This measure acknowledges that person-centered goals and patient satisfaction with their performance of a specific goal may be more helpful than standardized measures of outcomes and changes over time. GAS uses a five-point scale to measure whether the goal is achieved, and individual scores are developed (see Box 15.3 for tools used in setting goals).

Box 15.3 How to Set Goals?

There is no consensus on a gold standard for goal-setting methods. A widely used tool to set appropriate goals is called SMART. SMART stands for Specific (specifying the target activity), Measurable (quantifying the performance), Achievable (but challenging), Relevant (for the patient), and Timely (selecting the time period to achieve the desired state) (Wade, 2009). Another acronym that adds focus to the entire planning process is MEANING. It stands for Meaning (meaningful overall goals), Engage (engage to establish trust and communication), Anchor (anchor sub-goals to what is most significant for the patient as a tool for making sense of therapy), Negotiate (negotiate level/steps of progress), Intention-implementation gap (specific steps/coping plans are frequently needed to bridge intention-implementation gap), New goals (view goal-setting abilities as a strategy that be used over time), and Goals (goals requires behavior change).

Preferably the goal-setting process occurs within the first week of the rehabilitation episode starting with a conversation between the patient (including next of kin) and the rehabilitation team. The patient's social support, for example, family members or friends, is welcome because family and friends often possess important knowledge about the patient's life and are important resources for the patient. Patient's communication ability, cognition, and mood may be significantly impacted in the early phase of a rehabilitation episode, and patients may not know what to expect from a rehabilitation service.

15.4 Training as Part of Daily Life

Public health care is under pressure globally due to demographic changes, expansion of services, and increasing costs. There are consequently limits to how many resources can be invested in the neurorehabilitation of any individual and decisions to decline continuation of centralized training based on cost-benefit analyses are inevitable. Fortunately, it is not only cheaper for the health care system, but also highly desirable, advantageous, and even necessary for the individuals undergoing neurorehabilitation to be dismissed to their own homes as soon as possible and perform the training/rehabilitation as part of their daily life. The basic form of home-based training consists of a training program prescribed by a therapist and performed regularly and independently by the patient at home. Home-based training where the training is performed without the presence of an "expensive" therapist provides the possibility for extensive and frequent training. However, the responsibility for daily training rests with the individual, who may struggle to stay motivated. This may be overcome by different relatively cheap technical solutions (see Chap. 16) and the introduction of an enriched environment (EE). EE combines movement with sensory engagement, cognitive processing, and social interaction. Recovering in more physically, cognitively, and socially stimulating environments facilitates activity and enhances brain recovery, contributing to greater independence and potentially a better quality of life (see Box 15.4).

Box 15.4 Behind the Concept of Enriched Environment

In the mid-1940s, Donald O. Hebb (1904–1985) discovered that rats raised as pets in his home had better learning and memory capacity than those kept in standard laboratory cages. Decades later, in the 1960s, the concept of EE, where the brain is stimulated by its physical and social surroundings, was introduced. Adult rats that were allowed to share cages with toys, tunnels, and running wheels were found to develop heavier and thicker cerebral cortices than controls living in traditional impoverished laboratory cages in solitude. Since then, EE's effect and underlying mechanisms in promoting neurorehabilitation have been widely studied in animal models. Decades of preclinical research have established robust evidence that EE facilitates neuroplastic processes, such as structural changes, angiogenesis, neurogenesis, and the release of growth factors. Furthermore, EE has been shown to exhibit significant effects throughout the lifespan, from neonatal to aged animals, and the effect of EE on rehabilitation can be enhanced by adding more task-specific activities targeting the primary impairment (McDonald et al., 2018).

In humans, EE has been shown to effectively increase activity in patients and reduce time spent inactive and alone. However, novel ideas integrating activities that offer more strenuous exercise, like rodent running wheels, are to be invented. This highlights that replicating preclinical trials with standardized EE components in a human clinical setting is challenging. It has also been argued that humans, by default, live in an EE because everyday life is synonymous with complexity and variability. This, however, contrasts with the impoverished and isolated environment in which many patients with neurological impairments live. Furthermore, the rehabilitation setting is frequently reported as being unstimulating and boring, highlighting the need for paying attention to surroundings and settings at hospitals, rehabilitation units, and supportive living facilities. Based on preclinic studies, the ideal paradigm of EE encompasses a changing environment that encourages socialization, exercise, sensorimotor and cognitive stimulation, and task-specific therapy targeting the primary impairment (see Fig. 15.3)

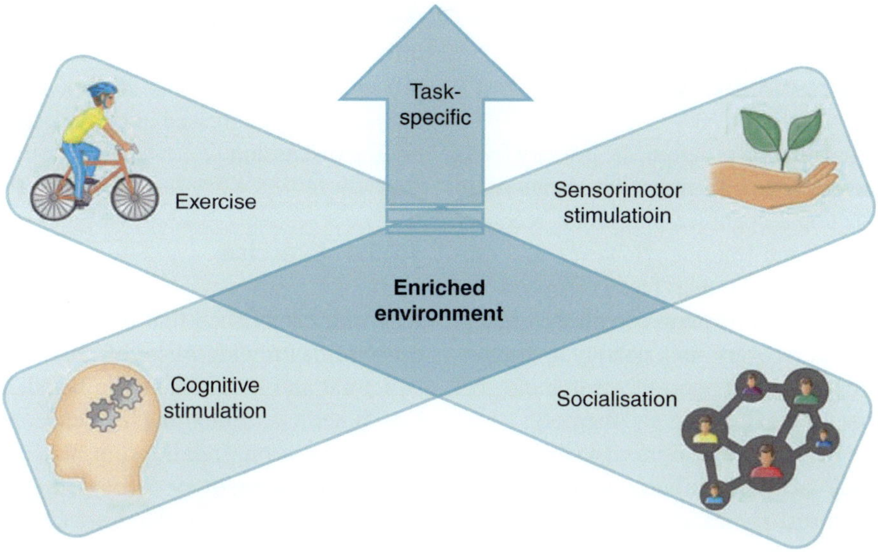

Fig. 15.3 Diagram illustrating the components of enriched environment: exercise, socialization, sensorimotor- and cognitive stimulation. The Arrow labeled "Task-Specific" emphasizes the value of activities targeting the primary impairment within the enriched environment

Environmental enrichment is not prescribed by a therapist; rather, it is based on the idea that exposure to the elements of such environments in daily life naturally encourages patients to be more active. Examples of activities that have been used in human experiments to create an EE are:

- Access to reading material (books, magazines, newspapers)
- Easily accessible computers/iPads with Internet connection
- Access to virtual reality and interactive gaming through computers or gaming consoles
- Access to board games (including puzzles and chess)
- Access to music and audiobooks
- Opportunity to be creative via art and craft (drawing, painting, and craft-work)
- Opportunity to participate in interactive recreational activities (e.g., Bingo)
- Access to exercise areas
- Opportunity to participate in shared meals
- Opportunity to participate in group sessions/ activity

Some of these activities may be supervised by a health professional (e.g., medical, nursing, or therapist) or a non-professional (family member, other volunteers) to enable participation in the available activity (for example, by setting up a game or playing a game with the patient).

Several attempts have been made to dissect EE into the relative importance of its components (exercise, sensorimotor stimulation, cognitive stimulation, and socialization). Theoretically, combining all four components in humans would have a cumulative beneficial effect on the recovery process. Most likely, adding any kind of enrichment will increase the amount and effect of training in daily life. Patients highlight that communal areas and outdoor spaces, which provide engagement opportunities, reduce boredom. Therefore, aspects from EE should be considered when designing and organizing environments such as hospitals, rehabilitation units, supportive living facilities, training- and recreational areas. Healthcare professionals must also consider each patient's unique needs when considering how training may become part of daily life and the potential risks of adverse events. By customizing the components of enrichment according to the individual needs and capabilities of the patient, a safe and efficient rehabilitation environment may be created in both the rehabilitation unit and at the home and workplace of the patient.

15.5 Beyond Training—Lifestyle Changes That May Promote Neuroplasticity

In a neurorehabilitation program, the primary focus naturally revolves around direct interventions to promote functional cognitive and motor recovery through training and learning. However, it is crucial to recognize additional factors beyond the training itself that contribute to overall well-being, aid in functional recovery, and, notably in the context of neuroplasticity, support the neurobiological processes involved in learning and memory.

For those who have experienced a stroke, their prior lifestyle often contributes to the insult's underlying causes. Therefore, it is logical for this patient group to receive lifestyle recommendations aimed at reducing associated risk factors. These recommendations may include actions such as quitting smoking, reducing fat intake, losing weight, and engaging in regular exercise. Importantly, these suggestions should not be limited to stroke patients; they can be structured and provided to all patient groups in an organized manner. This approach helps individuals comprehend the significance of lifestyle changes to promote general health, which is a prerequisite for functional recovery.

Patients with nervous system injuries face an elevated risk of developing lifestyle disorders due to various reasons. Their functional disabilities limit their ability to exercise and generate the necessary stimuli for optimal cardiovascular and metabolic regulation. Although they lead an involuntary sedentary lifestyle, it is crucial to emphasize factors associated with a healthier lifestyle. If regular exercise is not feasible due to functional disability, individuals can still adopt healthier habits such as quitting smoking, consuming nutritious food, and managing blood pressure and cholesterol through medication if needed. Additionally, efforts to enhance sleep quality or minimize factors disrupting sleep are equally important in this context.

Beyond their impact on general health, exercise, sleep, and nutrition also play pivotal roles in optimal brain function. These factors can significantly contribute to promoting functional cognitive and motor recovery after a brain injury by directly facilitating the molecular and cellular processes underlying learning and memory. This aspect will be addressed in more detail in the following discussion.

15.5.1 Exercise

It is well established that regular cardiovascular exercise has a wide range of positive effects on structural and functional brain health and cognitive functions. Emerging evidence particularly supports a strong relationship between exercise and enhanced memory formation and evidence also shows that Aerobic Exercise (AE) performed in close temporal proximity to the practice of a (cognitive and motor) task has a significant effect on the subsequent memory of what is learned (Roig et al., 2013). It is suggested that a single exercise bout induces plasticity-promoting effects on both the molecular and system level. These include an exercise-induced increase in arousal and cerebral blood flow, as well as a higher expression of catecholamines (e.g., dopamine, epinephrine, norepinephrine) or neurotrophic factors (e.g., BDNF, IGF-1, VEGF) (Wanner et al., 2020). In addition, increased corticospinal excitability, reduced intracortical inhibition, and beneficial effects on synaptic efficacy, particularly indicated by increased long-term potentiation (LTP)-like plasticity, have been demonstrated. Interestingly, studies suggest that the enhanced effect of practice appears to depend on the intensity of AE about learning/practice. Performing AE with moderate to vigorous intensity seems more effective than mild AE and performing high-intensity training seems more effective than moderate.

Thus, scheduling a session of AE temporal close to the practice of a (cognitive and motor) task might create an optimized environment for neuroplasticity, enhancing the outcome/memory of what has been learned/practiced. Studies suggest that exercise before skill practice mainly improves early skill consolidation, whereas bouts following motor practice appear to facilitate long-term, sleep-dependent stages (Wanner et al.,

2020). Although speculative, one potential reason for this finding might be the transient period of those mentioned above exercise-induced physiological effects. For example, elevated levels of catecholamines or neurotrophic factors and the sustainability of increased corticospinal excitability return to baseline shortly after exercise has ended and may thus only temporarily enhance neuroplastic mechanisms. Therefore, it seems conceivable that pre-practice exercise mainly affects the early stages of memory consolidation. In contrast, post-practice exercise allows a prolonged availability of physiological effects during later stages of memory consolidation. However, sleep and fatigue may also interact with the observed effects on memory.

Before initiating high-intensity exercise, preemptive medical screening is recommended, as well as monitoring of heart rate, blood pressure, and rating of perceived exertion (RPE) during exercise. In addition, because of the high occurrence of silent myocardial ischemia rates reported within the stroke population, exercise testing with electrocardiography is recommended before initiating cardiovascular exercise in this population.

It should be mentioned that resistance exercises referring to repetitive, monotonic, and effortful voluntary muscle contractions leading to increased muscle strength have been shown to enhance neuroplasticity. However, the functional transfer of resistance training-induced neuroplasticity to enhanced motor function across the lifespan in health and disease remains unclear. Further investigations must be performed before conclusions and recommendations can be summarized (Hortobágyi et al., 2021).

15.5.2 Sleep

Sleep plays a crucial role in the recovery of function following brain injury and should be a consideration in any neurorehabilitation program. Lack of sleep significantly impacts performance and attention, potentially undermining the effectiveness of well-designed training programs. Sleep deprivation is associated with various symptoms linked to reduced brain function, including decreased attention, prolonged reaction time, memory lapses, reduced learning rate, cognitive decline, motor skill deterioration, and increased fatigue.

Numerous studies have demonstrated that sleep is associated with improved consolidation of both cognitive and motor memory. In some cases, sleep may even enhance performance in a motor task beyond the previous day's training session, a phenomenon known as increased offline learning. Although the mechanisms behind this are not fully understood, research points to the significance of different sleep phases and activity in relevant neural networks at specific frequencies. Some studies suggest that sleep can help consolidate memory before interference from other tasks, and strategic planning of therapy sessions and sleep may optimize the benefits of therapy.

The growing problem of sleep difficulties, such as insomnia, in many countries is attributed to increased exposure to artificial light, particularly from electronic devices. Stress and worries that hinder mental calmness, along with the natural aging process affecting sleep-regulating mechanisms in the brain, contribute to this issue. Considering the crucial effects of sleep on learning and memory, it is unfortunate that patients undergoing neurorehabilitation often struggle with sleep. Prioritizing interventions that promote sleep in patients with brain injuries and neurological conditions should be a fundamental aspect of neurorehabilitation programs and incorporated as standard procedures in neurorehabilitation centers.

Implementing lighting regulations to closely mimic the day-night light cycle, even within intensive care units, is an easily achievable measure. It is advisable to include routine information for all patients, especially upon their return home, emphasizing the importance of avoiding bright artificial light, particularly from televisions, computer screens, or cell phones.

Patients should also be educated about the significant connection between regular exercise and sleep. It is crucial to clarify that it is not the exertion from a single exercise session that matters, but rather the consistency of regular exercise over an extended period. This consistency appears to contribute to stabilizing the internal biological clock, fostering a habitual bedtime. Maintaining consistent bedtime and wake-up times further supports the stability of the biological clock and aids in falling asleep.

While specific nutrients' impact on sleep remains uncertain, adhering to regular mealtimes contributes to stabilizing the biological clock and promoting a restful night's sleep. Eating right before bedtime is discouraged, but ensuring one is not hungry when attempting to sleep is essential, suggesting consumption of a meal a few hours before bedtime.

The primary barriers to sleep for many individuals are worries and stress, which can be challenging to address directly. However, various cognitive coping strategies are available, either through psychologists or self-help apps.

In the case of persistent sleep difficulties, sleep medication should generally be considered only when other interventions prove ineffective and should be used for a limited duration.

15.5.3 Nutrition

The brain, being the most metabolically active organ in the body, requires a continuous supply of energy (oxygen, glucose) and nutrients to function effectively. This ensures the everyday functioning of neurons and their supporting cells (microglia, oligodendrocytes), facilitating the transmission of electric and chemical signals throughout the nervous system's networks. Additionally, this supply is vital for maintaining or modifying connections based on experiences and learning. A consistent influx of nutrition is crucial for establishing new synapses with fresh neurotransmitters and receptors.

Evidence from animal experiments suggests that specific nutrients, such as the omega-3 fatty acid docosahexaenoic acid (DHA), may be more effective in aiding the formation of new synaptic connections related to learning and memory compared to other nutrients. While some refer to these nutrients as "brain food" or "superfood," it is essential to note that there is a lack of sufficient evidence to determine whether these nutrients are genuinely as vital for establishing new connections in the human brain as animal experiments imply.

Individuals undergoing neurorehabilitation after brain injuries may not require a specialized diet. However, available evidence suggests that, like everyone else, it is crucial for these individuals to follow official nutrition recommendations from health authorities. Diets recommended by health authorities, based on international consensus recommendations, are generally beneficial for both overall health and the brain's ability to form new connections related to learning and memory. Therefore, such diets are particularly recommended for individuals undergoing neurorehabilitation.

In essence, adhering to these recommendations involves consuming less saturated fat and more polyunsaturated fat, including omega-3 fatty acids found in vegetables, fish, and fruit.

15.6 That All Sounds Good, But How Will It Work in Practice?

The present chapter has outlined various principles, which should be considered when designing neurorehabilitation programs. However, to make it work in practice, their relevance and feasibility must be assessed thoroughly by the individual patient and the setting of the rehabilitation program. Prioritization of how a program should be designed must be based on the patient's goal and motivation, where the content of the rehabilitation is guided by the current understanding of neurobiology and plasticity. Due to large variability between patients in terms of impairments, both physically and cognitively, a large responsibility lies on the clinicians, neurorehabilitation units, and departments to ensure efficient interventions to improve function after neurological injuries. Incorporating content based on neurobiology and plasticity to the individual patient is therefore a cornerstone to ensure optimization of neurorehabilitation programs starting during admission shortly after the injury with lifelong progressions. From a neurobiological point of view, optimization of function is always possible. Whether the patient is motivated and able to make the necessary effort to reach continuous improvements will therefore be the limiting factor.

Review Questions
- What neurobiological knowledge can be applied to optimize a practice session?
- How can an understanding of neurobiology be utilized in the planning of a rehabilitation program?

References

Christiansen, L., & Perez, M. A. (2018). Targeted plasticity in the corticospinal tract after human spinal cord injury. *Neurotherapeutics, 15*(3), 618–627.

Cole, J. (1995). *Pride and a daily marathon*. Bradford Books.

Corbetta, D., Sirtori, V., Castellini, G., Moja, L., & Gatti, R. (2015, 2015). Constraint-induced movement therapy for upper extremities in people with stroke. *Cochrane Database of Systematic Reviews*, (10), CD004433. https://doi.org/10.1002/14651858.CD004433.pub3

Guadagnoll, M. A., & Lee, T. D. (2004). Challenge point: A framework for conceptualizing the effects of various practice conditions in motor learning. *Journal of Motor Behavior, 36*, 212–224.

Hortobágyi, T., Granacher, U., Fernandez-del-Olmo, M., et al. (2021). Functional relevance of resistance training-induced neuroplasticity in health and disease. *Neuroscience and Biobehavioral Reviews, 122*, 79–91.

Kleim, J. A. (2011). Neural plasticity and neurorehabilitation: Teaching the new brain old tricks. *Journal of Communication Disorders, 44*(5), 521–528. https://doi.org/10.1016/j.jcomdis.2011.04.006

Lang, C. E., MacDonald, J. R., Reisman, D. S., et al. (2009). Observation of amounts of movement practice provided during stroke rehabilitation. *Archives of Physical Medicine and Rehabilitation, 90*, 1692–1698. https://doi.org/10.1016/j.apmr.2009.04.005

Maier, M., Ballester, B. R., & Verschure, P. (2019). Principles of neurorehabilitation after stroke based on motor learning and brain plasticity mechanisms. *Frontiers in Systems Neuroscience, 13*, 74. https://doi.org/10.3389/fnsys.2019.00074

McDonald, M. W., Hayward, K. S., Rosbergen, I. C. M., et al. (2018). Is environmental enrichment ready for clinical application in human post-stroke rehabilitation? *Frontiers in Behavioral Neuroscience, 12*.

Nielsen, J. B., Willerslev-Olsen, M., Christiansen, L., Lundbye-Jensen, J., & Lorentzen, J. (2015). Science-based neurorehabilitation: Recommendations for neurorehabilitation from basic science. *Journal of Motor Behavior, 47*(1), 7–17. https://doi.org/10.1080/00222895.2014.931273

Perez, M. A., Lungholt, B. K., Nyborg, K., & Nielsen, J. B. (2004). Motor skill training induces changes in the excitability of the leg cortical area in healthy humans. *Experimental Brain Research, 159*(2), 197–205. https://doi.org/10.1007/s00221-004-1947-5

Roig, M., Nordbrandt, S., Geertsen, S. S., & Nielsen, J. B. (2013). The effects of cardiovascular exercise on human memory: A review with meta-analysis. *Neuroscience and Biobehavioral Reviews, 37*, 1645–1666.

Schneider, E. J., Lannin, N. A., Ada, L., & Schmidt, J. (2016). Increasing the amount of usual rehabilitation improves activity after stroke: A systematic review. *Journal of Physiotherapy, 62*, 182–187. https://doi.org/10.1016/j.jphys.2016.08.006

Taub, E., Uswatte, G., Mark, V. W., & Morris, D. M. (2006). The learned nonuse phenomenon: Implications for rehabilitation. *Europa Medicophysica, 42*(3), 241–256.

Thomas, R., Beck, M. M., Lind, R. R., Korsgaard Johnsen, L., Geertsen, S. S., Christiansen, L., et al. (2016). Acute exercise and motor memory consolidation: The role of exercise timing. *Neural Plasticity, 2016*, 6205452. https://doi.org/10.1155/2016/6205452

Turner-Stokes, L. (2009). Erratum: Goal attainment scaling (GAS) in rehabilitation: A practical guide. *Clinical Rehabilitation, 23*, 362–370. https://doi.org/10.1177/0269215509346900

Wade, D. T. (2009). Goal setting in rehabilitation: An overview of what, why and how. *Clinical Rehabilitation, 23*, 291–295.

Wanner, P., Cheng, F. H., & Steib, S. (2020). Effects of acute cardiovascular exercise on motor memory encoding and consolidation: A systematic review with meta-analysis. *Neuroscience and Biobehavioral Reviews, 116*, 365–381.

Warraich, Z., & Kleim, J. A. (2010). Neural plasticity: The biological substrate for neurorehabilitation. *PM & R : The Journal of Injury, Function, and Rehabilitation,* 2(12 Suppl. 2), S208–S219. https://doi.org/10.1016/j.pmrj.2010.10.016

Neurorehabilitation Technologies

16

Andrew J. T. Stevenson, Erika G. Spaich,
Prithvi Ravi Kantan, Lisbeth Højkjær Larsen,
Jakob Lorentzen, and Thomas Sinkjær

Abstract

Neurorehabilitation practices can be potentiated by incorporating neurorehabilitation technologies designed to facilitate personalized, engaging, focused, intense, varied, and task-specific training. A selected set of technologies that specifically target sensory-motor training are briefly presented, their use to potentiate activity-dependent neuroplasticity is described, and the clinical evidence of their use by individuals affected by different neurological conditions or injuries is summarized. These technologies encompass functional electrical stimulation (FES), robotic-assisted training, biofeedback, brain-computer interfaces (BCI), virtual reality (VR), augmented reality (AR), noninvasive brain stimulation (NIBS), body weight supported training (BWST), wearable sensors, and home-based training. When integrating neurorehabilitation technologies into rehabilitation scenarios, opportunities to improve outcomes and challenges associated with their use arise. These are presented along with a series of final reflections about future research directions and applications of neurorehabilitation technologies conclude this chapter.

Keywords

Neurorehabilitation · Technology · Intervention · Neuroplasticity · Neurological conditions

Box 16.1 Case Story: Foot Drop Following Stroke

It has now been two months since Elizabeth, a 62-year-old high school teacher, suffered from an ischemic stroke that originally left her unable to walk due to paralysis of her right leg. After the initial stay at the local hospital's acute stroke unit, Elizabeth was transferred to a specialized neurorehabilitation unit for intensive rehabilitation therapy. To date, Elizabeth's rehabilitation has

(continued)

The original version of the chapter has been revised. A correction to this chapter can be found at https://doi.org/10.1007/978-3-031-81120-3_26

A. J. T. Stevenson (✉) · E. G. Spaich
Department of Health Science and Technology, Aalborg University, Aalborg, Denmark

Center for Neurotechnology and Rehabilitation, Aalborg University, Aalborg, Denmark
e-mail: ajts@hst.aau.dk; espaich@hst.aau.dk

P. R. Kantan
Department of Architecture, Design and Media Technology, Aalborg University, Copenhagen, Denmark
e-mail: prka@create.aau.dk

L. H. Larsen · J. Lorentzen
Department of Neuroscience, University of Copenhagen, Copenhagen, Denmark
e-mail: lihl@sund.ku.dk; jlorentzen@sund.ku.dk

T. Sinkjær
Department of Health Science and Technology, Aalborg University, Aalborg, Denmark
e-mail: ts@hst.aau.dk

J. B. Nielsen et al. (eds.), *Neuroplasticity-based Neurorehabilitation*,
https://doi.org/10.1007/978-3-031-81120-3_16

Box 16.1 (continued)

been largely successful as she has now regained the ability to walk independently for short distances. However, Elizabeth is unable to lift her forefoot due to continued weakness of the muscles in her right leg, contributing to her asymmetric, slower, and more unsteady gait pattern. Because of this foot drop, Elizabeth has difficulty clearing her foot during the swing phase, often dragging or scuffing her foot along the ground. In compensation, Elizabeth attempts to lift her knee higher than usual to avoid dragging her toes. When she is tired, she will sometimes swing her straight leg to the side in a semicircle to move forward. These compensation strategies contribute to Elizabeth's slow gait and fatigue. She has also been close to falling trying to get between her bed and the bathroom. A couple of weeks ago, Elizabeth was fitted with an ankle foot orthosis, which helps to keep her ankle and foot in position to help the foot clear the ground. The orthosis has improved Elizabeth's confidence, posture, and walking speed. However, Elizabeth has complained about the orthosis limiting air circulation around the skin and having difficulty feeling the walking surface. At Elizabeth's latest therapy session, her physiotherapist tested an approach called functional electrical stimulation (FES) to target her foot drop problem. During the therapy session, an electrical stimulator delivered small pulses of electrical stimulation through electrodes placed on Elizabeth's leg to activate the ankle dorsiflexor muscles at strategic times during the gait cycle. While Elizabeth was initially skeptical and afraid that the electrical stimulation would be uncomfortable, her physiotherapist explained that FES can promote central motor recovery and other benefits include improved strength, walking speed, retraining ankle dorsiflexor muscle activation timing, lower energy expenditure, and reduced risk of falls. The electrical stimulation was not uncomfortable, and Elizabeth is looking forward to continuing the FES training in the coming therapy sessions.

16.1 Introduction

Neurorehabilitation technology refers to technological tools and interventions to aid in the rehabilitation of individuals with neurological conditions or injuries. This field encompasses a wide range of devices, systems, and techniques designed to improve motor, sensory, cognitive, and communication functions in individuals affected by conditions such as stroke, traumatic brain injury, spinal cord injury, multiple sclerosis, Parkinson's disease, and other neurological disorders.

While neurorehabilitation technology can include various types of devices, systems, and techniques, the focus of this chapter is to highlight examples of technologies with a proposed effect on neuroplasticity processes to improve sensory-motor neurorehabilitation. Selected neurorehabilitation technologies and their background in basic neuroscience will be described. The justification for these technologies will be discussed, considering how they may induce neuroplasticity.

The examples of neurorehabilitation technologies that will be described in this chapter include functional electrical stimulation (FES), robotic-assisted training, biofeedback, brain-computer interfaces (BCI), virtual reality (VR), augmented reality (AR), noninvasive brain stimulation (NIBS), body weight supported training (BWST), wearable sensors, and technology-supported home-based training (see Fig. 16.1).

Overall, these neurorehabilitation technologies play a crucial role in facilitating recovery, promoting independence, and enhancing the well-being of individuals with neurological impairments.

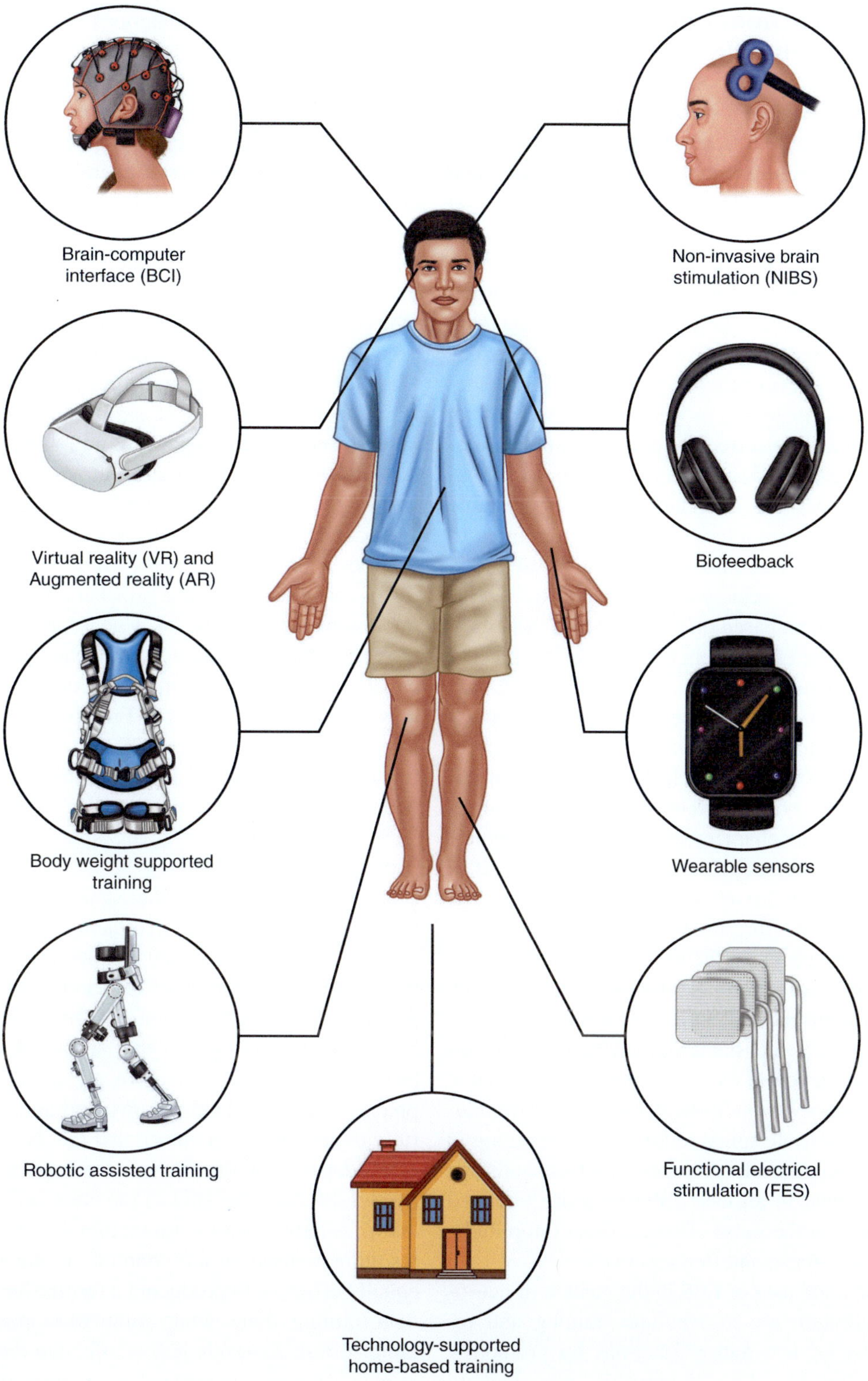

Fig. 16.1 Examples of sensory-motor neurorehabilitation technologies and locations where they can physically be applied

16.2 Functional Electrical Stimulation (FES)

Functional electrical stimulation (FES) is a technique that uses electronically generated electrical pulses to activate excitable body tissue to improve bodily functions. The simplest FES system is composed of an electrical stimulator connected through wires to a pair of electrodes placed on the surface of the skin above a nerve or muscle. FES can also be delivered through implanted electrodes that are in close contact with the excitable tissue. This could for example be a cuff electrode placed around a peripheral nerve or an epidural array electrode implanted on the lumbosacral spinal cord to deliver spinal cord stimulation. Deep brain stimulation uses implantable electrodes to stimulate deep brain structures to treat specific movement disorders. In all cases, the operating principle is similar, and it is explained here based on a surface FES system.

When the FES system is turned on, the electrical stimulator generates electrical pulses that result in an electric current that travels through the wires and is converted into an ion current at the electrode-skin interface. The ion current flows in the body between the electrodes and, if of appropriate characteristics, results in depolarization of the excitable underlying tissue. It is usually nerve tissue that depolarizes since its depolarization threshold is lower than that of muscle tissue. Once the nerve tissue depolarizes, the generated action potential propagates in both the orthodromic and antidromic directions. When the depolarized tissue is a motor nerve, the result is a contraction of the innervated muscles. When it is a sensory nerve instead, the sensory stimulation can activate spinal reflex circuits resulting in subsequent muscle responses and concomitant movements. In all cases, the response obtained depends on the pulse characteristics (amplitude, duration, shape, and frequency).

The main uses of FES in the context of neurorehabilitation are to facilitate training and relearning of lost motor functions by promoting neuroplasticity, i.e., therapeutic use, and to restore motor functions permanently, i.e., prosthetic use. Common therapeutic applications of FES focus on restoring functions such as reaching, grasping, or walking in a training context and during a limited time, aiming at achieving a level of functionality that will not require further FES assistance. The core concept is that intensive, personalized functional exercising with full engagement of the patient, who voluntarily attempts to execute the movements, is supported by FES to obtain the full execution of the task in training. Involvement of the patient, both in planning the functional movement and attempting to execute it, is crucial for motor re-learning (see Chap. 7). FES is then provided synchronously to facilitate the activation of single muscles or a range of coordinated agonistic and antagonistic muscles, to obtain the desired movement. FES-supported movement execution provides sensory feedback to the central nervous system and an experience of success, both of which are essential for motor re-learning. The prosthetic use of FES implies a sustained use of a neuroprosthesis to replace a lost or severely diminished function, under the premise that with no stimulation, no or very limited function exists. From a technological point of view, surface FES systems are used for both therapeutic and prosthetic purposes, while the span broadens to include implantable FES systems when prosthetic applications are considered.

Carry-over effects of therapeutic FES interventions outlasting the treatment period have been shown for various applications and target groups, such as training of gait and grasping in people with a stroke or spinal cord injury. The carry-over effect suggests that sustained neuroplastic changes had taken place, and although the precise neural mechanisms involved are still not fully understood, it is known that the therapeutic effect depends on the attempted voluntary activity and the characteristics of the electrical stimulation. Suprathreshold stimulation interventions resulting in fused muscle contractions are at least equally effective in producing a restorative effect than training alone, while stimulation at around motor-threshold levels is less effective (Howlett et al., 2015). To understand the central mechanisms behind these effects, research on healthy individuals has investigated how the stimulation parameters affect the excitability of the corticospinal pathways. For suprathreshold stimulation, the stimulation intensity, and to a lesser extent the stimulation duration, were the parameters that modulated most of the excitability of the corticospinal pathways; the same results were not consistently seen for low-intensity stimulation (Chipchase et al., 2011). Changes mainly in the somatosensory and motor brain areas, but also in the connections between brain areas and spinal projections, have been associated with the use of neuromuscular stimulation, but a definitive, causal relationship between said changes and functional gains, such as improved grasping and gait is still lacking.

16.3 Robotic-Assisted Training

Robotic devices are designed to assist movement execution by using external forces to drive body parts and/or counteract the force of gravity. Active robotic systems for movement training move the limb(s) of the patient through a predefined path mainly using electromechanical actuation, although pneumatic actuation can be found in some systems as well. Active robotic systems are operated using traditional position control schemes to move, for example, the arm of a patient from one position to another using a certain velocity profile. Interactive robotic systems react to the inputs from the patient to provide an optimal assistance strategy, facilitating the creation of dynamic rehabilitation tasks, where the patient becomes part of the control loop and receives support according to their abilities. Passive systems are not actuated, constrain the limb to a determined range of motion, and often consist of mechanical linkages, connected with spring mechanisms, that move easily when pushed and have an antigravity effect.

Robotic systems can be categorized according to how they control and drive the movement of the body into end-effector and exoskeleton systems. End-effector systems interact with the patient using a single distal attachment point. They control the kinematics of the endpoint but not that of the proximal segments and joints. For example, an end-effector system with a single attachment point near the wrist would result in several possible shoulder and elbow movements, while a system with a single attachment point at the foot, would result in movement of the entire leg with no control of the precise positioning of the knee joint. Exoskeleton-based systems encapsulate the body part to move, e.g., the arm, the hand, or the leg, providing the opportunity to fully control the orientation and velocity of the movement, by actuating all relevant segments. Exoskeletons can be made of rigid materials or soft materials to which exotendons are attached. Some soft exoskeletons have gained use as assistive devices.

In neurorehabilitation, robotic systems can provide highly repetitive movement training to address patients' nonuse issues and movement relearning, while simultaneously assisting physiotherapists in delivering the intervention. Basic principles of motor learning including movement repetition, training specificity, and intensity are thus targeted by robotic-assisted training (see Chap. 7). Some systems incorporate video gaming and virtual/augmented reality technology with haptic, visual, and audio feedback or cues to increase the motivation to train longer and more efficiently. Spinal and supraspinal plasticity-mediated effects might be partially responsible for the benefits experienced by the patients.

The post-training effect observed in the walking ability of stroke patients seems indistinct of the device used to train, but the likelihood of becoming an independent walker increases when training with a combination of robotic- and physiotherapy-based gait training. Best results were obtained when patients were nonambulatory at inclusion, when they trained in the subacute poststroke phase, and when they used end-effector robots instead of exoskeletons (Bruni et al., 2018). Regarding arm and hand training poststroke, improvements in arm function and muscle strength might be expected but results are not conclusive due to the large variability in training protocols (Mehrholz et al., 2018).

16.4 Biofeedback

Biofeedback, which has existed since the late 60s and is grounded in basic research on human self-regulation of physiology, is a form of technology used to modify human behaviors, (neuro-) physiological processes, and states of consciousness. Broadly, it uses electronic instruments to measure physiological processes in an individual and provide instantaneous or "real-time" feedback to enhance the individual's awareness of these processes, to help them gain voluntary control and modify their physiology. Technically, a biofeedback system is one that "senses, processes, and feeds a person's bodily functions, parameters and (or) states back to the person through one or more sensory modalities" (Kos & Umek, 2018). Due to the abundance of available electronic instruments for measuring various aspects of the body, it is practical to provide biofeedback for various purposes (e.g., motor rehabilitation, relaxation therapy, respiratory and cardiovascular regulation). Users can receive feedback on a wide range of physiological/biomechanical variables (e.g., muscle activity, posture, joint motion, heart rate variability) through sensory stimuli across a range of modalities (e.g., vision, audition, touch) (Kos & Umek, 2018). With the flexibility and power of modern digital technology, the feedback can be presented in a myriad of interesting and intuitive formats (e.g., 3-D virtual environments, synthesized sounds, and computer games), making biofeedback systems adaptable to suit the needs and capacities of a wide range of potential users (children and adults, cognitively impaired or otherwise) (Hribernik et al., 2022).

In neurorehabilitation, biofeedback is primarily used to support motor relearning by leveraging neuroplasticity (Sigrist et al., 2013). It has been established that timely and task-relevant sensory feedback is crucial to motor learning (see Chap. 7), and that multimodal feedback (i.e., distributed across multiple sensory modalities) is more effective than unimodal feedback due to increased precision of perception, neuronal activity, and neural representation (Sigrist et al., 2013) at the neural level. For instance, auditory biofeedback can be used during upper or lower limb rehabilitation to add a sonic feedback component to otherwise silent movements (e.g., sit-to-stand), helping reallocate perceptual and cognitive workload while providing useful concurrent feedback on movement (Sigrist et al., 2013). The integration of this novel *extrinsic* information channel with existing *intrinsic* channels (e.g., vision, proprioception) can lead to more robust internal representations of movement, serving to facilitate and accelerate motor relearning (Sigrist et al., 2013). Biofeedback can additionally improve patient motivation and engagement, reducing the need for ongoing contact with and monitoring by healthcare professionals. Biofeedback systems need to be set up and configured prior to training (mounting sensing hardware, configuring training goals and feedback stimuli) to cater to variability in terms of patient-specific needs and goals; most systems are therefore operated by therapists present during the training session, although systems for home-based independent use by patients have also been tested successfully (Hribernik et al., 2022).

In patient populations and various supervised clinical and home-based settings, biofeedback can bring about moderate-to-large effects immediately after treatment and larger effects than with conventional therapy. However, its potential is not fully realized due to a current lack of understanding of the "best" way to provide feedback on movement (e.g., direct simultaneous feedback on joint motion or error-based feedback relative to a target kinematic pattern) due to a lack of integration of motor learning principles into feedback design and a lack of systematic comparisons between feedback variants for the same movement (Sigrist et al., 2013). In general, real-time biofeedback is a relatively new area of research, and it is anticipated that biofeedback systems and applications will eventually become important training tools for patients in a variety of settings as the technology continues to improve and its production costs continue to fall (Hribernik et al., 2022). Given the rate of advancement in the field of multimodal interaction systems (especially virtual reality, tangible interfaces, and gesture-based interfaces), it is plausible to expect that biofeedback systems will become progressively more ubiquitous in clinical and home-based rehabilitation settings alike within the foreseeable future, serving as an important enhancement to conventional training protocols and benefiting a wide range of patients in the process.

16.5 Brain-Computer Interfaces (BCIs)

A brain-computer interface (BCI) is a direct communication pathway between the activity of the brain and an external output device, such as a computer, exoskeleton, robotic limb, or functional electrical stimulator. The primary components involved in most current BCI systems include recording neural signals from the brain (for example during motor imagery or actual movement intention by the user), processing these signals through a computer algorithm, and translating the processed signals into an intended action using an end-effector device. BCIs therefore do not use the normal neuromuscular output pathways, which may be damaged in neurological conditions such as stroke, spinal cord injury, cerebral palsy, or multiple sclerosis.

In terms of treating neurological patients and improving their quality of life, the two main strategies of BCI are to either (1) replace or (2) restore useful functions. Strategy one for replacing function, also named assistive BCI, aims to completely bypass the damaged neuronal pathways by providing a continuous and permanent alternative for communication and control of external devices, including exoskeletons or robotic limbs (Mane et al., 2020). Strategy two for restoring function, named rehabilitative BCI, aims for the functional recovery of damaged neuronal networks and thereby the restoration of impaired functional capabilities by effective facilitation of neuroplasticity (Mane et al., 2020). Since functional independence and a return to daily life without the need for any assistive devices are desired, rehabilitative BCIs are preferred in neurorehabilitation.

In general, there are different techniques for recording neural signals for BCIs, ranging from invasively implanted microelectrode arrays in the brain to noninvasive techniques, based on how close electrodes get to the neural tissue of the brain. Noninvasive recording techniques in rehabilitative BCI include electroencephalography (EEG), magnetoencephalography (MEG), electrooculography (EOG), and magnetic resonance imaging (MRI).

Primary implementations of external output devices for rehabilitative BCI focused on motor recovery include functional electrical stimulation (FES), virtual reality (VR), exoskeletons, and robotic devices. These have primarily been tested in stroke patients and to a lesser degree in spinal cord injury and cerebral palsy patients. The rationale for combining BCI systems with these therapies is to deliver high-repetition movement practice and potentially increase neuroplasticity by engaging Hebbian-type learning mechanisms by augmenting the sensorimotor feedback loop (Mane et al., 2020) (see Chap. 7).

A recent systematic review of randomized controlled trials found that EEG-based BCI has significant immediate and long-term effects in improving upper-limb motor functions after stroke compared to conventional therapies (Mansour et al., 2022). Specifically, the review found the highest effect sizes in BCIs utilizing the intention of movement as the user input and FES as the feedback technique.

16.6 Noninvasive Brain Stimulation (NIBS)

Noninvasive brain stimulation (NIBS) employs electrical or magnetically induced currents to stimulate the brain through the scalp and can temporarily excite or inhibit activity in target brain regions. Currently, the two most common NIBS techniques are transcranial magnetic stimulation (TMS) and transcranial direct current stimulation (tDCS).

While single- and paired-pulse TMS techniques can be used to assess neurophysiological processes, such as the integrity of the corticospinal and corticobulbar tracts, repetitive TMS (rTMS) techniques can be used as a neuromodulatory tool to influence brain function (Liew et al., 2014). rTMS induces frequency and intensity-specific after-effects. Low-frequency stimulation (≤1 Hz) induces a decrease in cortical excitability while high-frequency stimulation (≥5 Hz) results in an increase in cortical excitability for at least 30 min (Liew et al., 2014). Depending on the specific stimulation protocol used, the neuromodulatory effects of rTMS can outlast the stimulation period by several minutes to hours.

Another form of rTMS is patterned rTMS. It consists of the repetitive application of short rTMS bursts at a high stimulation frequency. Theta burst stimulation (TBS) is the most common paradigm, where short bursts of 50 Hz rTMS are applied at a rate in the theta range (5 Hz). As with low- and high-frequency rTMS, continuous TBS (cTBS) and intermittent TBS (iTBS) induce cortical depression and facilitation, respectively, for up to 70 min. Paired associative stimulation (PAS) is a related technique that involves the application of a peripheral nerve stimulus followed by a single TMS pulse at specific interstimulus intervals aimed at increasing the excitability of the corticospinal pathways.

tDCS is applied using a direct current (DC) generator connected to two anodal and cathodal sponge-enclosed rubber electrodes positioned over the scalp. It is thought that low-amplitude currents (ranging from 0.5 to 2.0 mA) applied at the scalp can partially penetrate and reach cortical tissues. In contrast to TMS, tDCS does not result in the induction of action potentials. tDCS seems to modify the threshold for the discharge of cortical neurons. tDCS can modulate cortical excitability in a polarity-dependent fashion. While anodal stimulation increases cortical excitability, cathodal stimulation is thought to decrease it. Both produce after-effects lasting 30–40 min, following 15–30 min of stimulation, with the after-effects strongly dependent on the duration and intensity of the stimulation.

Generally, NIBS is thought to modulate neural activity via differing mechanisms, such as the induction of LTP-like protocols (see Chap. 6). It has been proposed that modulation of these mechanisms induces motor plasticity, contributing to motor learning and secondarily impacting the neurorehabilitation process (Liew et al., 2014) (see Chap. 13). Although their mechanisms are different, these NIBS techniques can be used to induce plasticity at the systems level, to examine the neurophysiology of brain circuits, and have potential therapeutic use in psychiatric and neurological disorders. A recent review with meta-analysis found evidence suggesting that excitatory stimulation protocols are the most promising NIBS interventions in improving upper limb motor function and performance in activities of daily living poststroke (Ahmed et al., 2023).

16.7 Virtual Reality (VR) and Augmented Reality (AR)

Virtual reality (VR) and augmented reality (AR) are two related technologies that allow for the ability to create new and exciting interactive neurorehabilitation experiences. VR uses a headset to place the patient in a computer-generated world that can be explored, while AR takes digital images and layers them on the real world viewed by the patient using either a clear visor, tablet, or smartphone.

Both VR and AR technologies are growing at a rapid pace and are being implemented within neurorehabilitation in a variety of different ways. VR and AR can aid conventional therapeutic interventions by providing the opportunity for more varied and engaging tasks, thereby increasing patient motivation and dedication to completing the treatment (Kouijzer et al., 2023). Furthermore, neurorehabilitation in VR and AR environments can provide patients and therapists with an adaptable and customizable experience, since modifying the virtual components of a rehabilitation environment is much easier than doing the same for traditional, physical environments.

Together, VR/AR systems can be categorized into game-based and nongame-based subtypes (Kouijzer et al., 2023). Game-based systems offer combinations of patient exertion and video games, allowing for gamification principles to make traditionally repetitive and tedious rehabilitation programs more engaging for patients. Nongame-based systems typically mimic real-world training conditions more closely, potentially allowing for safer and more controlled rehabilitative environments. Both systems can provide objective information about the progress and quality of the task and encourage patients to be actively involved in the rehabilitation process. Therefore, VR/AR could be incorporated as a tool for assessing neurological recovery during the rehabilitation process. Moreover, VR/AR neurorehabilitation could be implemented remotely by a specialist for nearly immediate results available for interpretation, allowing for more flexible home-based training solutions.

VR and AR systems can target cognitive, motor, and sensory rehabilitation. Examples of these technologies include systems designed to focus selectively on discrete cognitive abilities, including attention, executive functions, and language and memory abilities. Many VR/AR systems are based on conventional neurorehabilitation treatments such as mirror therapy, reach and grasp movements, virtual nine-hole peg tests, and balance and gait-based training tasks like visually guided stepping.

Most of the initial studies investigating the use of VR/AR systems as an adjunct to conventional neurorehabilitation therapies show promising results and suggest that they are feasible and effective tools in the treatment of neurological disorders (Kouijzer et al., 2023). However, comprehensive research is still limited. The lack of standardization within clinical neurorehabilitation trials and across VR/AR systems may lead to differing results. Further, some individuals using VR/AR reported limited mobility and experiences of nausea and headaches. Despite these challenges, the continued development of VR/AR technologies may provide treatment options that enhance neuroplasticity and patient engagement in task-oriented, repetitive, and intensive training environments as well as offer more flexibility and independence for both therapists and patients throughout the rehabilitation process (see Chap. 15).

16.8 Body Weight Supported Training

Body weight support (BWS) systems are technologies that partially support the weight of the body to facilitate movement execution. Patients and therapists can then focus on training gait, balance, grasping, and releasing while reducing the percentage of body weight support as recovery and relearning happen. When training gait, BWS systems have the additional function of preventing falls and allowing patients with limited strength to exercise while providing as little support as possible, so the patient engages actively in producing varied movements. Active participation and training specificity and variability are crucial for motor learning (see Chap. 15).

Systems to provide arm weight support, also called gravity-compensated systems can facilitate movement excursion and work area by reducing the synergistic coupling of the shoulder and elbow during training, which benefits the upper limb functionality, e.g., people with multiple sclerosis.

Weight-bearing during hemiparetic treadmill gait training was introduced in the 80s and it was inspired by animal research on recovery of locomotion in spinal cord injured cats. Since then, subacute and chronic stroke patients, patients with incomplete spinal cord injuries, Parkinson's disease, cerebral palsy, and multiple sclerosis have been offered body BWS treadmill training. BWS can be provided by different technologies. In harness-based BWS systems, the patient wears a body harness that has an overhead attachment to a frame or a ceiling-mounted rail and provides a lifting force that can be static or dynamic. Static systems provide fixed unloading, which might perturb the natural physiological gait pattern characterized by vertical movements of the trunk throughout the gait cycle. Dynamic systems measure the vertical position or force and use them to control the position or force, providing a close-to-normal vertical trunk kinematic. Harness-based BWS systems are available for treadmill and overground training, and in the latter case, they can support training along a trajectory dictated by the position of a ceiling-mounted rail or free-walking when the harness is suspended from a movable structure on wheels. Harness-based BWS systems rely on the harness to partially unload the body weight and in many situations, physiotherapists must assist patients in controlling balance and mobilizing the legs. Robot-assisted BWS addresses the latter by counteracting the effect of gravity while simultaneously actuating on the lower limbs. Robot-assisted unloading and mobilization are addressed in the section about robotics, but a particular mention of saddle-based BWS systems is made here. Movement of the pelvis is natural during walking thus, facilitating pelvic movements during gait training is desirable to enhance motor relearning by training movements as close to normal as possible. This can be achieved by saddle-based BWS systems, which apart from unloading the body, support displacement of the pelvis in the vertical, transverse, and frontal directions, and rotation in the frontal and transverse planes.

Lower body positive pressure systems can also provide BWS during treadmill training. In this case, the treadmill and the lower body of the patient are placed in a bag-like compartment that is inflated to reduce the body weight, facilitating safe gait training. In poststroke, lower body positive pressure supported gait training resulted in increased walking velocity and functional ambulation, but more research is needed to understand, e.g., the relation between unloading and muscle activation.

Body weight unloading results in reduced muscle activity, energy cost, and ground reaction forces, and for a body weight unloading of up to 30%, the kinematic patterns remain roughly similar, which might be beneficial for gait training. In overground walking, and depending on the BWS system used, energy consumption might be affected by the need to carry the BWS system in the direction of walking. BWS during treadmill training has shown positive results on gait velocity and gross motor function in children and adolescents with cerebral palsy; and it has improved the clinical severity of patients with Parkinson's disease and the lower limb motor function of patients with spinal cord injury (for reviews, see Alotaibi et al., 2024; Lorenzo-García et al., 2021; Huang et al., 2024). For stroke patients, even though no superiority of BWS gait training on outcomes such as gait velocity and balance was shown, there are indications that people who can walk when starting training, seem to profit from BWS gait training (Mehrholz et al., 2017).

16.9 Wearable Sensors

Wearable motion sensors are small, light, noninvasive electronic devices that can be worn or mated with human skin/clothes to monitor physical activity continuously without interrupting or limiting movement. This technology provides objective and quantifiable information about functional capabilities and may allow interactive (bio) feedback. Because wearable sensors are easy to wear, they may also provide continuous long-term motion monitoring.

Various sensors can track physical activity. In the study of human motion, the most frequently used are accelerometers, inertial measurement units (IMUs), and surface electromyography (sEMG). IMUs combine data from accelerometers and gyroscopes and are often used because of their ability to detect motion accurately in time and space. Accelerometers and IMUs detect motion from the body segment they are attached to, whereas sEMG detects activity from the underlying muscle. Assessment of physical activity can be obtained by one or multiple sensors depending on the recording's purpose. For example, the use of a single accelerometer can track simple movements of the forearm, but tracking more complex motion requires either additional sensors or more advanced data analysis techniques (e.g., machine learning or artificial intelligence). Tracking motion during the execution of daily life is particularly difficult in neurological patients as movements are often slower, more segmented, and more variable than movements of healthy individuals. The use of a smartwatch to obtain valid measures such as steps may therefore be subjected to uncertainty because the algorithm used in such a device is based on regular walking patterns. To ensure valid and precise detection of performed movements among patients, the underlying algorithm must be adapted to these different movement patterns and/or combined with more sensors. For example, multiple sensors enable observation of limb neglect by looking at the symmetry (or lack thereof) in sensor readings from the affected and unaffected sides.

Quantifying motor ability by wearable sensors may have multiple purposes that can optimize the outcome of neurorehabilitation and induce neuroplasticity. For example, in the early (remote) diagnosis of a disease, a jumpsuit, equipped with movement sensors tracking infant spontaneous movements can provide early insight into movement abnormalities and enable early intervention optimizing impact on development (Airaksinen et al., 2022). In addition, IMUs may also objectively, and time efficiently assess hand and arm stages of clinical scores poststroke allowing clinicians to assess and monitor function and progress accurately (MacEira-Elvira et al., 2019). IMUs may also be useful in the prediction of rehabilitation outcomes and thereby improve the opportunity to tailor rehabilitation programs. Another possibility of application is continuous tracking (for days and weeks) assessing quality, range, and/or dose of movements. This provides an opportunity to evaluate rehabilitation as it occurs during daily life activities and the adherence to home-based rehabilitation. In this context, data ownership and ethical aspects of data use are important aspects to consider. Finally, wearables can be used to give interactive, timely, and meaningful feedback to patients guiding and motivating progressive skills practice, for example by delivering sensory cues or providing objective performance feedback (see Chap. 15). A variety of available systems combine wearable sensors with a gamification element, again to ensure and enhance motivation for (independent) practice.

The technical properties of modern wearable motion sensors demonstrate excellent test-retest reliability and validity for assessing movement. However, for wider-spread adoption of wearables in neurorehabilitation, understanding the end-use must go hand-in-hand with technology development. The efficacy of these sensors is primarily evaluated in short-term experiments. Routine and longer-term use of wearables introduces many challenges that are not addressed in short clinical studies, such as durability, power consumption, comfort, and usability. Although the transition toward the integration of these devices into clinical practice represents an extra effort, it can reduce costs once it becomes ubiquitous.

16.10 Technology-Supported Home-Based Training

The basic form of home-based training consists of a training program prescribed by a therapist and performed regularly and independently by the patient at home. With the increasing integration of information- and communications technology into the everyday lives of many people, new opportunities have emerged to facilitate home-based training. For example, technology may provide a sensory stimulus to promote a specific activity, e.g., an auditory stimulus to facilitate a certain rhythm or a visual stimulus to enhance motivation. Sensory stimuli may also motivate the individual to perform at a certain tempo. For example, it has been shown that treadmill training at home with feedback on gait speed and walking distance can effectively increase training volume for individuals with CP and induce significant functional improvements.

A further level of technology may be added to the home-based training by including interactivity between a sensory stimulus and the actions of the individual. This type of interaction is the basis of video gaming and is therefore achievable by modifying video games into exercise sessions through special sensors or controllers, also sometimes referred to as exergaming. Elements from e.g., biofeedback and VR may be adopted, and motivation and neuroplastic changes may be promoted by the embedded necessity of active participation and through different types of feedback and rewards (see Chaps. 7 and 15).

Finally, communication technology may facilitate interaction between the patient training at home and the therapist in the clinic. With recent developments in computer technology, the possibility of delivering and supervising individually targeted training through the Internet has emerged. For example, a web-based system called Mitii enables the transfer of an individualized training program through the Internet. It consists of a server-based interactive training system using Flash technology. These improvements in technology also allow the therapist to act as a remote personal coach. It has been demonstrated that it is possible to provide a large amount of training with positive results and at low costs (Comans et al., 2017). Another system with a similar methodology that can provide effective home-based training is called CareToy (Sgandurra et al., 2017). This system is based on an interactive enriched environment individually designed to meet the needs of infants born prematurely with an increased risk of developing CP. Mitii, CareToy, and similar internet-based training methods have shown great potential in incorporating important recommendations for neurorehabilitation such as intensifying training dose, individualizing training, setting goals, assessing progress, enabling immediate feedback to facilitate performance during the training, and providing long-term feedback to facilitate motivation.

To sum up, home-based training, with the addition of technological solutions, can be of notable value to neurorehabilitation by promoting various factors of neuroplasticity. Generally, home-based training can promote a larger training volume and more flexible scheduling according to the needs of the individual. With the addition of technology, important neuroplastic factors such as goal setting, feedback, rewards, and motivation can be stimulated, enabling better results (see Chap. 15). However, factors such as progressive challenges, variation, and ensuring the highest level of active participation most often, require a therapist to interact with the system and ensure that these factors are regularly aligned, making it more expensive and labor-intensive. Identifying the most important factors of the specific neurorehabilitation program is key to implementing technology-supported home-based training.

16.11 Opportunities, Challenges, and Future Directions

16.11.1 Opportunities

Neurorehabilitation technologies offer numerous opportunities to improve the outcomes and quality of life for individuals with neurological conditions.

- **Enhanced Rehabilitation Outcomes:** Neurorehabilitation technologies can provide targeted, intensive, and personalized interventions to facilitate recovery and functional improvement in individuals with neurological impairments. The neurorehabilitation technologies addressed in this chapter can promote neuroplasticity, restore motor function, enhance sensory perception, and improve cognitive abilities.
- **Personalized Interventions:** Neurorehabilitation technologies can tailor interventions to individual patient characteristics, preferences, and needs, optimizing treatment efficacy and engagement.
- **Hybrid Solutions:** Hybrid neurorehabilitation technology solutions combining multiple modalities may leverage the strengths of different technologies to enhance rehabilitation outcomes. For example, combining robotic assistance with functional electrical stimulation and virtual reality exercises can provide immersive, engaging, and task-specific training that promotes motor learning and recovery.
- **Augmentation of Traditional Therapies:** Neurorehabilitation technologies complement traditional rehabilitation approaches by providing additional modalities for motor learning, sensory retraining, and functional task practice. Integrating technology-enhanced interventions into existing rehabilitation programs may therefore enhance therapeutic outcomes, motivate patients, and diversify treatment options.
- **Early Intervention:** Advances in neuroimaging, wearable sensors, and mobile health technologies enable early detection of neurological changes and monitoring of disease progression. Neurorehabilitation interventions delivered at the earliest stages of injury or disease onset have the potential to prevent secondary complications, mitigate disability, and optimize long-term outcomes.
- **Home-Based and Remote Rehabilitation:** Telemedicine, mobile apps, and wearable devices enable the delivery of neurorehabilitation interventions in the comfort of patients'

homes, extending access to care, reducing healthcare costs, and overcoming geographical barriers. Remote monitoring and telerehabilitation platforms also facilitate continuity of care, ongoing assessment, and support for self-management and adherence to treatment regimens.
- **Research and Innovation:** Neurorehabilitation technologies drive advancements in basic science, clinical research, and technological innovation, fostering collaboration among researchers, clinicians, engineers, and industry partners. By elucidating the underlying mechanisms of recovery, identifying novel therapeutic targets, and developing innovative interventions, these technologies contribute to the continuous improvement of rehabilitation practice and the development of next-generation treatments.

16.11.2 Challenges

While neurorehabilitation technologies offer promising opportunities for improving outcomes and quality of life for individuals with neurological conditions, they also face several challenges that need to be addressed in the future.

- **Complexity and Customization:** Neurological conditions vary widely in their manifestations and severity, requiring personalized approaches to rehabilitation. Designing technologies that can adapt to individual needs and provide effective interventions for diverse conditions is a significant challenge.
- **Understanding the Neurophysiological Mechanisms:** By understanding the underlying mechanisms of neurorehabilitation, the overall effectiveness of technologies may improve. However, there are several challenges including the complexity of the nervous system, heterogeneity of neurological conditions, the temporal dynamics of recovery, the limitations of current research methods including neuroimaging and neurophysiological techniques, and translations into clinical practice.
- **Translation into Clinical Practice:** Implementing neurorehabilitation technologies into clinical settings requires overcoming barriers such as regulatory approval, reimbursement issues, and clinician training. Adoption may be slow due to skepticism, cost concerns, or lack of awareness about the benefits of these technologies. Furthermore, technology often requires expert knowledge to maintain and utilize the systems effectively, posing challenges for both clinicians and users.
- **Evidence-Based Validation:** Despite growing interest and investment in neurorehabilitation technologies, robust scientific evidence supporting their effectiveness is often lacking. Conducting well-designed clinical trials and longitudinal studies to evaluate the outcomes and long-term impacts of these interventions is essential for establishing their efficacy and guiding clinical practice. This includes discovering best practices within the specific technologies (for example stimulation parameters in FES and NIBS) and knowing when to use different neurorehabilitation technologies and for how long to maximize their effects.
- **Ethical and Privacy Considerations:** Neurorehabilitation technologies may involve the collection and analysis of sensitive data related to patients' neurological function and health status. Ensuring the privacy, confidentiality, and ethical use of patient information while leveraging technology for rehabilitation purposes is a significant concern that requires careful attention and regulatory oversight.
- **User Acceptance and Adherence:** Acceptance and adherence to neurorehabilitation technologies by patients and caregivers can be influenced by factors such as usability, comfort, perceived benefits, and motivation. Ensuring that technologies are user-friendly, engaging, and compatible with patients' needs and preferences is critical for maximizing their effectiveness. It is therefore important to consider the opinions of the end users when designing and testing neurorehabilitation technologies.

- **Interdisciplinary Collaboration:** Effective neurorehabilitation often requires a multidisciplinary approach involving professionals from diverse fields such as neuroscience, rehabilitation medicine, engineering, psychology, and computer science. Facilitating collaboration and communication among experts with different backgrounds and expertise can be challenging but is essential for developing comprehensive and integrated rehabilitation strategies.

16.11.3 Future Directions

The future of neurorehabilitation technologies holds tremendous promise. Embracing the opportunities and addressing the challenges posed by neurorehabilitation technologies in the future will require concerted efforts from researchers, clinicians, engineers, and patients to advance the field of neurorehabilitation and harness the full potential of technology to improve outcomes for individuals with neurological conditions.

A one-size-fits-all approach to neurorehabilitation does not work, and neurorehabilitation technologies will provide personalized precision neurorehabilitation tailored to individual patient characteristics. Advances in big data analytics, machine learning, and artificial intelligence will enable the analysis of large datasets to identify biomarkers, predict treatment responses, and optimize rehabilitation strategies. Data-driven approaches will facilitate precision medicine in neurorehabilitation, guide clinical decision-making, personalize treatment plans, and improve patient outcomes through evidence-based practice.

It should be noted that all the above does not mean that neurorehabilitation technologies will fully replace traditional methods of neurorehabilitation. However, neurorehabilitation technologies occupy an important place within the field and can effectively complement traditional therapies.

Overall, the future perspectives of neurorehabilitation technologies hold immense potential to revolutionize the field of rehabilitation, transform the care of individuals with neurological conditions, and promote recovery, independence, and quality of life. By embracing innovation, collaboration, and interdisciplinary approaches, researchers, clinicians, and engineers can harness the power of technology to address the complex challenges of neurological rehabilitation and reveal new opportunities for patient-centered care and functional recovery.

Review Questions

- How may neurorehabilitation technologies induce neuroplasticity?
- How can neurorehabilitation technology improve motivation for training in patients with neurological disorders?
- How can technology be used to make neurorehabilitation more individualized for both the patient and clinician?
- How should the efficiency of new neurorehabilitation technologies be demonstrated? (Stevenson et al., 2024)

References

Ahmed, I., Mustafaoglu, R., Rossi, S., et al. (2023). Non-invasive brain stimulation techniques for the improvement of upper limb motor function and performance in activities of daily living after stroke: A systematic review and network meta-analysis. *Archives of Physical Medicine and Rehabilitation, 104*(10), 1683–1697. https://doi.org/10.1016/j.apmr.2023.04.027

Airaksinen, M., Gallen, A., Kivi, A., et al. (2022). Intelligent wearable allows out-of-the-lab tracking of developing motor abilities in infants. *Communications Medicine, 2*(1), 69. https://doi.org/10.1038/s43856-022-00131-6

Alotaibi, A., Ibrahim, A., Ahmed, R., et al. (2024). Effectiveness of partial body weight-supported treadmill training on various outcomes in different contexts among children and adolescents with cerebral palsy: A systematic review and meta-analysis. *Children (Basel), 11*(1), 9. https://doi.org/10.3390/children11010009

Bruni, M. F., Melegari, C., De Cola, M. C., et al. (2018). What does best evidence tell us about robotic gait rehabilitation in stroke patients: A systematic review and meta-analysis. *Journal of Clinical Neuroscience, 48*, 11–17. https://doi.org/10.1016/j.jocn.2017.10.048

Chipchase, L. S., Schabrun, S. M., & Hodges, P. W. (2011). Peripheral electrical stimulation to induce cortical plasticity: A systematic review of stimulus parameters.

Clinical Neurophysiology, 122(3), 456–463. https://doi.org/10.1016/j.clinph.2010.07.025

Comans, T., Mihala, G., Sakzewski, L., et al. (2017). The cost-effectiveness of a web-based multimodal therapy for unilateral cerebral palsy: The Mitii randomized controlled trial. *Developmental Medicine and Child Neurology, 59*(7), 756–761. https://doi.org/10.1111/dmcn.13414

Howlett, O. A., Lannin, N. A., Ada, L., et al. (2015). Functional electrical stimulation improves activity after stroke: A systematic review with meta-analysis. *Archives of Physical Medicine and Rehabilitation, 96*(5), 934–943. https://doi.org/10.1016/j.apmr.2015.01.013

Hribernik, M., Umek, A., Tomazic, S., et al. (2022). Review of real-time biomechanical feedback systems in sport and rehabilitation. *Sensors-Basel, 22*(8), 3006. https://doi.org/10.3390/s22083006

Huang, L., Huang, H. L., Dang, X. W., et al. (2024). Effect of body weight support training on lower extremity motor function in patients with spinal cord injury: A systematic review and meta-analysis. *American Journal of Physical Medicine & Rehabilitation, 103*(2), 149–157. https://doi.org/10.1097/PHM.0000000000002320

Kos, A., & Umek, A. (2018). *Biomechanical biofeedback systems and applications*. Springer International Publishing.

Kouijzer, M. M. T. E., Kip, H., Bouman, Y. H. A., et al. (2023). Implementation of virtual reality in healthcare: A scoping review on the implementation process of virtual reality in various healthcare settings. *Implementation Science Communications, 4*(1), 67. https://doi.org/10.1186/s43058-023-00442-2

Liew, S. L., Santarnecchi, E., Buch, E. R., et al. (2014). Non-invasive brain stimulation in neurorehabilitation: Local and distant effects for motor recovery. *Frontiers in Human Neuroscience, 8*, 378. https://doi.org/10.3389/fnhum.2014.00378

Lorenzo-García, P., Cavero-Redondo, I., Torres-Costoso, A., et al. (2021). Body weight support gait training for patients with Parkinson disease: A systematic review and meta-analyses. *Archives of Physical Medicine and Rehabilitation, 102*(10), 2012–2021. https://doi.org/10.1016/j.apmr.2021.02.016

MacEira-Elvira, P., Popa, T., Schmid, A. C., et al. (2019). Wearable technology in stroke rehabilitation: Towards improved diagnosis and treatment of upper-limb motor impairment. *Journal of Neuroengineering and Rehabilitation, 16*(1), 142. https://doi.org/10.1186/s12984-019-0612-y

Mane, R., Chouhan, T., & Guan, C. (2020). BCI for stroke rehabilitation: Motor and beyond. *Journal of Neural Engineering, 17*(4), 041001-2552/aba162. https://doi.org/10.1088/1741-2552/aba162

Mansour, S., Ang, K. K., Nair, K. P. S., et al. (2022). Efficacy of brain–computer interface and the impact of its design characteristics on poststroke upper-limb rehabilitation: A systematic review and meta-analysis of randomized controlled trials. *Clinical EEG and Neuroscience, 53*(1), 79–90. https://doi.org/10.1177/15500594211009065

Mehrholz, J., Thomas, S., & Elsner, B. (2017). Treadmill training and body weight support for walking after stroke. *Cochrane Database of Systematic Reviews, 2017*(8). https://doi.org/10.1002/14651858.CD002840.pub4

Mehrholz, J., Pohl, M., Platz, T., et al. (2018). Electromechanical and robot-assisted arm training for improving activities of daily living, arm function, and arm muscle strength after stroke. *Cochrane Database of Systematic Reviews, 2018*(9), CD006876. https://doi.org/10.1002/14651858.CD006876.pub5

Sgandurra, G., Lorentzen, J., Inguaggiato, E., et al. (2017). A randomized clinical trial in preterm infants on the effects of a home-based early intervention with the 'CareToy System'. *PLoS ONE, 12*(3), e0173521. https://doi.org/10.1371/journal.pone.0173521

Sigrist, R., Rauter, G., Riener, R., et al. (2013). Augmented visual, auditory, haptic, and multimodal feedback in motor learning: A review. *Psychonomic Bulletin & Review, 20*(1), 21–53. https://doi.org/10.3758/s13423-012-0333-8

Stevenson, A. J. T., Spaich, E. G., Kantan, P. R., Larsen, L. H., Lorentzen, J., & Sinkjær, T. (2024). Neurorehabilitation technologies chapter: complete list of references. https://doi.org/10.54337/aau720743491

Part III

Neurorehabilitation of Specific Neurological Disorders

Stroke

17

Carolynn Patten, Daniel Neudorf,
Ryan L. Nguyen, and Kwan L. Ng

Abstract

Stroke is leading cause of disability and second leading cause of death worldwide. Advances in acute and peri-acute stroke management have decreased stroke mortality by at least 65% such that there are currently more than 101 million people living with stroke sequelae representing a near doubling of the number of stroke survivors over the last 30 years. As a result, more effective and efficient rehabilitation interventions are needed to promote recovery of function following stroke, especially for younger individuals in the most vital and productive years of their lives. To this end, the field of neurorehabilitation has acknowledged neuroplasticity as the basis of neurorehabilitation and begun to incorporate knowledge from basic science demonstrating the central nervous system's capacity for experience-driven adaptation.

Neurorehabilitation incorporates a wide range of strategies and interventions aimed at promoting recovery of function. Rehabilitation practitioners play a key role in this process. Therefore, understanding the intersection between rehabilitation and neuroplasticity is important for developing effective rehabilitation interventions that optimize neural recovery and reorganization following stroke. The success of rehabilitation strategies in inducing neuroplasticity after a stroke depends not only on the type of interventions but also on their intensity, dose, and timing within the post-stroke recovery period.

Keywords

Stroke · Recovery · Neuroplasticity · Rehabilitation · Compensation · Poststroke-sensitive period · Capacity · Comorbidities

C. Patten (✉)
Biomechanics, Rehabilitation, and Integrative Neuroscience (BRaIN) Lab, Center for Neuroengineering and Medicine, Department of Physical Medicine & Rehabilitation, School of Medicine, VA Northern California Health Care System, University of California, Davis, Davis, CA, USA
e-mail: cpatten@ucdavis.edu

D. Neudorf
Inpatient Rehabilitation, Dominican Hospital, Santa Cruz, CA, USA
e-mail: Dr.Neurdorf@Daniel.Neudorf.com

R. L. Nguyen
Biomechanics, Rehabilitation, and Integrative Neuroscience (BRaIN) Lab, Department of Physical Medicine & Rehabilitation, School of Medicine, University of California, Davis, Davis, CA, USA
e-mail: rmqnguyen@ucdavis.edu

K. L. Ng
Department of Neurology, School of Medicine, University of California, Davis, Davis, CA, USA
e-mail: klng@ucdavis.edu

J. B. Nielsen et al. (eds.), *Neuroplasticity-based Neurorehabilitation*,
https://doi.org/10.1007/978-3-031-81120-3_17

Box 17.1 Case Study

Michelle, a 49-year-old right-hand dominant woman, presented to the emergency department of a community hospital with new onset left-sided weakness and neglect and right-sided gaze preference. Her medical history revealed: hypertension, coronary artery disease, 3-vessel coronary artery bypass graft (CABG), acute myocardial infarction, congestive heart failure, atrial fibrillation (without use of blood thinners), 30 pack-year history of tobacco use, and methamphetamine abuse. Michelle was found at home after failing to appear at work last known to be well (LKW) at 21:30 the prior evening. Initial CT imaging revealed an acute occlusion in the right middle cerebral artery (MCA) at the M1/M2 artery junction. The National Institutes of Health Stroke Scale (NIHSS) (Box 17.2) was 18/42. Tele-neurology consultation with a regional academic comprehensive stroke center determined LKW exceeded the temporal window for thrombolytic therapy but considered her a good candidate for mechanical thrombectomy.

On **transfer** and **admission** to the academic stroke center, Michelle was able to speak and follow commands. Examination revealed: no movement in either left upper or lower extremities, upgoing Babinski reflexes, left-sided facial droop, right-sided gaze deviation, dysarthria, diminished sensation in the left hemibody, extinction to double simultaneous stimulation, and left-sided neglect. The NIHSS had increased to 19/42 corresponding with moderately severe stroke. CT head perfusion imaging revealed a large perfusion mismatch. Michelle was taken for mechanical thrombectomy; complete perfusion was restored (i.e., TICI3) after one pass. Repeat CT showed moderate right MCA ischemic infarct. MRI revealed a moderate acute infarction on the right involving the basal ganglia, frontal lobe, temporal lobe, and insular cortex with additional small foci of acute infarction within the medial right frontal lobe and temporoparietal region, and a region of petechial hemorrhage in the right basal ganglia. The NIHSS was improved to 14/42 while the clinical exam was largely unchanged. She was admitted to the Neuro Intensive Care Unit (ICU).

Michelle's **right MCA stroke** was considered to result from cardioembolic etiology, secondary to atrial fibrillation. CT angiography of her neck revealed no carotid stenosis or significant atherosclerotic disease. She was not diabetic. Echocardiogram was unremarkable revealing an ejection fraction of 65% with normal atrial dimensions. During her acute hospital admission, she was started on apixaban and atorvastatin for secondary stroke prophylaxis, received smoking and substance use cessation counseling, and received physical, occupational, and speech therapies.

At **2 days poststroke** Michelle was downgraded from the ICU; she was discharged from the hospital and **admitted to acute inpatient rehabilitation on day 6.** She was nonambulatory, requiring maximum assistance for bed mobility and dressing and moderate assistance for transfers. She tolerated a soft diet and thin liquids. She revealed mild impairment in memory, thought organization, and problem-solving. During **inpatient rehabilitation,** she was seen by physicians and participated in 3 h of combined therapies (PT/OT/ST) daily, 6 days weekly. Her inpatient rehabilitation hospitalization was notable for a bout of suicidal ideation first noted on **day 11 poststroke**. A serotonin-epinephrine reuptake inhibitor (SNRI), duloxetine, was initiated, followed by an escalating dose regimen. Michelle worked with neuropsychology and her suicidal ideation was resolved.

Following 21 days of inpatient rehabilitation (**day 27 poststroke),** she was **discharged to home**. At discharge, her clinical

(continued)

Box 17.1 (continued)
examination was notable for improved left facial droop, left lower extremity weakness (4/5 proximally, 1/5 distally), antigravity strength in the left upper extremity, improved dysarthria, and NIHSS 12/42. Michelle tolerated a regular diet, performed bed mobility and transfers independently, and required contact guard assistance when performing ADLs and ambulating up to 25 m on level surfaces.

Per phone follow-up at **90 days post-stroke,** a Modified Rankin Score (mRS) of 2 (of 5) reflected slight disability.[1]

17.1 Epidemiology

Stroke is the leading cause of disability and second leading cause of death worldwide. The World Stroke Organization (WSO) reports stroke incidence of 12.2 million new strokes annually, an increase of 18.5% between 1990 and 2019 (Feigin et al., 2022). The risk of stroke has increased leading to the current expectation that one in four people aged 25 or more is likely to experience stroke in their lifetime. A somewhat greater proportion of all strokes occurs in women (53%) than men (47%). Historically, stroke was considered a neurological disorder of the elderly, but current data reveal that over 62% of all strokes occur in people younger than 70 years of age. Among these, more than 16% of strokes occur in people aged 15–49 years of age. Together these data underscore the markedly increasing incidence of stroke in younger people, including children. Worldwide, there are currently more than 101 million people living with stroke sequelae, representing a near doubling of the number of stroke survivors over the last 30 years. This change has been driven, in part, by a 65% decrease in stroke mortality emphasizing the need for and importance of effective neurorehabilitation strategies.

Changes in stroke incidence rates, estimated at ±2% per 5 years of age, are likely to result from increased exposure to, or conversely, better control of, major stroke risk factors including *metabolic* (e.g., high systolic blood pressure, high body mass index, high fasting plasma glucose, high total cholesterol, and low glomerular filtration rate), *behavioral* (e.g., tobacco use, poor diet, low physical activity levels), and *environmental* (e.g., air pollution, lead exposure) risk factors which account for 71.0%, 47.0%, and 37.8% of global stroke burden (GSB), respectively (Tsao et al., 2023). High systolic blood pressure is the largest single risk factor for stroke (55.5% GSB), followed by high body mass index (24.4% GSB), high fasting plasma glucose (20.2% GSB), ambient particulate matter pollution (20.1% GSB), and tobacco use, specifically smoking (17.7% GSB). Combined, these risk factors account for 87% of the global burden of stroke. These statistics argue strongly for increased primary stroke prevention and management of modifiable risk factors, especially in younger individuals (Tsao et al., 2023). Socioeconomic determinants of health, particularly poor dietary quality, environmental exposure, tobacco use, and low physical activity, coupled with suboptimal access to healthcare and inadequate health literacy point to a rapidly escalating problem of immense public health importance with serious economic and social consequences.

For the vast majority of individuals, stroke recovery will be incomplete leaving them with persistent, residual functional impairments. At least half of stroke survivors will require assistance in activities of daily living including mobility, personal care, and speech and communication (see Chap. 10). Instrumental activities of daily living (IADL), the more complex tasks critical to self-management that enable independence, may be further impacted by impairments of cognitive and executive function (Truelsen et al., 2006). As a result, a considerable proportion of all stroke-related healthcare costs are attributed to rehabili-

[1] When used for outcome prediction in clinical trials, the mRS is often dichotomized where scores 0–2 predict good functional outcomes and scores 3–6 predict poor functional outcomes.

tation, nursing, lost productivity, and long-term care (Rudberg et al., 2018). More effective and efficient rehabilitation interventions are needed to promote recovery of function following stroke, especially for younger individuals in the most vital and productive years of their lives. To this end, the field of neurorehabilitation has acknowledged neuroplasticity as its foundational basis and has begun to incorporate knowledge from basic science demonstrating the central nervous system's capacity for experience-driven adaptation (Kleim & Jones, 2008). Understanding the relationship between neurobiological mechanisms of recovery, principles of neural plasticity, and behavioral change is important to advancing the scientific understanding and clinical basis of stroke rehabilitation (Kreisel et al., 2007).

17.2 Pathophysiology

A stroke is the brain's equivalent of a heart attack, and thus is commonly referred to as "brain attack." Stroke occurs when a blood vessel within the brain is blocked by a clot (ischemic stroke) or bursts (hemorrhagic stroke). Interrupted blood flow prevents the circulation of oxygen and nutrients to brain tissue. Interruption lasting more than a few seconds leads to cell death and brain damage that impacts the functions controlled by the affected brain region. Even temporarily interrupted circulation followed by revascularization as occurs with a transient ischemic attack (TIA) (i.e., <24-h duration) or revascularization procedures (i.e., thrombolysis, thrombectomy) compromises brain tissue impacting its long-term potential for recovery. Interrupted brain circulation persisting for more than 24 h causes more extensive tissue damage and cell death, lasting brain damage, long-term disability, and even death (Osa Garcia et al., 2022).

Stroke is both a cardiovascular and neurological disease—cardiovascular because it occurs in people with **poor cardiometabolic function**; and neurological because it disrupts circulation in vessels within the brain. Brain attacks emerge from two primary causes: (i) *ischemia*—resulting from either occlusion (clots) or narrowing in arteries leading to and within the brain, or (ii) *hemorrhage*—blood vessel rupture. The majority (>62%) of strokes are ischemic and stem from vascular conditions (e.g., atherosclerosis, coronary artery disease, hyperlipidemia). Acknowledging these cardiometabolic underpinnings, in common with heart disease, hypertension is the leading cause of stroke. Increased systolic blood pressure damages the arterial linings, increases susceptibility to plaque accumulation, and effectively narrows the arteries that supply the heart and brain.

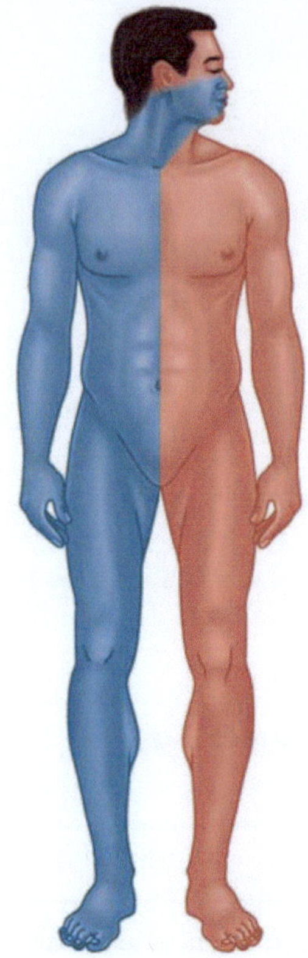

Fig. 17.1 Stroke affects the contralateral hemibody. Using a left middle cerebral artery stroke as example, effects (weakness, dyscoordination, impaired sensory integration, and in some cases hyperreflexia) are primarily unilateral, affecting the contralateral leg, arm, hand, and lower two-thirds of the face

In the **motor domain**, stroke manifests in **primarily unilateral impairment** affecting the limbs and hemibody contralateral to the affected brain hemisphere (Fig. 17.1). The classical presentation of stroke is a large ischemic infarct affecting the middle cerebral artery (MCA) which supplies the primary motor cortex (M1). As depicted in Fig. 17.2, the somatotopy of M1 is arranged such that the contralesional face, hand, arm, and leg may all be affected. The severity of hemiparetic impairment in each body segment differs based on the extent and specific locus of the vascular infarct and the duration of interrupted blood flow.

Strokes can occur in any blood vessel and therefore affect any brain region. Smaller strokes affecting smaller blood vessels and subcortical areas may induce more focal impacts, affecting, for example, motor but not speech function or vice versa. While advanced neuroimaging makes it possible to identify the anatomical locus of the primary infarct, the **penumbra**—defined as viable tissue surrounding the irreversibly damaged ischemic core—is of importance (Fig. 17.3). Both the degree of perfusion mismatch between the ischemic core and the penumbra, and the extent (dimensions) of the penumbra are important considerations for neural recovery and neuroplastic potential (Osa Garcia et al., 2022). Additionally, due to extensive network connectivity within and between brain regions, the effects of stroke are typically more widespread than the ischemic core. For example, ischemic damage to primary cortical areas leads to reorganization in remote brain regions well beyond the peri-infarct area and the magnitude of these remote changes is greater in the presence of more severe primary ischemic damage.

Improved acute and peri-acute stroke management procedures, such as intravenous thrombolytic agents (i.e., "clot busters") and mechanical thrombectomy, are now routinely performed when indicated and available (Jan & Chong, 2024). These revascularization procedures can salvage penumbral tissue reducing the extent of impaired brain function and mitigating functional impairments. It is expected that the reactivation of penumbral tissue offers an important substrate for neuroplasticity. In combination, the duration of interrupted brain circulation, infarct dimensions, size, and condition of the penumbra determine whether subsequent neuroplasticity involves ***reactivation*** of the primarily affected

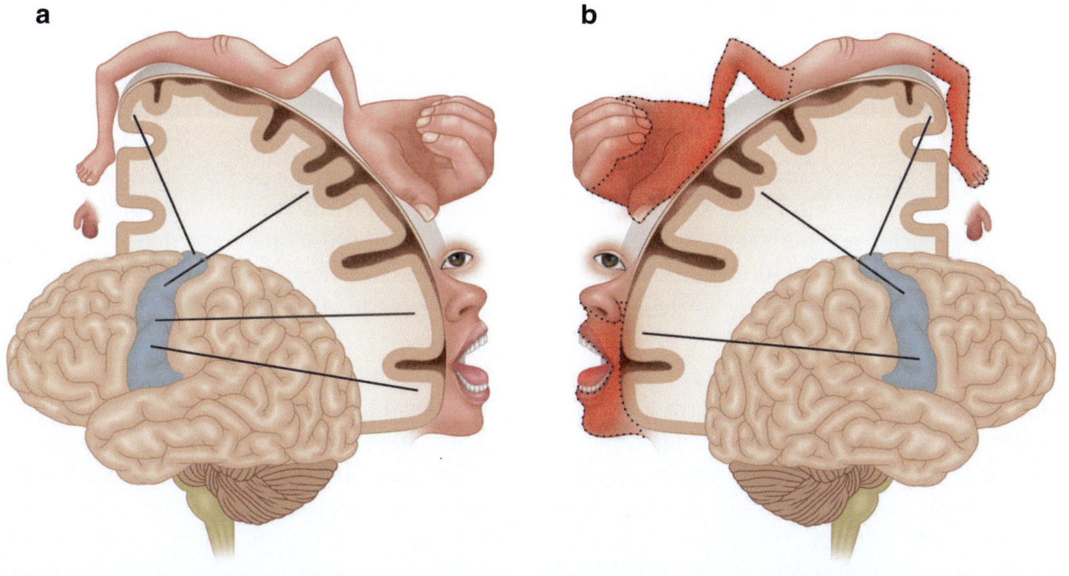

Fig. 17.2 (**Panel a**) Somatotopic arrangement of body representations in the primary motor cortex. Face, hand, arm, and leg representations are localized from lateral-to-medial. (**Panel b**) Mapping illustrates how stroke location can induce differential effects across functional systems depending on the blood vessel affected and the extent of lesion. Large relative representations of hand, arm, and face illustrate the more common impact of stroke on these functional systems. Actual location and dimensions should be considered illustrative, as neural representations vary by individual and use

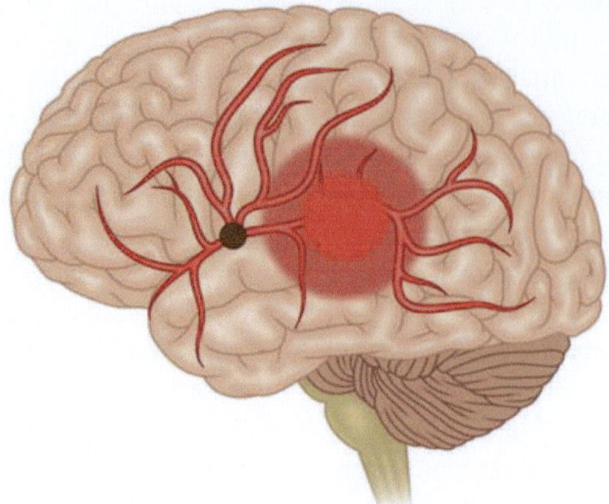

Fig. 17.3 The penumbra is a region of viable tissue (lighter red zone) surrounding the ischemic core (dark red zone) resulting from partially retained perfusion representing a labile zone that can either improve or exacerbate outcome in the early period following stroke. If blood flow is restored within a critical window of time, the penumbra has the potential to quickly recover, improving outcomes. However, penumbral tissue is vulnerable to the same metabolic processes (excitotoxicity, oxidative stress, inflammation) as the ischemic core, thus further compromise can expand the primary stroke core. The penumbra is considered viable for up to 24 h following stroke establishing the temporal window for reperfusion interventions. Due to maintained circulation/perfusion, tissue in the penumbral region is considered capable of neuroplasticity thus offering substrate for recovery through recruitment and restitution

tissue, ***recruitment*** of adjacent tissue (penumbra), or ***retraining*** of alternate brain areas with the representation of the function affected by the stroke (Warraich & Kleim, 2010).

17.3 Improvement of Function

The primary goal of stroke rehabilitation is recovery of function. However, significant discrepancies remain regarding how "function" is defined. From a rehabilitation clinician's perspective, function pertains to the behavioral manifestations of a given neurologic system. In the context of upper-extremity motor function, it refers to the ability to move the arm and hand; interact with the environment to reach, grasp, and manipulate objects; integrate sensory signals; and perform meaningful tasks ranging from grooming and self-care, to writing, drawing, playing a musical instrument, tool use. Such activities underlie one's autonomy and self-expression, and are the essence of being human.

In the clinical domain, motor function is typically assessed using validated measurement scales such as the: Fugl-Meyer Motor Assessment (FMA), Action Research Arm Test (ARAT), or Wolf Motor Function Test (WMFT) (Box 17.2), and recovery is inferred from an improved score. Such instruments are typically scored on an ordinal scale which leaves gaps in the ability to capture small, but important, functional changes and produces discontinuities in the significance of incremental changes. More importantly, these scales evaluate motor performance on the basis of *task completion* rather than differentiating whether improved scores occur due to compensation or true recovery. The conundrum is that following rehabilitation, improved clinical scores may *suggest* reduced motor impairment, yet fail to inform *how* the score improved or the specific aspect of impairment that was reduced.

Distinction of recovery phenotypes is key to evaluating the impact of rehabilitation. ***Recovery*** is defined as the capacity to perform a movement in the same manner as before the stroke. In contrast, ***Compensation*** is defined as the emergence of new motor patterns resulting from substitution or adaptation of residual motor elements. By way of example, a stroke survivor producing change in the upper extremity (UE) Fugl-Meyer score (Box 17.2) from 48 to 54 (of 60) points might be char-

Box 17.2 Clinical Evaluation of Function Poststroke

Assessment tools in clinical neurorehabilitation span World Health Organization International Classification of Functioning (ICF) model framework (see Fig. 1.1) which distinguishes between the underlying *pathophysiology* of the **Health Condition** (stroke); *impairments* at the **Body Function/Structure** level (e.g., weakness, spasticity, muscle activation patterns, dyscoordination); *disability* at the **Activity** level (e.g., impaired task performance—reaching, grasping, walking); and *handicap* at the **Participation** level (i.e., an individual's ability to perform their desired life roles and activities of self-care). Restoration of nervous system structure and function, neuroplasticity, occurs at the pathophysiological level and is measured using myriad approaches: neuroimaging, EEG, TMS, electrophysiology, EMG, and others. It remains a question, however, whether neuroplastic changes measured thusly translate to meaningful behavioral changes. Important to addressing this question is to understand commonly used clinical assessments and their intended purpose. The items below represent a small subset of tools commonly used for clinical assessment of motor function and recovery following stroke.

ICF Body Structure/Function Domain

National Institutes of Health Stroke Scale

The National Institutes of Health Stroke Scale (NIHSS) is a quantitative measure of stroke-related neurological deficits accounting for the severity of symptoms associated with cerebral infarcts. The 15-item scale assesses the level of consciousness, extraocular movements, visual fields, facial muscle function, extremity strength, sensory function, coordination (ataxia), language (aphasia), speech (dysarthria), and hemi-inattention (neglect). The total NIHSS score ranges from 0 to 42, where higher scores indicate greater severity of neurological impairment. An NIHSS score <6 is associated with good recovery while scores >16 forecast a high probability of death or severe disability. Each additional point >6 decreases the likelihood of a good prognosis by 17%. NIHSS scores are interpreted to represent: **0,** no stroke symptoms; **1–4,** minor stroke; **5–15,** moderate stroke; **16–20,** moderate to severe stroke; and **21–42,** severe stroke. The NIHSS was originally designed to assess the efficacy of thrombolytic interventions (i.e., tPA), thus is particularly useful for determining initial stroke severity, guiding treatment decisions for individuals arriving at the hospital with stroke sequelae, and evaluating acute response to interventions (e.g., thrombolysis, thrombectomy) administered within hours poststroke. NIHSS at 24-h post-onset is a strong predictor of functional outcome at 90 days. Importantly, the NIHSS is not responsive to change over longer time frames (i.e., days to weeks) and thus is not well suited to assess rehabilitation outcomes that occur in the postacute period.

Time to administer—10 min.

Fugl-Meyer Motor Assessment

The Fugl-Meyer Assessment of Motor Recovery after Stroke (FMA) is one of the most widely used measures for the evaluation of **motor impairment** following stroke and is often used to document motor recovery. The FMA is a performance-based measure testing five domains: motor, sensory, balance, joint range of motion, and joint pain with the motor domain subdivided into individual scales for the upper (22 items, 66 points) and lower (17 items, 34 points) extremities.

The FMA was originally developed based on an underlying conceptual model that assumed recovery of motor function after stroke follows a definable stepwise

(continued)

Box 17.2 (continued)

course. Important in this progression was the assumption that the re-emergence of reflexes precedes the onset of volitional motor action. Contrasting with the reflex-hierarchical model of motor control that informed development of the original FMA, current models of motor control acknowledge task-, phase-, and context-dependent influences of reflexes on motor activity during movement. From this perspective, reflexes tested at rest are unlikely to yield meaningful information regarding volitional motor control. Consistent with this neurobiological understanding, systematic evaluation of measurement properties of the upper-extremity (UE) FMA revealed that resting-state reflex items assess a different underlying construct from the remainder of the test items. A modified 30-item version of the UE FMA (absent reflex items) demonstrates a unidimensional measure of volitional movement, construct validity, and stability over time. Of practical concern for current clinical and research use, is the importance of noting which UE FMA version is used, verifying the full scale of scores produced by the instrument used, and appropriate interpretation of the aggregate score.

Time to administer—30 min (all five domains).

ICF Activity Domain

Wolf Motor Function Test

The Wolf Motor Function Test (WMFT) is a quantitative measure of upper-extremity motor function. The WMFT augments observation of basic movements with a combination of timed (WMFT-TIME) and functional tasks (WMFT-FAS, 0–5 ordinal score) to assess dexterity, strength, and functional ability. Six test items involve timed tasks, eight items measure strength, and nine items evaluate coordination. Both arms are tested starting with the less affected side. Timed tasks are allowed a maximum of 120 s. The most widely used version of the WMFT includes 17 items producing a maximum score of 75. Lower scores are indicative of worse motor function.

Time to administer—35 min.

Action Research Arm Test

The Action Research Arm Test (ARAT) is a performance-based assessment of upper-extremity motor function involving observation of motor tasks ranging from easy to difficult. Nineteen items are scored on a four-point ordinal producing a maximum score of 57. Higher scores indicate better UE function. Test items can be divided into four subdomains: grasp, grip, pinch, and gross arm movement affording improved interpretability regarding which items are easy, difficult, or optimally challenging compared to the aggregate score. Within each subdomain, items are ranked by difficulty such that achieving a score of 3 on the first item credits the performer as having scored 3 on all subsequent items. If a score of <3 is achieved on the first item, testing proceeds to the second item, which is the easiest item on the scale. If the performer scores 0 on this item, they are unlikely to score better on the remainder and thus can be credited with 0 for the other items. This item-difficulty hierarchy affords efficiency when conducting the assessment. The ARAT is a modified version of the Upper Extremity Function Test. The ARAT and WMFT are highly correlated.

Time to administer—5–15 min.

ICF Participation Domain

Stroke Impact Scale

The Stroke Impact Scale (SIS) is a 59-item Patient Reported Outcome (PRO) questionnaire used to assess self-perceived handicap and health-related quality of life by probing eight domains: strength, hand function, ADL/IADL, mobility, communication, emotion, memory and thinking, participation and life role function (Duncan,

(continued)

Box 17.2 (continued)
1999). Scores from the domains of strength, hand function, mobility, and ADL/IADL can be summed to produce a *physical dimension score*. A separate question asks the individual to rate (scale of 0–100) how much they feel they have recovered from their stroke. To assure validity, respondents must be able to follow 3-step commands and score at least 16/30 on the Mini-Mental Status Exam. SIS scores are moderately to strongly related to commonly used performance-based outcomes including the FMA, WMFT, and ARAT.

Time to administer—15–20 min.

Modified Rankin Scale

The Modified Rankin Scale (mRS) is a single-item **global outcomes rating scale** used to categorize a person's level of independence relative to premorbid status. Assessment is conducted via clinical examination and personal interaction/interview probing all functional domains including physical, mental, and speech. One grade (range 0–5) is assigned making the mRS time efficient to administer by the clinician at bedside or by telephone. Specific levels are: **0, no disability**; **1, no significant disability** despite symptoms, able to carry out all usual duties and activities; **2, slight disability**, unable to perform *all* premorbid activities but able to look after own affairs independently; **3, moderate disability**, requiring some help, but able to walk without assistance; **4, moderately severe disability**, unable to walk or attend to bodily needs (i.e., feeding bathing, toileting, dressing) without assistance; **5, severe disability**, bedridden/incontinent/requiring constant nursing care and attention. Information regarding the patient's neurological function should be obtained by examination. Due to its simplicity, efficiency, and reproducibility, the mRS is used extensively by medical disciplines to document outcomes for clinical trials at 60 and 90 days poststroke.

acterized as a partial recovery phenotype, that is if changes stem from increased ability to perform individuated (vs. synergistic) movements, increased strength enabling effective grasp(s), and increased speed of movement execution with the more involved side. Alternatively, improved clinical scores can result from the individual's ability to produce some volitional activity versus none (i.e., UE FMA), from executing a dysfunctional movement pattern faster or more consistently (i.e., WMFT-Time), or by substituting with other body parts (i.e., increased trunk flexion to substitute for incomplete elbow extension during reaching). While manifestations in the latter cases would contribute to improved clinical scores, they are considered compensations since they differ from premorbid movement strategies. Equally important, these compensatory strategies are likely to interfere with the reacquisition of normal movement and may even promote maladaptive neuroplasticity (Levin et al., 2009).

Regardless of the recovery phenotype expressed, it is neither possible, nor appropriate, to infer the nature of neurobiological recovery solely from clinical and behavioral assessments. Neuroplasticity is defined as any change at the level of neuron structure or function which is observed directly from measures of individual neurons or inferred from measures taken across populations of neurons (Warraich & Kleim, 2010). Accordingly, behavioral measures and changes in behavior are not, of themselves, direct measures of neural plasticity.

17.3.1 Plasticity Poststroke

While distinct from behavioral manifestations, neurobiological changes following stroke also involve both recovery and compensation. It has been argued that true neural recovery is not possible since, once neural tissue has been compromised, it cannot be fully restored. Despite ischemic compromise, inherent functional redundancy retained within the brain affords a basis for neuroplasticity. Damaged neural tissue initially compromised by ischemia may undergo reestablishment of its function, also referred to as **restoration**. Restoration is a *recovery* mechanism and would most likely occur in the case where perfusion is restored, in areas immediately surrounding the brain lesion (penumbra), and in the diaschisis. When stroke leads to the death of neurons, engagement of residual brain areas not directly affected by the stroke are recruited. Through *reorganization* of neural connections, other brain regions may *compensate* and take over the function previously performed by the affected area either by utilizing preexisting connections or by establishing new connections via intensive motor rehabilitation (see Chap. 13) (Warraich & Kleim, 2010).

Given the classical presentation of stroke affecting the primary motor cortex (M1), neuroplastic changes often involve reorganization of the M1 representation—incorporating adjacent or related/associated anatomical areas (see Chaps. 5 and 13). In some cases, most typically in severe strokes, homologous pathways ipsilateral to the involved limb(s) are recruited. This form of compensatory neural reorganization involves unmasking of existing, uncrossed corticospinal pathways or may reveal bilateral/hemispheric activity present in health that remains viable and can be recruited to subserve motor function following stroke.

17.3.2 Methods Poststroke

Neurorehabilitation incorporates a wide range of strategies and interventions aimed at promoting recovery of lost function. Rehabilitation practitioners play a key role in this process by devising interventions that are specific to real-life activities and incorporate appropriate feedback, instructions, rewards, and goal attainment. Specific motor training induces a spectrum of changes in the brain, influencing gene expression, synaptic efficacy, dendritic spine dynamics, and motor map expansion. These changes are task-specific, distinguishing them from rote movement repetition and showcasing the brain's ability to adapt and reorganize based on learning a specific skill (see Chap. 7). Neurorehabilitation interventions that effectively leverage such behavioral adaptations can drive changes in the central nervous system and successfully induce neuroplasticity (see Chap. 15) (Kleim & Jones, 2008).

Various approaches tap into the brain's adaptive capacity thus offering potential for rehabilitation to promote recovery following a stroke. Among these, task-specific motor training is viewed as a foundational approach. Through repetition of targeted exercises designed to address individual motor deficits, task-specific motor training ostensibly contributes to cortical neuroplasticity. Conceptually, techniques like Constraint-Induced Movement Therapy (CIMT, see Box 15.2) and locomotor training utilize key principles of task-specific motor training in the context of intensive, challenging, and motivating activities intended to stimulate changes in the motor cortex. Importantly, these strategies offer opportunities for high doses of repetition, a critical factor to induce adaptation and enhance motor function.

The efficacy of rehabilitation strategies in inducing neuroplasticity after a stroke depends not only on the type of intervention but also on the **timing, intensity, and dose**. Enriched, motivating, and engaging rehabilitative environments have been linked to the positive influence of neurotrophic factors stimulating neuroplasticity which fluctuates over the period of poststroke recovery. Understanding the critical, **optimal time windows** for effective rehabilitation is extremely important to increasing the success of achieving recovery (Fig. 17.4). Equally important is delivering interventions of **adequate intensity**. As a general principle, a system must be taxed *toward* its capacity to adapt and improve. In this regard, an important challenge for rehabilitation practitioners to recognize is that capacity varies both across individuals and within individuals over time. Low-intensity activities, assisted activities, and passive movements, while necessary components of a rehabilitation program, may not be sufficiently intense to stimulate adaptation. A closely related concept is **dose**, the quantity of therapeutic intervention delivered. By way of example, considering intensity and dose together, a therapist might oversee a *dose* of 20 reaching movements 5 days a week for 3 weeks equating to

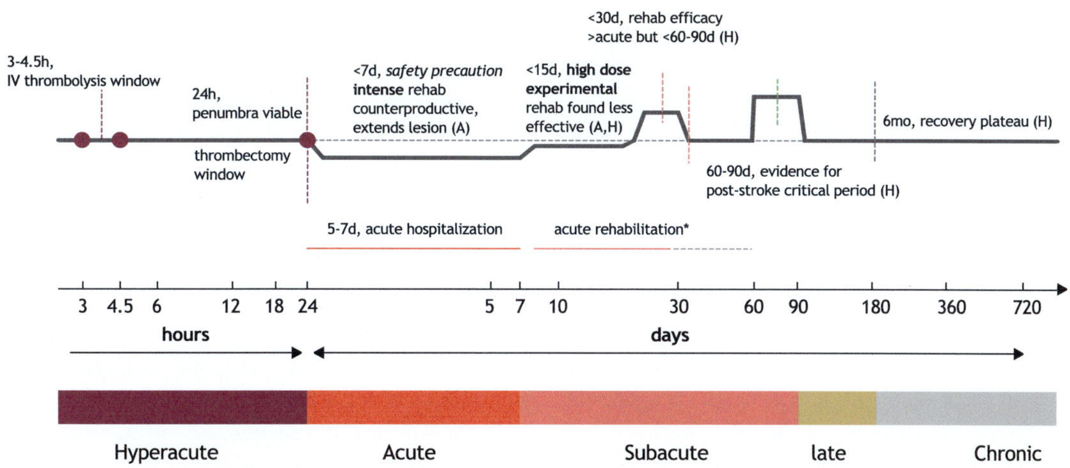

Fig. 17.4 Conceptual timeline of neurobiological recovery poststroke spanning hyperacute (up to 24 h), acute (7 days), subacute (90 days), late subacute (180 days), and chronic (6–24 months) periods. **Acute** phase typically corresponds with hospitalization for medical management, stabilization, and revascularization procedures, if indicated. Acute inpatient rehabilitation typically occurs during the **subacute** phase with variable length of stay depending on stroke severity, functional status, home discharge setting, and regional differences in practice patterns. Vertical deflections in the trajectory illustrate epochs of heightened or blunted neural responsiveness, referenced to premorbid brain state (dashed gray line) signaling potential for neurorehabilitation to optimize neuroplasticity. Premorbid brain state differs by individual on the basis of age, health, activity, nutrition, etc. Annotations on trajectory reflect evidence from animal (A) or human (H) models regarding the safety and efficacy of motor rehabilitation. A critical/sensitive period has been demonstrated in human stroke survivors (60–90 days) during which rehabilitation efficacy is enhanced. **Chronic** phase, noted as 6 months, accompanied by a recovery plateau reflects the return of neurobiological processes to a premorbid state and reduced capacity for neuroplasticity. Functional gains are still noted during the chronic period

300 movements. But it is difficult to determine the potential utility of this intervention without understanding the intensity required to perform these reaches. By contrast, a therapist might deliver 10–15 reaches per session using the schedule above but instead, challenge the patient to perform at, or near, their capacity while monitoring for fatigue and reaching their performance limit. The intensity achieved by the intervention in this scenario of 150–225 movements is more likely to trigger adaptation and increase the patient's capacity. As a corollary point, not only will the patient's capacity adapt to a more intense intervention, but the threshold of adequate intensity changes concurrently. As a result, the specific activities performed within an intervention require ongoing adjustment to ensure adequate intensity of subsequent activities. Highly skilled rehabilitation practitioners play a key role in producing effective rehabilitation by balancing the timing, intensity, and dose of their interventions to leverage the highly dynamic recovery process.

Intervention approaches incorporating neuromodulation, that is peripheral and brain stimulation, are strong potential tools for neurorehabilitation, especially when used in combination with active rehabilitation therapies. Techniques, such as repetitive transcranial magnetic stimulation (rTMS) and transcranial direct current stimulation (tDCS) (see Chap. 16), have been investigated as either standalone therapies or as a primer for traditional activity-based therapies. The neuromodulatory effects are argued to impact cortical activation and promote axonal sprouting following a stroke. Notably, greater therapeutic efficacy has been detected when neuromodulatory therapies are combined with volitional intervention techniques (i.e., rTMS combined with task-specific training; locomotor training combined with tDCS, etc.). The combination appears to maximize neuroplasticity and functional improvements in individuals recovering from a stroke.

Vagal Nerve Stimulation (VNS) is an emerging neuromodulation therapy with great promise for neuroplasticity-based neurorehabilitation. Briefly, VNS involves stimulation of Cranial Nerve X—delivered either percutaneously or through an implanted cuff electrode. In rehabilitation applications, VNS has been found most effective when triggered in close temporal proximity to the execution of volitional movements. The putative effects of VNS leverage two hypothesized mechanisms of action: (i) neuroprotection—via reducing inflammation, enhancing cerebral blood flow, inhibiting glutamate release, and reducing oxidative stress; and (ii) stimulating neuroplasticity through activation of cholinergic, noradrenergic, and serotonergic networks that regulate synaptic plasticity. Studies of VNS to date in both animal models and humans have targeted upper-extremity recovery poststroke demonstrating positive, reproducible outcomes that in many cases far exceed the effects of motor rehabilitation alone and approach premorbid levels of function (Andalib et al., 2023). Thus, VNS delivered at the optimal time poststroke, combined with the appropriate dose of volitional task-specific practice appears to be a restorative intervention. Evidence demonstrating the true neuroplastic effects of VNS will emerge from ongoing and future research.

17.3.3 Is All Plasticity "Good"?

While neuroplasticity typically infers beneficial changes that promote recovery, not all forms of plasticity are advantageous. Neuroplastic changes can also be maladaptive (Byl et al., 1996). For example, in the context of severe sensory loss, alterations in the motor and somatosensory cortex have been associated with diminished pinch-grip performance, impaired two-point discrimination, and reduced intracortical inhibition. These unfavorable changes suggest a counterproductive relationship between brain reorganization and functional recovery. Maladaptive plasticity might also be manifest in the context of compensatory movement patterns and delayed-onset abnormal movements, and may involve recruitment of the ipsilateral motor pathway. Maladaptive changes can hinder recovery or introduce unwanted symptoms, undermining the intended effects of rehabilitation (Jang, 2013). Thus, while neuroplasticity can support recovery, maladaptive forms of neuroplasticity do occur and can impede the rehabilitation process. These insights emphasize the importance of accurate recognition of nonproductive intervention approaches and differentiation of intended outcomes to develop more successful treatments (Alaverdashvili et al., 2008).

17.4 Special Circumstances Affecting Stroke Rehabilitation

Understanding the intersection between rehabilitation and neuroplasticity is important for capitalizing on the brain's adaptive potential and informing the development of effective rehabilitation interventions that optimize neural recovery and reorganization following stroke (Zeiler & Krakauer, 2013).

Acutely poststroke, a brief period of heightened neural plasticity has been observed marked by significant changes in gene expression, altered dendritic spine plasticity, and reduced inhibitory neurotransmission. These electrophysiological changes render neurons more receptive to forming new synaptic connections leading to structural reorganization and boosting the potential for neurorehabilitation to induce true recovery of function through neuroplasticity. This **poststroke-sensitive period** is observed in the first month in animal models and the first 3 months in humans (see also Chap. 13). There is general concordance between animal and human models that the majority of true recovery occurs in this poststroke-sensitive period (PSSP). Moreover, rehabilitation in the PSSP is critical to overcome stroke-related impairments and, if appropriately administered, can play a crucial role in directing brain reorganization, especially in the peri-infarct cortex (i.e., penumbra). Indeed, near complete recovery can be attained if intense, task-specific motor retaining is offered within this critical window. Over time, the enhanced neuroplastic milieu observed in the PSSP normalizes and the brain's capacity for plasticity gradually diminishes. Not only is rehabilitation delivered outside of this critical window less effective, but stroke survivors may adopt compensatory movement strategies that become reinforced with repeated use over time. Environmental enrichment can further assist by providing a more stimulating and varied environment to facilitate recovery. Once this sensitive period closes, the brain's plasticity resembles that of the uninjured brain. Furthermore, it is important to account for how the premorbid neurobiological state of the brain (e.g., aging, tobacco use, substance use, vascular condition) influences neuroplastic potential prior to superposition with stroke. The relative differences in neuroplastic capacity demonstrate the critical role of timing and the type of interventions that can influence recovery poststroke.

Conceptually, intervention initiated early (i.e., hours-to-days poststroke) when biochemical processes are elevated might be argued to promote plasticity and optimize recovery. However, there are safety concerns. Forced overuse of the impaired limb too early poststroke (i.e., within the first 7 days postlesion) has been found to *extend the neural injury* and interfere with recovery (Humm et al., 1998; Kozlowski et al., 1996). Initially observed in animal models, this phenomenon has been confirmed in humans through clinical trials. Intense, high-repetition experimental intervention initiated within 9.7 (±4.5) days of stroke reveals an inverse dose-response relationship compared to lower-intensity, standard therapy (Dromerick et al., 2009). Of note, in the human condition, counterproductive effects of too much intense experimental therapy too soon impacted motor recovery without evidence of lesion enlargement on MR imaging. Nonetheless, any intervention that interferes with overall recovery poses an important safety concern and consideration for the design of rehabilitation interventions.

Outcomes combined across studies provide evidence for a critical period after stroke and enable the construction of a conceptual timeline of recovery (Fig. 17.4). At 1-year poststroke, the motor outcome is significantly better when intense rehabilitation is delivered between 60 and 90 days (subacute), compared to <30 days (acute), or ≥6 months (chronic) (Dromerick et al., 2021). In this context, it is important to appreciate that functional gains continue to be demonstrated when intense rehabilitation is delivered at ≥6 months following a stroke, although the effects may be smaller and require longer epochs of intervention to achieve the same result. Taken together, these and emerging findings point to the subacute period (i.e., 2–3 months poststroke) following the resolution of immediate, acute sequelae as the window when rehabilitation paradigms can be optimally synergistic with the critical, sensitive period of heightened neuroplasticity. Further research is needed to demonstrate the precise timing of this sensitive period with greater accuracy and resolution in the human condition.

While it is desirable to leverage neurobiological windows of opportunity by delivering rehabilitation interventions at the optimal timing, rehabilitation prescription can be challenged by real-world circumstances such as motivation, cognitive and executive function, and clinical practice patterns. **Depression** is a common comorbidity following stroke compromising motivation to participate in rehabilitation activities and address necessary lifestyle changes including diet, substance use, physical activity, and stress management. As described in the case study that frames this chapter (Box 17.1), the need to manage depressive symptoms, both behaviorally and pharmacologically, can supersede traditional rehabilitation goals and, potentially, interfere with leveraging the critical window for neuroplasticity. Equally important are stroke-related impairments of cognitive and executive function that impact stroke survivors' abilities to fully participate in and comply with their treatment programs, thus compromising rehabilitation efficacy. Finally, the end of the subacute period (i.e., 2–3 months poststroke) coincides with discharge from inpatient rehabilitation and transition to delivery of rehabilitation services in the home or outpatient settings. Many individuals are lost to follow-up in this period either due to administrative challenges, disparities, and social determinants influencing access to health care, or motivation to make significant lifestyle changes. As a result, many stroke survivors end up receiving little, if any, rehabilitative care during this period (Young et al., 2023) instead of the intense, high-dose interventions that have demonstrated meaningful, persistent functional effects (Dromerick et al., 2021).

17.5 Conclusions and Perspectives

Returning to Michelle's case at the beginning of this chapter, given her NIHSS score on admission, she could be considered to have a poor overall prognosis with a high likelihood of severe, persistent disability. Instead, contemporary approaches to acute stroke management dramatically altered her outcome. By the time Michelle was found at home, she was outside of the temporal window for intravenous thrombolytic therapy. However, the penumbra remains viable until 24-h poststroke onset (Fig. 17.4). Increased availability of mechanical thrombectomy (i.e., clot removal) procedures expands the opportunity for brain tissue salvage with downstream implications for neural plasticity and functional recovery. Following mechanical thrombectomy and reperfusion, Michelle's NIHSS improved markedly (14/42) indicating a better likelihood of survival and somewhat reduced, although moderate, disability.

In Michelle's case, characteristics favoring good recovery and neuroplastic potential include her relatively young age (49) and early, time-efficient tele-stroke consultation leading to mechanical thrombectomy that fully restored circulation. As mentioned in Sect. 17.1, the incidence of stroke in young(er) people has increased dramatically. Approximately 16% of strokes occur in individuals between ages 15 and 49; the majority of these result from poor control of *modifiable* risk factors: metabolic, behavioral, and environmental. To underscore this point, several factors in Michelle's health history compromise her potential for good recovery and neuroplasticity: significant prior cardiac history that was not well managed; extensive history of tobacco use (30 pack-years); and active methamphetamine use. In addition to increased stroke risk, these factors alter the premorbid state of the brain and its intrinsic potential for neuroplasticity. As a result, the expectation for Michelle's brain to recover and produce a robust neuroplastic response is much less than a healthier 49-year-old adult. Finally, chronic substance use, in this case methamphetamine, is an important risk factor for secondary stroke. Education and management of stroke risk factors (i.e., cardio-metabolic, behavioral, environmental) are key to the prevention of recurrent stroke.

Particularly important to effective rehabilitation and neuroplasticity is the patient's active engagement and participation in all forms of intervention, whether for motor, speech, cognitive, or other forms of therapy. Impairments of cognitive and executive function can negatively impact active engagement in rehabilitation. In Michelle's case, her acute rehabilitation process was compromised by a serious bout of depression. Her case is not unique. Indeed, depression is a frequent comorbidity following stroke and is recognized to undermine active engagement and participation in therapies. Rehabilitation outcomes improve when depression is managed effectively. Whether drugs used to manage depression in humans produce synergistic neuroplastic effects remains unclear. Equally important is managing conditions affecting cognition, executive function, and thought disorders—each set of conditions has its unique impact on motivation and engagement. The critical point is to manage this serious condition, mitigate more serious co-occurring effects, and promote active participation in rehabilitation therapies.

Despite challenges encountered during the inpatient rehabilitation admission, Michelle made significant functional gains enabling her discharge to home at approximately 1-month poststroke. Ideally, Michelle would have accessed outpatient rehabilitation therapies taking particular advantage of the opportunity for frequent, intense evidence-based treatments during the poststroke-sensitive period (60–90 days poststroke). As they become more available and demonstrate evidence of their potential to optimize the brain's inherent capacity for plasticity during this critical period, active therapies are more likely to be combined with neuromodulation, including Vagal Nerve Stimulation.

Beyond the critical period, ongoing participation in therapies including directed exercise groups is strongly recommended. There are myriad cases of stroke survivors who persist in their quest for recovery well beyond 6–or even 12-months poststroke demonstrating significant gains with regular, intense training.

Review Questions

- Why is it more difficult to obtain functional recovery if neurorehabilitation is not initiated soon after stroke?
- Discuss how knowledge and understanding of neuroplasticity may help to point toward solutions for the challenges in stroke neurorehabilitation. What are the possibilities of existing and/or new training treatments? What are the problems?

References

Alaverdashvili, M., Foroud, A., Lim, D. H., & Whishaw, I. Q. (2008). "Learned baduse" limits recovery of skilled reaching for food after forelimb motor cortex stroke in rats: a new analysis of the effect of gestures on success. *Behavioural Brain Research, 188*(2), 281–290.

Andalib, S., Divani, A. A., Ayata, C., Baig, S., Arsava, E. M., Topcuoglu, M. A., Caceres, E. L., Parikh, V., Desai, M. J., Majid, A., Girolami, S., & Di Napoli, M. (2023). Vagus nerve stimulation in ischemic stroke. *Current Neurology and Neuroscience Reports, 23*(12), 947–962.

Byl, N. N., Merzenich, M. M., & Jenkins, W. M. (1996). A primate genesis model of focal dystonia and repetitive strain injury: I. Learning-induced dedifferentiation of the representation of the hand in the primary somatosensory cortex in adult monkeys. *Neurology, 47*(2), 508–520.

Dromerick, A. W., Lang, C. E., Birkenmeier, R. L., Wagner, J. M., Miller, J. P., Videen, T. O., Powers, W. J., Wolf, S. L., & Edwards, D. F. (2009). Very Early Constraint-Induced Movement during Stroke Rehabilitation (VECTORS): a single-center RCT. *Neurology, 73*(3), 195–201.

Dromerick, A. W., Geed, S., Barth, J., Brady, K., Giannetti, M. L., Mitchell, A., Edwardson, M. A., Tan, M. T., Zhou, Y., Newport, E. L., & Edwards, D. F. (2021). Critical Period After Stroke Study (CPASS): A phase II clinical trial testing an optimal time for motor recovery after stroke in humans. *Proceedings of the National Academy of Sciences of the United States of America, 118*(39), e2026676118.

Duncan PW, Wallace D, Lai SM, Johnson D, Embretson S, Laster LJ. (1999). The stroke impact scale version 2.0. *Evaluation of reliability, validity, and sensitivity to change. Stroke; a journal of cerebral circulation. 30*(10):2131–40.

Feigin, V. L., Brainin, M., Norrving, B., Martins, S., Sacco, R. L., Hacke, W., Fisher, M., Pandian, J., & Lindsay, P. (2022). World Stroke Organization (WSO): global stroke fact sheet 2022. *International Journal of Stroke, 17*(1), 18–29.

Humm, J. L., Kozlowski, D. A., James, D. C., Gotts, J. E., & Schallert, T. (1998). Use-dependent exacerbation of brain damage occurs during an early post-lesion vulnerable period. *Brain Research, 783*(2), 286–292.

Jan, K., & Chong, J. Y. (2024). Treatment of acute ischemic stroke: the last 30 years of trials and tribulations. *Cardiology in Review, 32*(3), 203–216.

Jang, S. H. (2013). Motor function-related maladaptive plasticity in stroke: a review. *NeuroRehabilitation, 32*(2), 311–316.

Kleim, J. A., & Jones, T. A. (2008). Principles of experience-dependent neural plasticity: implications for rehabilitation after brain damage. *Journal of Speech, Language, and Hearing Research, 51*(1), S225–S239.

Kozlowski, D. A., James, D. C., & Schallert, T. (1996). Use-dependent exaggeration of neuronal injury after unilateral sensorimotor cortex lesions. *The Journal of Neuroscience, 16*(15), 4776–4786.

Kreisel, S. H., Hennerici, M. G., & Bazner, H. (2007). Pathophysiology of stroke rehabilitation: the natural course of clinical recovery, use-dependent plasticity and rehabilitative outcome. *Cerebrovascular Diseases, 23*(4), 243–255.

Levin, M. F., Kleim, J. A., & Wolf, S. L. (2009). What do motor "recovery" and "compensation" mean in patients following stroke? *Neurorehabilitation and Neural Repair, 23*(4), 313–319.

Osa Garcia, A., Brambati, S. M., Desautels, A., & Marcotte, K. (2022). Timing stroke: a review on stroke pathophysiology and its influence over time on diffusion measures. *Journal of the Neurological Sciences, 441*, 120377.

Rudberg, A. S., Berge, E., Gustavsson, A., Nasman, P., & Lundstrom, E. (2018). Long-term health-related quality of life, survival and costs by different levels of functional outcome six months after stroke. *European Stroke Journal, 3*(2), 157–164.

Truelsen, T., Piechowski-Jozwiak, B., Bonita, R., Mathers, C., Bogousslavsky, J., & Boysen, G. (2006). Stroke incidence and prevalence in Europe: a review of available data. *European Journal of Neurology, 13*(6), 581–598.

Tsao, C. W., Aday, A. W., Almarzooq, Z. I., Anderson, C. A. M., Arora, P., Avery, C. L., Baker-Smith, C. M., Beaton, A. Z., Boehme, A. K., Buxton, A. E., Commodore-Mensah, Y., Elkind, M. S. V., Evenson, K. R., Eze-Nliam, C., Fugar, S., Generoso, G., Heard, D. G., Hiremath, S., Ho, J. E., Kalani, R., Kazi, D. S., Ko, D., Levine, D. A., Liu, J., Ma, J., Magnani, J. W., Michos, E. D., Mussolino, M. E., Navaneethan, S. D., Parikh, N. I., Poudel, R., Rezk-Hanna, M., Roth, G. A., Shah, N. S., St-Onge, M.-P., Thacker, E. L., Virani, S. S., Voeks, J. H., Wang, N.-Y., Wong, N. D., Wong, S. S., Yaffe, K., & Martin, S. S. (2023). Heart disease and stroke statistics—2023 update: a report from the American Heart Association. *Circulation, 147*(8), e93–e621.

Warraich, Z., & Kleim, J. A. (2010). Neural plasticity: the biological substrate for neurorehabilitation. *PM & R, 2*(12), S208–S219.

Young, B. M., Holman, E. A., Cramer, S. C., & Investigators, S. S. (2023). Rehabilitation therapy doses are low after stroke and predicted by clinical factors. *Stroke, 54*(3), 831–839.

Zeiler, S. R., & Krakauer, J. W. (2013). The interaction between training and plasticity in the poststroke brain. *Current Opinion in Neurology, 26*(6), 609–616.

Spinal Cord Injury

18

Sina Sangari and Monica A. Perez

Abstract

About 20.6 million individuals suffer from complete or incomplete motor and/or sensory disability following spinal cord injury (SCI) worldwide. Natural neurologic recovery may occur, but it is limited and predicted by the clinical assessment (i.e., level and severity of the injury). Therefore, promoting recovery beyond what is expected is of high priority. Physical rehabilitation activities have focused on strengthening and compensating for identified motor deficits to support independence. In contrast, many neurorehabilitation strategies aiming to promote motor control of the paralyzed limbs by enhancing the plasticity of the damaged neural circuits following SCI have emerged. Although it is difficult to determine whether one approach is superior to another, a combination of different strategies have been shown to achieve greater benefit than individual therapy alone. In this chapter, the following topics will be reviewed: (1) SCI epidemiology and the challenge of neurorehabilitation following SCI; (2) the evidence showing that most injuries to the spinal cord in humans are anatomically incomplete; and (3) neuroplasticity-based neurorehabilitation strategies aiming to promote and/or enhance recovery of motor function through the strengthening of residual connections following SCI.

Keywords

Spinal cord injury · Neuroplasticity · Neurostimulation · Cell therapy · Exercise rehabilitation

S. Sangari
Shirley Ryan AbilityLab, Arms + Hands Lab, Chicago, IL, USA

Northwestern University, Department of Physical Medicine & Rehabilitation, Chicago, IL, USA
e-mail: ssangari@sralab.org

M. A. Perez (✉)
Shirley Ryan AbilityLab, Arms + Hands Lab, Chicago, IL, USA

Northwestern University, Department of Physical Medicine & Rehabilitation, Chicago, IL, USA

Edward Hines Jr., VA Hospital, Hines, IL, USA
e-mail: mperez04@sralab.org

Box 18.1 Case Story

David and Stephen were two males of 54 and 58 years old, who sustained a traumatic injury for about 40 years. Both were classified by the International Standards for Neurological Classification of Spinal Cord Injury (ISNCSCI) examination as having a T10 and T11 level SCI, respectively, and by the American Spinal Injury Association Impairment Scale (AIS) as AIS A (i.e., sensory and motor complete injury) (Box 18.2). Neither of them were able to exert voluntary electromyography (EMG) activity in the quadriceps femoris and soleus muscles. Percutaneous electrical stimula-

(continued)

J. B. Nielsen et al. (eds.), *Neuroplasticity-based Neurorehabilitation*,
https://doi.org/10.1007/978-3-031-81120-3_18

Box 18.1 (continued)

tion of the femoral and posterior tibial nerves revealed motor evoked responses in both muscles, reflecting the absence of lower motor neuron damages. Although they exhibited similar injury features, David showed severe spasticity (defined as a velocity-dependent increase in muscle tone due to the exaggeration of stretch reflexes) in the knee extensors and ankle plantar flexors, whereas Stephen showed flaccidity in both muscles. Interestingly, transcranial magnetic stimulation delivered over the leg representation of the primary motor cortex and transcutaneous electrical stimulation of the spinal cord above the level of the injury elicited motor evoked potentials (MEPs) in both muscles in David, indicating residual descending motor connectivity. Conversely, no responses were elicited in Stephen. Further investigations confirmed the existence of concomitant patterns of spared corticospinal connectivity and spasticity in humans with motor complete SCI (i.e., AIS A and B) and that most injuries to the spinal cord were anatomically incomplete. This evidence of some degree of continuity of the central nervous system tissue throughout the damaged spinal segments may provide the neural substrate required to support motor recovery.

18.1 Prevalence and Incidence of SCI

In 2019, it was estimated that 20.6 million individuals were living with a spinal cord injury (SCI) worldwide. The global incidence of SCI was 0.9 million new cases. Injury at the neck level represented 10.8 million cases of SCI, compared to 9.7 million cases below the neck level. Falls were the main cause of injury, particularly among older adults, followed by road injuries and interpersonal violence. The age-standardized incidence rate for women was 10.3 per 100,000, compared to 12.6 per 100,000 for men. The incident rates for both sexes amongst those under 70 years old were comparable. However, the incidence rate increased sharply with age for people over 70, with women exhibiting higher rates (GBD Spinal Cord Injuries Collaborators, 2023).

18.2 Pathophysiology of SCI

SCI disrupts the structural and functional connections between cortical and spinal structures, resulting in motor, sensory, and autonomic dysfunction. The pathophysiology of SCI results from both primary and secondary injuries. Primary injury is caused by acute mechanical trauma resulting in vascular disruption, ruptures of the blood-spinal cord barrier, cell degeneration including neurons, glial, and endothelial cells, and interruption of central nervous system (CNS) tracts in the spinal cord. Secondary injury refers to subsequent pathological mechanisms resulting from the primary injury, including hemorrhage, excitotoxicity, neuroinflammation, demyelination, astrogliosis, and extracellular remodeling. The ISNCSCI and the ASIA are standardized neurological examinations used to evaluate the extent of the injury through assessment of the sensory and motor functions (see Box 18.2). Individuals may be graded as sensory and motor complete (AIS A), sensory incomplete (AIS B), motor incomplete (AIS C, D), and normal (AIS E). Consequently, the extent and severity of the injury evaluated by these clinical exams are the most recognized predictors of recovery after injury (Kirshblum et al., 2021).

The most common injuries in humans involve contusions and compressions. As a result, the CNS tissue may exhibit varying degrees of continuity across the lesion, resulting in different patterns of descending connection to muscles below the injury. Anatomical analysis provided evidence of such CNS continuity in >60% of individuals with SCI, even in those with a diagnosis of clinically complete SCI. This is consistent with electrophysiological studies in people with motor complete SCI, which demonstrate their ability to generate electromyographic (EMG) signals in some but not all

Box 18.2 Classification and Clinical Scales

The International Standards for Neurological Classification of Spinal Cord Injury (ISNCSCI) in association with the American Spinal Injury Association (ASIA) Impairment Scale (AIS) are standardized neurological examinations commonly used to evaluate the extent of the injury. The ISNCSCI exam includes grading of motor and sensory functions throughout 10 pairs of myotomes and 28 pairs of dermatomes to determine the neurological level of the injury (Fig. 18.1). The AIS is grading the severity of the injury as sensory and motor complete (AIS A), sensory incomplete (AIS B), motor incomplete (AIS C and D) and normal (AIS E).

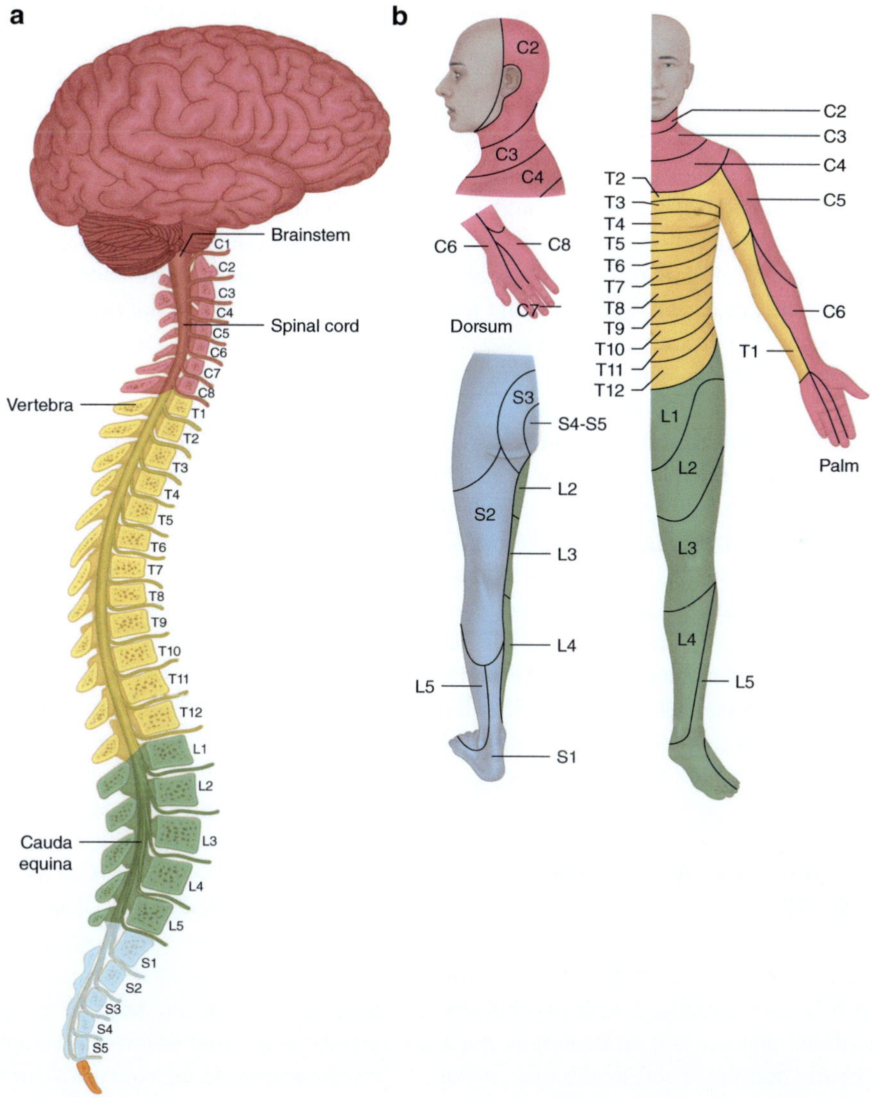

Fig. 18.1 Extent of the motor and sensory areas affected by the level of the injury. The spinal cord is organized into four main levels: cervical (C), thoracic (T), lumbar (L), and sacral (L). Each level is further divided into segments, each aligned with specific vertebrae (**a**), and associated with distinct motor and sensory functions (**b**). Therefore, an SCI will disrupt both the descending motor and ascending sensory pathways to all limb areas located at or below the level of the injury

muscles below the level of injury, implying preservation of some supraspinal control in these muscles. A combination of these and other methods indicated that a rather large proportion (80%) of humans with clinically complete SCI showed one or more signs of spared descending connections to isolated populations of motor units (Dimitrijevic & Kakulas, 2020). The category "discomplete" was introduced to designate such cases. This observation signifies that the absence of voluntary motor output in humans with a diagnosis of clinically complete SCI does not necessarily imply that spinal motoneurons caudal to the lesion are entirely deprived of descending innervation.

More recently, concomitant patterns of residual corticospinal responses and spasticity in muscles below the injury have been documented in humans with motor complete SCI, suggesting that a clinical examination of spasticity could represent a valuable predictor of residual descending motor connectivity following severe paralysis. Furthermore, the presence of spasticity and residual corticospinal connection has been associated with motor recovery in patients with subacute, clinically complete SCI following inpatient rehabilitation (Sangari et al., 2023). Similarly, those individuals with chronic injuries who are receiving epidural or transcutaneous spinal cord stimulation combined with motor training exhibited functional recovery (Hachmann et al., 2021). It is noteworthy that only a small percentage of individuals with severe SCI progress from motor complete to motor incomplete (Kirshblum et al., 2021; Sangari et al., 2023), which contrasts with the rather large fraction of discomplete patients who theoretically could develop meaningful motor behaviors.

18.3 Special Challenges Related to SCI

SCI impacts survivors' quality of life and lifespan, but it is also associated with psychological and emotional distress and an economic burden on the family and the social health care system. Although natural recovery primarily occurred during the first 6–9 months following the injury (Kirshblum et al., 2021), it is limited and highlights the need for neurorehabilitation strategies to promote further recovery. However, the first aspect of neurorehabilitation to consider is the timing of its implementation (e.g., acute, subacute, or chronic stage of the injury). Although observational and retrospective studies have suggested an association between delayed access to rehabilitation and poor functional recovery, this aspect requires further investigation.

The second aspect of neurorehabilitation to consider is identifying which patients may benefit from different neurorehabilitation strategies. Indeed, there is no standard lesion as every injury is unique, making each case distinct. The patient's characteristics and injury significantly impact rehabilitation and influence the selection of patients who are most likely to benefit from a specific rehabilitation strategy.

The third aspect of neurorehabilitation to consider is the effectiveness of various rehabilitation strategies. Since significant recovery of motor function is generally not expected beyond what is predicted by the clinical assessments (i.e., ISNCSCI and ASIA), conventional physical rehabilitation activities have focused on compensating for identified impairment and deficits. Although this approach results in the strengthening of muscles above the level of the lesion and strategies to move weak or paralyzed parts of the body, it does not promote recovery throughout the CNS for the motor control of the paralyzed limbs. In contrast, activity-based therapy refers to interventions that result in neuromuscular activation below the level of the injury, engaging the plasticity of the nervous system to promote recovery of motor function. This includes exercise training and neurostimulation strategies (Behrman & Harkema, 2007). Another rehabilitation approach is to promote recovery through neural repair using biological agents that enhance neuronal and/or glial plasticity. Although neuroplasticity-based strategies appear to be the most effective when used in conjunction with conventional rehabilitation, a better definition of how to determine the superiority of one approach over another is still needed and requires further investigation. However, evidence has shown that individual treatments are insufficient in restoring significant motor function, whereas combinatory approaches are thought to facilitate functional recovery in humans with SCI. Since most SCI in humans are anatomically incomplete, indicating the existence of residual corticospinal connections that could support neurological recovery, the next sections will discuss how strengthening transmission in these spared connections—through neuroplasticity-based approaches using neurostimulation, repair strategies, and exercise rehabilitation—might open avenues for motor recovery.

18.4 Neuroplasticity-Based Approaches

18.4.1 Neurostimulation

To date, promising functional restoration in humans with SCI has been demonstrated through neurostimulation approaches targeting the spinal cord and/or the brain, generally combined with exercise training. It has been reported that people with complete or incomplete injuries may regain some voluntary control over the paralyzed muscles. Though safe, these methods fail to fully restore independence, and some of them rely on perpetual stimulation to achieve the most substantial functional gains. Neurostimulation strategies aiming to reactivate or strengthen the cortical and spinal circuits above, at, and below the lesion to restore volitional movement are discussed in Box 18.3. Spinal cord approaches target the spinal neural network by either applying inputs at a distance that travel toward the spinal cord (i.e., paired associative stimulation) or by applying inputs more directly over the spinal cord (i.e., epidural stimulation and transcutaneous spinal cord stimulation). Brain approaches aim to involve cortical circuits and residual descending motor pathways by using either electrical or magnetic stimulation over the primary motor cortex (i.e., transcranial direct current stimulation and repetitive transcranial magnetic stimulation).

Box 18.3 The Spinal Cord as a Target for Neurostimulation

Paired associative stimulation or paired corticospinal-motoneuronal stimulation (PCMS) is a strategy aiming to enhance connectivity at corticospinal-motoneuronal synapses, thereby exploiting the naturally occurring adaptation in neuronal connections based on the principles of spike-timing-dependent plasticity—"neurons that fire together, wire together" (see Chap. 13). This mechanism relies on precisely timed stimulation of presynaptic neurons just prior (within a few milliseconds) to stimulation of their postsynaptic neurons to engage endogenous synaptic plasticity. A single session (200 pairs of stimuli) of PCMS targeting muscles innervated by motoneurons located below the lesion results in a transient increase in physiological outcomes measured as larger corticospinal responses and voluntary motor outputs (Urbin et al., 2017). In addition to improve physiological outcomes, there appears to be a threshold for the functional effects of the PCMS. Changes in functional outcomes, measured as time to complete the Graded and Redefined Assessment of Strength, Sensibility, and Prehension (GRASSP) and the 10-m walk tests, were found after 20 but not after 10 sessions of PCMS combined with exercise training. These improvements were preserved for several months after the interventions. Furthermore, 40 sessions of PCMS combined with exercise training showed to be an adequate dose to detect the minimal clinically important difference in most participants. Improvements in sensory and motor function and bladder and bowel function were also reported (Jo et al., 2023). Note that the effect of 20 to 40 sessions of PCMS on walking speed was two to three times higher than those reported

(continued)

Box 18.3 (continued)

after a similar number of sessions of exercise training alone, and similar to those obtained by invasive neurostimulation (Hachmann et al., 2021), highlighting the potential of noninvasive approaches for functional restoration.

Other approaches aim to influence spinal networks that project transsynaptically to motoneurons through stimulation of the spinal cord, either noninvasively (transcutaneous spinal cord stimulation, tcSCS) or invasively (epidural stimulation). When receiving tcSCS over the thoracolumbar spinal cord, individuals with motor complete and incomplete SCI showed enhanced voluntary control of lower limbs during treadmill stepping, regaining self-assisted standing, and postural control of upright sitting. Similarly, when receiving tcSCS over the cervical spinal cord, individuals with motor complete and incomplete SCI improved arm and hand function as measured by the time to complete the GRASSP test. This regain of function could be maintained for several months after the intervention (Taylor et al., 2021). Recent evidence showed that the effects of tcSCS are mediated through changes in the excitability of the cortical and spinal neuronal networks. Additional benefits of tcSCS have been reported including improvements in cardiovascular and bladder functions, and spasticity. Similarly, epidural stimulation applied over the lumbosacral spinal cord in conjunction with exercise training promoted recovery of voluntary lower limb function, independent standing, and assisted walking in individuals with motor complete SCI. Some individuals with incomplete SCI also maintained the ability to walk even without stimulation, reflecting neurological recovery. In addition, epidural stimulation has been shown to improve cardiovascular, bladder, and bowel functions in individuals with SCI. Although tcSCS and epidural stimulation demonstrated some functional efficacy, recovery remains limited due to the small number of participants tested. Moreover, functional improvements without stimulation may be observed but require intensive rehabilitation.

The Brain as a Target for Neurostimulation

Noninvasive brain stimulation approaches aim to modulate cortical excitability. Repeated transcranial magnetic stimulation (rTMS) over the motor cortex enhances sensory and motor recovery after SCI through long-term potentiation and depression of corticospinal synaptic transmission. rTMS over the hand representation of the motor cortex in individuals with incomplete SCI resulted in improvements in grasp function as measured by the time to complete the nine-hole-peg-test. rTMS over the leg representation of the motor cortex has been shown to improve motor scores and gait function as assessed by the 10-m walk test in individuals with subacute to chronic cervical and thoracic incomplete SCI. These motor improvements lasted for several weeks after the stimulation. In addition, rTMS has been shown to decrease neuropathic pain and reduce symptoms of spasticity (Tazoe & Perez, 2015). Although the effects promoted by rTMS are variable and rely on diverse stimulation parameters (e.g., intensity, frequency, number of stimuli/sessions, and cortical region targeted), and despite limited knowledge about the neuronal changes occurring along the corticospinal pathway, rTMS represents a promising approach to promote aspects of recovery after SCI. Another approach is transcranial direct current stimulation (tDCS), which consists of low-intensity continuous electric currents applied over the scalp. Anodal tDCS (i.e., anode located over the motor cortex) transiently raised the corticospinal excitability and improved

(continued)

Box 18.3 (continued)
sensory perception. When combined with exercise training, tDCS has been shown to improve arm and hand strength, and grasp function as measured by the time to complete the nine-hole-peg-test, but also locomotion outcomes and motor scores in individuals with incomplete SCI. These improvements persisted over several months after the stimulation. However, note that the same studies also reported changes after placebo stimulation. In addition, tDCS seems to affect neuropathic pain and symptoms of spasticity (Chen et al., 2023). Similar to rTMS, tDSC effects are limited and variable. Overall, brain and spinal cord stimulation strategies shows promising, yet limited, effects on functional restoration, which might be strengthened by other repair strategies.

18.4.2 Repair Strategies

New biological agents can enhance neuronal and/or glial plasticity. Animal models of SCI have shown that intraspinal transplants of Schwann cells, mesenchymal stromal cells, olfactory ensheathing cells, or oligodendrocyte precursor cells can protect neurons, increase vasculature, and mediate axonal growth and re-myelination. For example, neural stem cells differentiated from human pluripotent stem cells can facilitate axonal regeneration in the injured spinal cord. Additionally, the transplanted cells differentiate into neurons that establish a relay between supraspinal motor neurons and spinal cord neurons (Assinck et al., 2017). Several of these agents have undergone phase I/II/III clinical trials and the results from these studies varied from some improvements in motor and sensory scores, no significant effects, or a comparable or even less pronounced improvement compared to a control group. Though it is clear that cell transplantation in humans with SCI is generally feasible, the mechanisms by which these cell therapies promote functional restoration and the efficacy and long-term safety remain to be tested.

Growth factors (i.e., nerve growth factor, neurotrophin-3, brain-derived neurotrophic factor, glial cell-derived neurotrophic factor) administered to the damaged spinal cord by injection, release from biomaterials, or through genetic modification of spinal cord cells can protect neurons and result in axonal regeneration. Agents that interfere with endogenous axon growth-inhibitory molecules [i.e., chondroitin-sulfate proteoglycans (CSPGs), reticulon 4 (Nogo)] enable axon regrowth in the damaged spinal cord. With most of these agents (but not all), axons do not grow long distances or establish functional synaptic connections with host spinal cord neurons (Awad et al., 2015). Research is focused on overcoming these limitations, and phase I and phase I/II clinical trials in humans with SCI using CSPGs and Nogo are in progress.

Bioengineering is a rapidly growing component of neuroregeneration research. Solid or injectable biocompatible materials can provide platforms that enhance the survival of transplanted cells. Biomaterials can also enhance the targeted delivery of growth factors that stimulate neural repair and functional recovery. Though biomaterials are often combined with cell transplants or growth factors, some can on their own trigger tissue formation, angiogenesis, and axonal regeneration (Guijarro-Belmar et al., 2022). In addition to issues that limit the clinical practice of repair strategies, including ethical controversy, cell source, intervention time, uncontrolled cell proliferation, and long-term safety; some limitations make it difficult to compare patient developments and the effectiveness of protocols and treatments. Indeed, clinical studies employed a variety of protocols, the majority of which were not controlled, randomized or blinded. While some studies had modest sample sizes, others enrolled larger groups, but they were more heterogeneous. In addition, the outcomes reported and patient characterizations also displayed heterogeneity. Spinal cord repair therapies that are safe and effective for SCI patients have not yet been identified.

18.4.3 Exercise Rehabilitation

Exercise rehabilitation strategies designed to improve upper and lower limb function are commonly employed in individuals with motor incomplete injuries who demonstrate preserved descending motor control. For example, strategies using repetitive and intense gait practice have been shown to be effective in improving walking ability. Body weight supported treadmill training (BWSTT), robotic-assistive devices (see Chap. 16), and orthosis help therapists control and assist with both trunk and extremities kinematics, aiming to achieve a gait pattern that is close to that of control subjects during locomotion. Although the intention is to promote better outcomes, studies showed that both BWSTT and conventional overground gait training resulted in similar improvements in walking ability as measured by walking speed and the Walking Index for Spinal Cord Injury. In contrast, robotic-assisted gait training has been shown to improve the Walking Index for Spinal Cord Injury compared to overground gait training. However, it is unclear if BWSTT and robotic-assisted gait training showed better or similar improvement in walking distance compared to overground gait training (Duan et al., 2021).

18.5 Final Remarks

In addition to evidences indicating that a combination of different neurorehabilitation strategies achieves greater benefits than individual therapy alone, the effectiveness of neurorehabilitation relies on several factors, including the characteristics of the recipient, the timing of the intervention, the selected approaches, and the dosage administred. Consequently, determining if some neurorehabilitation approaches provide greater benefits than others requires further investigation.

Review Questions

- What are the neurorehabilitation strategies available for individuals with spinal cord injury?
- What characterizes effective neurorehabilitation following spinal cord injury?

References

Assinck, P., Duncan, G. J., Hilton, B. J., Plemel, J. R., & Tetzlaff, W. (2017). Cell transplantation therapy for spinal cord injury. *Nature Neuroscience, 20*, 637–647.

Awad, B. I., Carmody, M. A., & Steinmetz, M. P. (2015). Potential role of growth factors in the management of spinal cord injury. *World Neurosurgery, 83*, 120–131.

Behrman, A. L., & Harkema, S. J. (2007). Physical rehabilitation as an agent for recovery after spinal cord injury. *Physical Medicine and Rehabilitation Clinics of North America, 18*, 183–202, v.

Chen, J.-M., Li, X.-L., Pan, Q.-H., Yang, Y., Xu, S.-M., & Xu, J.-W. (2023). Effects of non-invasive brain stimulation on motor function after spinal cord injury: A systematic review and meta-analysis. *Journal of Neuroengineering and Rehabilitation, 20*, 3.

Dimitrijevic, M. R., & Kakulas, B. A. (2020). Spinal cord injuries, human neuropathology and neurophysiology. *Acta Myol, 39*, 353–358.

Duan, R., Qu, M., Yuan, Y., Lin, M., Liu, T., Huang, W., Gao, J., Zhang, M., & Yu, X. (2021). Clinical benefit of rehabilitation training in spinal cord injury: A systematic review and meta-analysis. *Spine (Phila Pa 1976), 46*, E398–E410.

GBD Spinal Cord Injuries Collaborators. (2023). Global, regional, and national burden of spinal cord injury, 1990-2019: A systematic analysis for the Global Burden of Disease Study 2019. *The Lancet Neurology, 22(11)*, 1026–1047. https://doi.org/10.1016/S1474-4422(23)00287-9. Erratum in: Lancet Neurol. 2024;23(4):e8. https://doi.org/10.1016/S1474-4422(24)00095-4.

Guijarro-Belmar, A., Varone, A., Baltzer, M. R., Kataria, S., Tanriver-Ayder, E., Watzlawick, R., Sena, E., Cunningham, C. J., Rajnicek, A. M., Macleod, M., Huang, W., Currie, G. L., & McCann, S. K. (2022). Effectiveness of biomaterial-based combination strategies for spinal cord repair—A systematic review and meta-analysis of preclinical literature. *Spinal Cord, 60*, 1041–1049.

Hachmann, J. T., Yousak, A., Wallner, J. J., Gad, P. N., Edgerton, V. R., & Gorgey, A. S. (2021). Epidural spinal cord stimulation as an intervention for motor recovery after motor complete spinal cord injury. *Journal of Neurophysiology, 126*, 1843–1859.

Jo, H. J., Kizziar, E., Sangari, S., Chen, D., Kessler, A., Kim, K., Anschel, A., Heinemann, A. W., Mensh, B. D., Awadalla, S., Lieber, R. L., Oudega, M., & Perez, M. A. (2023). Multisite Hebbian plasticity restores function in humans with spinal cord injury. *Annals of Neurology, 93*, 1198–1213.

Kirshblum, S., Snider, B., Eren, F., & Guest, J. (2021). Characterizing natural recovery after traumatic spinal cord injury. *Journal of Neurotrauma, 38*, 1267–1284.

Sangari, S., Chen, B., Grover, F., Salsabili, H., Sheth, M., Gohil, K., Hobbs, S., Olson, A., Eisner-Janowicz, I., Anschel, A., Kim, K., Chen, D., Kessler, A., Heinemann, A. W., Oudega, M., Kwon, B. K., Kirshblum, S., Guest, J. D., & Perez, M. A. (2023). Spasticity predicts motor recovery for patients with subacute motor complete spinal cord injury. *Annals of Neurology*. https://doi.org/10.1002/ana.26772

Taylor, C., McHugh, C., Mockler, D., Minogue, C., Reilly, R. B., & Fleming, N. (2021). Transcutaneous spinal cord stimulation and motor responses in individuals with spinal cord injury: A methodological review. *PLoS One, 16*, e0260166.

Tazoe, T., & Perez, M. A. (2015). Effects of repetitive transcranial magnetic stimulation on recovery of function after spinal cord injury. *Archives of Physical Medicine and Rehabilitation, 96*, S145–S155.

Urbin, M. A., Ozdemir, R. A., Tazoe, T., & Perez, M. A. (2017). Spike-timing-dependent plasticity in lower-limb motoneurons after human spinal cord injury. *Journal of Neurophysiology, 118*, 2171–2180.

Cerebral Palsy

19

Jens Bo Nielsen, Helle Hüche Larsen, and Andrea Guzzetta

Abstract

This chapter describes Cerebral Palsy (CP), a neural developmental disorder impacting 2–3 out of 1000 newborns globally. The cause of CP is often unknown, but factors such as compromised oxygen in the third trimester or prenatal infections may be involved. CP exhibits diverse motor dysfunctions, delaying motor milestones and introducing impairments in speech, communication, vision, and cognitive abilities. Early diagnosis is pivotal, given CP's dynamic nature, subject to fluctuations leading to either improvement or deterioration throughout an individual's life. The emphasis on early detection aims to capitalize on interventions during critical developmental phases when neuronal plasticity is most potent. Family-based, goal-directed, and engaging interventions for infants with CP are recommended, utilizing tools like abnormal MR brain scans and General Movement Analysis (GMA) for early and timely intervention. Ongoing support for continued development involves monitoring progress, engaging the child in goal setting, and seamlessly integrating therapy into daily life. Transition from youth to adulthood is addressed, underscoring the importance of maintaining physical activity and reducing dependency on hospitals. Challenges faced by adults with CP, including premature aging-related changes, are discussed, with recommendations for health practitioners to support a healthy, active lifestyle. This chapter consistently underscores the significance of early intervention, continuous support, and adaptive strategies to enhance the quality of life for individuals with CP throughout their lifespan.

Keywords

Cerebral palsy (CP) · Neural developmental disorder · Early diagnosis · Motor dysfunctions · Intervention strategies · Lifelong support

Box 19.1 Case Story

The pregnancy had been normal, but labor started suddenly in the 32nd week of pregnancy and Lisa was born 8 weeks prematurely. She therefore spent the first 4 weeks of life in an incubator before the doctors decided that it was safe for her to breathe and eat herself. Following the initial shock of the premature birth, Lisa's parents now looked forward to taking their newborn daughter home and starting their new family. However, before the doctors would allow Lisa to be sent home, they insisted on

(continued)

J. B. Nielsen (✉) · H. H. Larsen
Department of Neuroscience, University of Copenhagen, Copenhagen, Denmark
e-mail: jbnielsen@sund.ku.dk; hmhlarsen@sund.ku.dk

A. Guzzetta
University of Pisa, Fondazione Stella Maris, Pisa, Italy
e-mail: andrea.guzzetta@fsm.unipi.it

J. B. Nielsen et al. (eds.), *Neuroplasticity-based Neurorehabilitation*,
https://doi.org/10.1007/978-3-031-81120-3_19

Box 19.1 (continued)
having more tests on Lisa. One was an MR scan of the brain, which revealed a lesion on the right side of Lisa's brain. Although the doctors emphasized that this need not have any significance for Lisa's future development, it nevertheless made her parents worried. In the following months when they had finally got Lisa home, they observed her carefully and continued to worry that she would not develop normally. When Lisa was 5 months old (that is 3 months after the expected birth) they were offered a General Movement Analysis performed on Lisa. This revealed the absence of fidgety movements and Lisa's parents were explained that this would mean that Lisa was at very high risk of cerebral palsy. Although this was news that Lisa's parents had feared, they were nevertheless happy that it was now clear that something had to be done to help Lisa's development as much as possible. They agreed to be part of an intensive early intervention program, which required that they encourage Lisa through play to make movements and explore her surroundings and movement abilities several times per day for the next 6 months with monthly supervision from the therapists. This was not experienced as hard work for the parents. They enjoyed interacting with their daughter and being able to do something that could make a change in Lisa's development. Lisa is now 4 years old, and she has been diagnosed with very mild CP. She has some trouble using her left hand, but otherwise, she is functioning very well. Lisa started walking when she was 15 months old and now runs and jumps like any other 4-year-old child. Lisa started talking around 2 years of age and now speaks fluently. She is a bright girl who quickly learns new things. Apart from visits to an occupational therapist every 2 weeks, who helps her train her left hand, Lisa and her family are living a normal life. Her parents are certain that it is the early training that Lisa received that has made it possible.

19.1 Introduction

Cerebral Palsy (CP) is caused by a disturbance in neural development occurring before or around birth (Rosenbaum et al., 2007). It affects approximately 2–3 out of 1000 newborns, resulting in an estimated global prevalence of 17 million affected individuals (Graham et al., 2016).

The exact cause of CP is often difficult or impossible to clarify. However, many different risk factors and causal pathways have been suggested (Evans et al., 2023). The beginning of the third trimester of pregnancy appears to be a vulnerable period where compromised oxygen and nutritional supply to the fetus are likely to play a pathophysiological role. In some cases, infections, exposure to toxic substances, or medical health conditions of the mother may be identified as prenatal causes. Improved techniques for genetic diagnostics have shown that genetic factors play a role in many cases and continued development in this field is likely to reveal underlying genetic factors in an increasing number of cases. CP is more frequent among children born prematurely (50% of all cases of CP are related to premature birth) and in multifetus pregnancies, consistent with a role of compromised oxygen and nutritional supply to the fetus. Complications in relation to birth (asphyxia) are overall rare, but CP is a possible consequence. After birth, CP may be caused by head trauma, infections, and other medical conditions.

CP is highly diverse and varies widely clinically depending on type and severity, but the hallmark is some degree of motor dysfunction with difficulties in motor control and coordination, leading to abnormal or involuntary movements (see Box 19.2). Difficulty maintaining posture and balance is frequent and gait may be abnormal with foot drop, toe-walking, and

Box 19.2 Types of Cerebral Palsy

Spastic Cerebral Palsy

Spastic CP is the most common type, affecting approximately 70–80% of individuals with CP. It is characterized by muscle paresis, impaired muscle growth, weak muscles, and challenges in muscle coordination, posture, and gait. Contractures and joint malformations are common (see Box 19.3). This type of CP results from damage to the motor cortex or corticospinal tracts. Spastic CP is further divided based on the distribution of affected muscles:

Spastic Hemiplegia: One side of the body is affected, typically the arm and leg on the same side. Children with spastic hemiplegia may have difficulty with fine motor skills and may walk on their toes on the affected side.

Spastic Diplegia: Both legs are primarily affected, while the arms may have minimal or no involvement. Children with spastic diplegia often have difficulty walking due to tightness in the hip and leg muscles, leading to a scissoring gait or toe-walking.

Spastic Quadriplegia: All four limbs are affected, often along with the trunk and face. This is the most severe form of spastic CP and is frequently associated with other impairments, such as intellectual disability, seizures, and difficulties with speech and swallowing.

Dyskinetic Cerebral Palsy

Dyskinetic CP, which accounts for 5–10% of CP cases, is characterized by involuntary movements, which can be dystonic (slow and writhing) or choreoathetotic (rapid and jerky). This type results from damage to the basal ganglia. Children with dyskinetic CP may have difficulty maintaining posture and coordinating movements, which can affect their ability to sit, stand, and walk. Speech and swallowing may also be impaired due to involuntary movements of the face and tongue.

Ataxic Cerebral Palsy

Ataxic CP affects about 5–10% of individuals with CP. It is characterized by problems with balance and coordination (ataxia), resulting from damage to the cerebellum. Children with ataxic CP may have unsteady, shaky movements, and difficulties with tasks that require precise coordination, such as writing or buttoning a shirt. They may also have a wide-based gait to compensate for their balance issues.

crouched gait as the most frequent disturbances. Children with CP often show delays in reaching motor milestones such as sitting up, crawling, and walking. Development of muscle contractures and abnormal joint positions are common as an early complication to the affected control of movement. Additional impairments are commonly seen in association with motor disorders (Delacy & Reid, 2016). Speech and communication may be affected depending on the type of CP and some may show difficulties in eating and swallowing leading to nutritional challenges. Vision is impaired in one in three children with CP, while hearing in about one in ten. Cognitive abilities such as attention, learning, and memory may be affected in some individuals. Seizures are seen in 20% to 50% of individuals with CP and may contribute to further reduction of cognitive abilities.

CP is a lifelong condition. The primary disturbance of neural development may lead to a variety of life trajectories that depend not only on the time, location, and size of the primary lesion but also on repair mechanisms and plastic responses of the surrounding nervous system, secondary reactions in other parts of the body (i.e., muscles, tendons, etc. with possible development of contractures; see Box 19.3), environmental stimuli, interventions, and many other factors. Consequently, CP is not a stable chronic condition, but rather a dynamic state, subject to fluctuations that may manifest as either deterioration or improvement over the individual's lifespan. There is widespread international agreement that early diagnosis and intervention play a pivotal role in steering individuals toward the most favorable developmental path throughout their entire life.

19.2 Early Diagnosis of CP to Harness Early Neuroplasticity

CP is typically diagnosed during the second year of life in most developed countries (Boychuck et al., 2019). Consequently, many children with CP may not receive specific intervention until more than a year after the nervous system injury occurred. This contrasts sharply with the immediate intervention that adults receive following injuries to the nervous system, such as stroke, spinal cord injury, or traumatic brain injury. The delayed diagnosis and intervention are particularly concerning because the first 6–12 months after birth are likely a critical period for the development of motor abilities.

Identifying children at risk of CP shortly after birth is feasible, as per international guidelines, by using a combination of diagnostic tools (Novak et al., 2017). Before the age of 5 months, a combination of abnormal MR brain scan results and the absence of fidgety movements (characteristic fine, quick, and irregular movements of the extremities, especially visible in hands and fingers during the infant's active, awake state between 3 and 5 months of age) indicates a high risk of CP. This should prompt immediate initiation of intervention and continuous monitoring of the infant's development. After 5 months of age, if a neurological examination shows paresis, altered muscle tone, or other signs of abnormal motor development in conjunction with abnormal MR findings, it provides sufficient diagnostic certainty to start intervention and continued surveillance.

The strong interest in early detection is based on the opportunity to initiate intervention at an early phase of development, at a time when mechanisms of neuronal plasticity are most powerful. To that end, perinatal brain lesions offer a particularly insightful model for understanding neuroplasticity. The concept of the advantageous effects of early as opposed to later brain damage was initially proposed by Paul Broca in 1865 (Berker et al., 1986) and further investigated by Margaret Kennard in the late 1930s (Kennard & Fulton, 1942). Subsequent studies across various species have consistently supported the overarching principle of the efficacy of early damage and rehabilitation, provided that other factors such as the location, extent, or type of injury distribution (focal vs. diffuse), and clinical correlates (e.g., presence of seizures or genetic susceptibility of the child) are carefully considered (Anderson et al., 2005).

In language, research following Paul Broca's early observations supports the principle of early damage advantages. Recent advancements, employing fMRI language tasks, have revealed a striking similarity in the activation patterns between the left hemisphere in normal controls and the right hemisphere in brain-injured patients following early left brain periventricular lesions. This indicates a near-equipotentiality of the two hemispheres at birth regarding language development. As development progresses, this option diminishes, leading to intrahemispheric reorganization and varying degrees of language disturbance with later lesions. Similarly, in cases of cerebral lesions affecting the motor system, neuroplastic mechanisms play a crucial role in the recovery of voluntary movements by restoring cortical impulses to spinal motor neurons and interneurons. The use of fMRI can offer insights into the nature of reorganization in each patient, but it must be complemented by techniques with high temporal resolution, such as Transcranial Magnetic Stimulation (TMS), which help document the plastic reorganization of corticospinal connections. Analogous mechanisms of early neuroplasticity can be observed when exploring the somatosensory or visual systems after early brain damage. This observation reinforces the notion that the comprehensive network of connections, often referred to as the connectome, undergoes significant reshaping when damage occurs during the early phases of development.

19.3 Early Intervention in Infants with CP

Growing evidence supports the notion that early intervention, grounded in principles of neuroplasticity and motor learning, can profoundly impact the long-term motor and cognitive development of children with CP, although controlled studies are difficult to perform in this domain (Morgan et al., 2021). Internationally, there is a shared consensus that successful early interventions aimed at fostering motor and cognitive development in children with CP and other neurodevelopmental disorders should incorporate some essential elements that are outlined below.

19.3.1 The Intervention Should Be Family-Based

The success of early intervention depends more than anything on the active involvement of parents, siblings, and other members of the extended family. It is a shock for the parents to realize that their newborn child has a brain injury and most—if not all—will need help and guidance to tackle all the uncertainties and questions that this unexpected new situation has created. Reactive depression is not uncommon, and the risk of divorce is high among parents of children with CP. These signs of parental stress are not helpful for the development of the child and should be handled before they occur—if necessary, with the help of a psychologist. The family—and especially the parents—will also need guidance on how to best take care of their child and stimulate development as optimally as possible. This will require that the parents are made active members of a "therapeutic team" together with doctors, occupational therapists, physical therapists, speech therapists, and others if needed. In this way, the parents may achieve ownership of the therapeutic plan for their child and under the guidance of therapists be able to promote the motor and cognitive development of the child in daily life. At this stage of life, the parent-child interaction is key to optimal development. It cannot and should not be replaced by formalized training carried out by a professional therapist. The parents should spend as much time as possible with their child to create a mutual bond and stimulate the child according to the advice and guidance from the therapists. The short time a therapist has available to work with the child makes little difference for the child's development, but should rather be used to guide and instruct and most importantly support the parents. It is their daily interaction with the child that will make a difference for the child later in life.

19.3.2 The Intervention Should Activate and Engage the Child: Physically and Mentally

Learning skills and optimizing motor abilities require active involvement and engagement. This is equally true for small infants as for older children and adults. Passive stimulation may give the child comfort and help establish the all-important bonds between child and parent, but when it comes to facilitating and optimizing the child's motor development, it is necessary to engage the child and encourage the active movement of affected body parts. In this regard, an enriched environment which makes it easy to engage the child in active play will help. This can and should be adapted to individual families and their homes. There are limitless possibilities of finding unique solutions that can activate the individual infant optimally. It will be up to the therapists and families to find what works best and addresses the challenges of the individual child most efficiently. The family needs to be thought of as a whole and supported in the best way possible so that they themselves have the resources to make informed decisions on behalf of their child.

19.3.3 The Intervention Should Be Goal-Directed and Monitor Progress

It is crucial for parents and therapists to collaboratively establish clear and realistic intervention goals. This process allows parents to experience success when these goals are attained, fostering a sense of hope and reassurance that their efforts in stimulating their child are making a meaningful impact. Additionally, breaking down a seemingly insurmountable challenge into achievable tasks helps to instill confidence, motivation, and possibly relief from parental stress. Oftentimes parents feel overwhelmed and afraid that they are not doing enough for their child. Clear goals and a plan may help handle this feeling. In cases where the set goals are not achieved, it can serve as a valuable opportunity for constructive analysis. This enables the identification of areas that need improvement and allows for refining the intervention in the future.

Box 19.3 Contractures

Contractures develop in most children with spastic CP and are the most important secondary cause of reduced motility. The term "contracture" is often confused with "contraction," but they are not the same. Contracture is not caused by active muscle contraction but by changes in the muscle and surrounding tissue, leading to increased stiffness, reduced muscle length, joint misalignment, and deformity.

Contractures develop due to a lack of neural activation and use of the muscles during development, possibly in combination with involuntary muscle overactivity. Without proper neural signals and usage, the muscles fail to grow appropriately, while bones may continue to grow at an almost normal rate, creating significant tension in the muscles. This tension causes an accumulation of connective tissue in and around the muscles, leading to increased stiffness, reduced joint mobility, and eventual joint deformity. Increased involuntary muscle activity can also contribute to this process.

Preventing contractures involves promoting muscle growth through physical activity and exercise and reducing involuntary muscle activity with antispastic therapies. Fully developed contractures are challenging to treat, and orthopedic surgery is often the only effective option.

19.4 Facilitating Continued Development in Children with CP

After the initial early intervention, it is crucial to provide ongoing monitoring of the child's development and offer support to parents for continued stimulation of the child's motor skills and abilities. Additionally, specialized medical assistance, such as medication or surgery, should be offered when deemed necessary.

The principles of continued therapy and intervention for children with cerebral palsy are similar to when they were infants, with parents as primary caregivers and therapists providing essential guidance and support. However, as the child grows older, new challenges and opportunities arise.

As communication with the child becomes more accessible, goal setting can gradually involve the child, eventually making them a central participant in their own training and development. Involving professional pedagogues and teachers from kindergartens and schools can further facilitate the child's ongoing motor and cognitive growth. Effective coordination among healthcare professionals, parents, and educators becomes crucial for optimizing the child's development.

Encouraging the child's involvement in play, social activities with other children, and sports during leisure time is vital. Also, the natural integration of movement activities in everyday life, such as walking, biking or even cleaning one's room may help reduce sedentary time. As the child grows older, the incorporation of various games and sports, including interactive computer games, becomes increasingly feasible and significant in promoting motor and cognitive abilities.

However, it is equally essential to prevent experiences of failure when compared to other children, or when facing scorn due to their disability. Deliberate activities to foster communication and understanding among peers and families may be necessary to ensure a positive and supportive environment.

The medical management of cerebral palsy typically involves pharmacological interventions to address involuntary movements and muscle overactivity (see Chap. 5), seizures, pain, and other symptoms. Baclofen, administered orally or via an intrathecal pump, is commonly used to reduce involuntary muscle overactivity. Botulinum toxin injections directly into muscles block neuromuscular transmission and are used to suppress focal involuntary muscle overactivity and improve passive range of movement. Antiepileptic drugs are prescribed for children with CP who experience seizures, while medications like gabapentin or diazepam may be used to manage pain and discomfort. When using these medical treatments, it is important to consider that they may suppress not only involuntary movements and unwanted muscle overactivity but also the child's ability to perform voluntary movements. Additionally, the centrally acting medications (baclofen and diazepam) can affect the mechanisms underlying learning and memory, either directly or by causing drowsiness. These negative effects should be weighed against their benefits and the therapeutic goals set by therapists. This highlights the importance of a multidisciplinary approach in treating children with CP, involving therapists and other healthcare professionals in the clinical decision-making process.

Surgical interventions are considered when medical treatments and therapies are insufficient to manage symptoms or improve function. Orthopedic surgeries are among the most common, addressing musculoskeletal deformities such as contractures, scoliosis, and hip dislocations. Procedures like tendon lengthening, muscle release, and osteotomies aim to correct abnormal postures and alignments, thus enhancing mobility and reducing pain. Postoperative rehabilitation is crucial to maximize the benefits of these surgical interventions. This involves intensive physical therapy to strengthen muscles and improve motor skills.

Understanding the different types, severities, and distributions of CP is crucial for developing personalized treatment plans. Each child's specific needs and abilities must be considered to maximize their functional independence and quality of life (see Box 19.4). Multidisciplinary approaches involving physical therapy, occupational therapy, speech therapy, and medical or surgical interventions are essential to addressing the diverse challenges faced by children with CP.

Box 19.4 Classification and Clinical Scales

A number of classification systems and scales are used to characterize the abilities of children with CP in different domains from the least affected (Level I) to the most severely affected (Level V).

Gross Motor Function Classification System (GMFCS)

The Gross Motor Function Classification System (GMFCS) is used to classify the severity of CP based on the child's ability to perform gross motor functions and focuses on gait and posture.

Manual Ability Classification System (MACS)

The Manual Ability Classification System (MACS) complements the GMFCS by classifying how children with CP use their hands to handle objects in daily activities.

Communication Function Classification System (CFCS)

The Communication Function Classification System (CFCS) assesses the communication abilities of individuals with CP.

Eating and Drinking Ability Classification System (EDACS)

The Eating and Drinking Ability Classification System (EDACS) classifies

(continued)

Box 19.4 (continued)
how children with CP eat and drink safely and effectively.

Visual Function Classification System (VFCS)

The Visual Function Classification System (VFCS) assesses the visual abilities of individuals with CP, focusing on the functional use of vision in daily activities.

19.5 Transition from Youth to Adult

For many young individuals with CP, a natural desire to become increasingly independent from their parents may lead them to turn away from therapy offerings provided by public institutions. Having spent a significant portion of their lives in hospitals or physiotherapy clinics, some may feel compelled to take control of their own lives, which could result in neglecting the training and therapy they have received thus far, in favor of spending leisure time with friends or on their own.

Furthermore, only a few countries can afford to continue offering free regular therapy and surveillance as children with CP grow into teenagers or young adults. Consequently, therapy aimed at maintaining a certain functional level and promoting physical activity may no longer take place, contributing to a relatively early decline in function. To counter this, it is essential to integrate therapy and training into everyday leisure and sports activities during childhood. Ideally, young individuals with CP would continue to be physically active as a natural part of daily life and build friendships through sports and leisure activities. Reducing the number of visits to hospitals and clinics and focusing on facilitating enjoyable and motivating activities in daily life are key to achieving this goal.

As young adults with CP face the same challenges as their peers—striving for independence, pursuing education, careers, and potentially starting families—it becomes evident that they share the same dreams and hopes for the future. However, the reality is that a significant portion of young people and adults with CP may not receive education, engage in employment, or have partners and children (Michelsen et al., 2014).

Recognizing the importance of addressing the transition from childhood to adulthood, there is a growing focus on transition programs and clinics designed for adolescents and young adults with CP. These programs aim to promote a healthy lifestyle throughout adulthood and help individuals address the obstacles hindering their access to education, employment, and family life.

19.6 Adults

Due to advancements in medical care, rehabilitation, and new technologies, individuals with CP now generally have a life expectancy comparable to the general population. However, aging with a disability presents unique challenges, and many individuals with CP experience premature aging-related changes in their health and functioning, alongside typical age-related concerns like arthritis, osteoporosis, and cardiovascular issues (Kemp, 2005).

Upon entering adulthood, approximately 60% of adults with CP are capable of walking, but this ability commonly declines in early to middle adulthood, along with a reduction in balance and an increased risk of falling. These changes can significantly impact their everyday life, leading to potential self-restriction of activities. It is crucial to address these challenges, as individuals with CP often lead sedentary lifestyles, putting them at risk of developing lifestyle-related diseases (Verschuren et al., 2016).

Health practitioners play a crucial role in supporting adults with CP as they age and managing coexisting and age-related conditions. Empowering individuals to take responsibility for their training and goal setting is important, with an emphasis on promoting and maintaining physical activity. Everyday activities like walking or taking the stairs can contribute to a normal, active lifestyle. Additionally, engaging in moderate to vigorous activities should be encouraged, and therapists can assist by providing alternative solutions, using technologies, or adapting the environment to enhance accessibility.

Incorporating social activities with others can be motivational and combat feelings of isolation. As individuals with CP and their families plan for ongoing care, health practitioners need to be knowledgeable about age-related changes in CP to provide high-quality supervision and support. By addressing these aspects proactively, the overall health and well-being of individuals with CP can be improved, allowing them to lead fulfilling lives throughout their lifespan.

19.7 Conclusions

In conclusion, CP presents a formidable challenge stemming from early disruptions in neural development, impacting millions worldwide. The condition's clinical diversity underscores the need for a nuanced comprehension of its effects on motor, cognitive, and sensory functions. Early diagnosis and intervention, pivotal for leveraging neuroplasticity, stand as fundamental pillars guiding individuals toward positive developmental paths. Family-centered, goal-oriented interventions, initiated in infancy and sustained throughout life, are indispensable elements and should be implemented worldwide, accommodating variations in the economic means of individual countries.

Review Questions

- How do prematurity and prenatal factors contribute to the risk of developing CP in newborns?
- What are the key principles and components of effective early intervention strategies for infants diagnosed with cerebral palsy, and how do they impact long-term outcomes?

References

Anderson, V., Catroppa, C., Morse, S., Haritou, F., & Rosenfeld, J. (2005). Functional plasticity or vulnerability after early brain injury? *Pediatrics, 116*(6), 1374–1382. https://doi.org/10.1542/peds.2004-1728

Berker, E. A., Berker, A. H., & Smith, A. (1986). Translation of Broca's 1865 report. Localization of speech in the third left frontal convolution. *Archives of Neurology, 43*(10), 1065–1072. https://doi.org/10.1001/archneur.1986.00520100069017. PMID: 3530216.

Boychuck, Z., Bussières, A., Goldschleger, J., Majnemer, A., & Prompt Group. (2019). Age at referral for diagnosis and rehabilitation services for cerebral palsy: A scoping review. *Developmental Medicine and Child Neurology, 61*(8), 908–914. https://doi.org/10.1111/dmcn.14034. PMID: 30273970.

Delacy, M. J., & Reid, S. M. (2016). Profile of associated impairments at age 5 years in Australia by cerebral palsy subtype and Gross Motor Function Classification System level for birth years 1996 to 2005. *Developmental Medicine and Child Neurology, 58*, 50–56. https://doi.org/10.1111/dmcn.13012

Evans, M. I., Britt, D. W., & Devoe, L. D. (2023). Etiology and ontogeny of cerebral palsy: implications for practice and research. *Reproductive Sciences, 31*(5), 1179–1189. https://doi.org/10.1007/s43032-023-01422-6. PMID: 38133768.

Graham, H. K., Rosenbaum, P., Paneth, N., Dan, B., Lin, J. P., Damiano, D. L., Becher, J. G., Gaebler-Spira, D., Colver, A., Reddihough, D. S., Crompton, K. E., & Lieber, R. L. (2016). Cerebral palsy. *Nature Reviews Disease Primers, 7*(2), 15082. https://doi.org/10.1038/nrdp.2015.82

Kemp, B. J. (2005). What the rehabilitation professional and the consumer need to know. *Physical Medicine and Rehabilitation Clinics of North America, 16*(1), 1–18, vii.. https://doi.org/10.1016/j.pmr.2004.06.009

Kennard, M., & Fulton, J. F. (1942). Age and reorganization of central nervous system. *Mount Sinai Journal of Medicine, 9*, 594–606.

Michelsen, S. I., Flachs, E. M., Damsgaard, M. T., Parkes, J., Parkinson, K., Rapp, M., Arnaud, C., Nystrand, M., Colver, A., Fauconnier, J., Dickinson, H. O., Marcelli, M., & Uldall, P. (2014). European study of frequency of participation of adolescents with and without cerebral palsy. *European Journal of Paediatric Neurology, 18*(3), 282–294. https://doi.org/10.1016/j.ejpn.2013.12.003

Morgan, C., Fetters, L., Adde, L., Badawi, N., Bancale, A., Boyd, R. N., Chorna, O., Cioni, G., Damiano, D. L., Darrah, J., de Vries, L. S., Dusing, S., Einspieler, C., Eliasson, A. C., Ferriero, D., Fehlings, D., Forssberg, H., Gordon, A. M., Greaves, S., Guzzetta, A., Hadders-Algra, M., Harbourne, R., Karlsson, P., Krumlinde-Sundholm, L., Latal, B., Loughran-Fowlds, A., Mak, C., Maitre, N., McIntyre,

S., Mei, C., Morgan, A., Kakooza-Mwesige, A., Romeo, D. M., Sanchez, K., Spittle, A., Shepherd, R., Thornton, M., Valentine, J., Ward, R., Whittingham, K., Zamany, A., & Novak, I. (2021). Early intervention for children aged 0 to 2 years with or at high risk of cerebral palsy: International clinical practice guideline based on systematic reviews. *JAMA Pediatrics, 175*(8), 846–858. https://doi.org/10.1001/jamapediatrics.2021.0878

Novak, I., Morgan, C., Adde, L., Blackman, J., Boyd, R. N., Brunstrom-Hernandez, J., Cioni, G., Damiano, D., Darrah, J., Eliasson, A. C., de Vries, L. S., Einspieler, C., Fahey, M., Fehlings, D., Ferriero, D. M., Fetters, L., Fiori, S., Forssberg, H., Gordon, A. M., Greaves, S., Guzzetta, A., Hadders-Algra, M., Harbourne, R., Kakooza-Mwesige, A., Karlsson, P., Krumlinde-Sundholm, L., Latal, B., Loughran-Fowlds, A., Maitre, N., McIntyre, S., Noritz, G., Pennington, L., Romeo, D. M., Shepherd, R., Spittle, A. J., Thornton, M., Valentine, J., Walker, K., White, R., & Badawi, N. (2017). Early, accurate diagnosis and early intervention in cerebral palsy: advances in diagnosis and treatment. *JAMA Pediatrics, 171*(9), 897–907. https://doi.org/10.1001/jamapediatrics.2017.1689

Rosenbaum, P., Paneth, N., Leviton, A., Goldstein, M., Bax, M., Damiano, D., Dan, B., & Jacobsson, B. (2007). A report: the definition and classification of cerebral palsy April 2006. *Developmental Medicine and Child Neurology. Supplement, 109*, 8–14. Erratum in: Dev Med Child Neurol. 2007 Jun;49(6):480. PMID: 17370477.

Verschuren, O., Peterson, M. D., Balemans, A. C., & Hurvitz, E. A. (2016). Exercise and physical activity recommendations for people with cerebral palsy. *Developmental Medicine and Child Neurology, 58*(8), 798–808. https://doi.org/10.1111/dmcn.13053

Multiple Sclerosis

20

Ulrik Dalgas and Lars G. Hvid

Abstract

Multiple sclerosis (MS) is a chronic progressive demyelinating autoimmune disorder of the central nervous system, that over time causes accumulating disability and worsening of a diverse range of symptoms. Currently, a number of disease-modifying treatments exist, capable of slowing the progression of MS. In addition, pharmacological treatments aimed at alleviating symptoms exist for some symptoms, whereas they have limited or no efficacy on others while causing frequent adverse effects. Therefore, nonpharmacological interventions with the potential to further slowdown disease progression or treat symptoms are highly warranted in MS. Over the past three decades, a paradigm change has taken place establishing exercise as a cornerstone of MS rehabilitation as opposed to previously where it was considered damaging. Today exercise studies have established exercise as an effective symptomatic treatment (i.e., tertiary prevention), but recent studies have evaluated the disease-modifying effects (i.e., secondary prevention) of exercise as well as the impact on the risk of developing MS (i.e., primary prevention) showing promising results here as well. Moreover, tailored training can help people with MS increase their muscle strength, cardiorespiratory fitness, balance, and coordination, while simultaneously reducing core symptoms such as fatigue and gait impairments. Furthermore, training may have positive effects on (preserving) cognition, but the evidence is not conclusive.

This chapter describes the prevalence, incidence, prognosis, and pathophysiology of MS. In addition, characteristic symptoms associated with the disease are presented and treatment of many of these symptoms is discussed with a special focus on exercise and physical activity as interventions for people with MS. Finally, the chapter discusses the possible mechanisms, the available options, and the current challenges.

Keywords

Multiple sclerosis · Exercise · Rehabilitation · Prevention · Treatment

Box 20.1 Case Story

Susan, a 40-year-old woman was diagnosed with multiple sclerosis (MS) 2 years ago, after experiencing numbness and tingling in her legs and arms. She also had problems with her vision and balance. Susan has relapsing-remitting MS, which

(continued)

U. Dalgas (✉)
The Danish MS Hospitals, Ry and Haslev, Denmark
e-mail: dalgas@ph.au.dk

L. G. Hvid
The Danish MS Hospitals, Haslev, Denmark

Exercise Biology, Department of Public Health, Aarhus University, Aarhus, Denmark
e-mail: lhvid@ph.au.dk

J. B. Nielsen et al. (eds.), *Neuroplasticity-based Neurorehabilitation*,
https://doi.org/10.1007/978-3-031-81120-3_20

Box 20.1 (continued)
means that she has periods of relapses, followed by periods of remission or recovery. During a relapse, she may experience new or worsening symptoms, such as weakness, spasticity, pain, bladder problems, or mood changes. During remission, she may have no symptoms or some residual symptoms.

One of Susan's main challenges is walking impairment. Furthermore, she often feels stiffness, and pain in her legs, which makes it difficult for her to walk long distances or climb stairs. Susan also has trouble with balance and coordination, which increases her risk of falling. Another challenge is cognitive impairment. Susan sometimes has problems with memory, attention, concentration, and information processing. She may forget names, appointments, or tasks. Also, she has trouble following instructions, multitasking, or solving problems. Susan finds it hard to cope with the demands of her job and the expectations of her colleagues. She uses strategies such as writing notes, using reminders, organizing her work, and prioritizing her tasks to help her with her cognitive functioning.

Susan also struggles with fatigue (see Box 9.5), which is one of the most common and disabling symptoms of MS. Enough sleep does not help her feel less weary and drained. Keeping up her enthusiasm and vigor throughout the day is therefore often hard for her. Heat sensitivity is another problem for her, as it makes her feel more fatigued and worsens her other symptoms. She copes with her fatigue by taking breaks, setting a reasonable pace, reducing stress, and cooling down.

Susan takes disease-modifying medication, that disrupts the immune system's attack on myelin. This specific therapy, along with all other existing disease-modifying therapies, does not cure MS, but it can reduce the number and severity of relapses, prevent new brain lesions, and slow down the progression of disability. In addition to medical treatment, Susan attends weekly physiotherapy mainly to improve her muscle strength, endurance, and flexibility.

20.1 Prevalence and Incidence of Multiple Sclerosis

MS is a common neurological disease that affects the nervous system. The number of patients worldwide is increasing every year. In 2020, there were 2.8 million persons with MS (PwMS), a 30% increase from 2013 (Walton et al., 2020). This increase may be due to better diagnosis and counting methods, a longer lifespan of PwMS, and a growing global population. Today, one in three PwMS is older than 60 years.

Women are more likely to get MS than men, and worldwide, women are diagnosed with MS about twice as often as men (Walton et al., 2020). The reasons for this are unclear but may involve hormonal and genetic differences as well as environmental and social factors.

The prevalence of MS varies across continents (Walton et al., 2020), being 36 per 100,000 people worldwide, 133 per 100,000 in Europe, and only 5 per 100,000 in Africa.

The average age of the first MS symptoms is around 35 years without major differences between men and women. Importantly, the incidence of MS has risen over the past decades as has the gap between men and women (Walton et al., 2020).

20.2 Pathophysiology of Multiple Sclerosis

The cause of MS is unknown but likely involves both environmental and genetic factors (Compston & Coles, 2008; Jakimovski et al., 2023). Living in certain geographical regions (e.g., Europe and America), low sunlight exposure, being female, and smoking are well-known risk factors. Moreover, people who are exposed to viruses like Epstein-Barr virus and Human herpesvirus 6 (HHV-6) have a higher risk. Another genetic factor is the antigen HLA-DR2, which has been linked to MS for many years (Compston & Coles, 2008).

Although there is ongoing debate about whether subtypes of MS exist and how they should be characterized (Thompson et al., 2023), several different types of MS have traditionally been considered, each with distinct clinical characteristics. The "traditional" five main types include *Relapsing-Remitting MS* (RRMS) which is the most common form of MS at onset. Individuals with RRMS experience episodes of new or worsening symptoms (relapses or exacerbations) followed by periods of partial or complete recovery (remission). Over time, some individuals with RRMS may transition to *secondary progressive MS* (SPMS) with a gradual worsening of neurological function. SPMS is characterized by a more stable and progressive accumulation of disability, with or without occasional relapses and remissions. *Primary Progressive MS* (PPMS) is characterized by a gradual, steady progression of disability from the onset of symptoms, without distinct relapses or remissions. PPMS is less common than RRMS and SPMS and is often diagnosed in individuals over the age of 40. *Progressive-Relapsing MS* (PRMS) is characterized by a steady progression of disability from the onset, with occasional acute relapses. PRMS is a relatively rare form of MS. Finally, *Benign MS* is also present in a subset of patients, where individuals experience a mild course of the disease with minimal disability progression over an extended period. It is important to note that the classification of MS types can evolve over time for an individual, and some may experience features of different types at various points in their disease course (McGinley et al., 2021).

Independent of subtypes, MS is a condition where the immune system attacks the myelin sheaths that cover the axons in the CNS. Axons carry signals from the neurons in the CNS. The myelin sheaths help speed up the propagation of the signaling. When the myelin sheaths are damaged or destroyed, the signal from the CNS to the target can be slowed down or even blocked, which can cause impairments and disability. MS is an autoimmune disease, which means that the body's defense system mistakes normal cells for foreign cells and attacks them (see Box 20.2).

Box 20.2 Pathogenesis

T-helper cells are important immune cells that release cytokines to activate other immune cells when they find foreign antigens. In MS, the antigens could be Epstein-Barr virus or HHV-6. These antigens look like proteins on the oligodendrocytes, which are the cells that produce myelin for the axons. The T-helper cells confuse the myelin proteins on the oligodendrocytes for antigens and release cytokines such as IL-1, IL-6, IL-17, IL-22, TNF-α, and INF-γ. These cytokines cause changes in the blood-brain barrier, such as making it more permeable and dilated, which allows granulocytes to enter the area, where the T-helper cells are. The cytokine INF-γ also enters the bloodstream and activates macrophages, which are then also directed to the area. Plasma cells make antibodies that are specific to the proteins on the oligodendrocyte and attach to them. This makes the activated macrophages eat the oligodendrocyte. When the oligodendrocyte is damaged, other cells try to repair it by putting scar tissue on the damaged areas. These are called plaques or sclera. This happens on many neurons and axons, explaining the name "multiple sclerosis." When this happens, T-regulatory cells also come to the area and secrete IL-10 and TGF-β to stop the reaction. This can lead to some healing caused by the oligodendrocytes remyelinating the axon. If the demyelination lasts for a long time, the axon can eventually be lost. Further information can be found elsewhere (Compston & Coles, 2008; Jakimovski et al., 2023; McGinley et al., 2021).

20.3 Symptoms

MS is characterized by a variety of symptoms often presented in a unique combination. Common symptoms include fatigue, walking impairments, muscle weakness, pain, numbness and tingling in the extremities, visual impairments, bladder dysfunction, depression (and other mental health issues), and cognitive dysfunction. In general, symptoms worsen over time along with their detrimental influence on everyday life. Some symptoms are deemed "invisible" (e.g., fatigue, pain, and cognitive dysfunction), and are often somewhat overlooked. Each symptom is quite complex, as exemplified by walking impairments and cognitive dysfunction. The former include preferential problems with walking endurance and walking balance/coordination (Skjerbaek et al., 2023), whereas the latter mainly include problems with executive function, attention, memory, and information processing speed (DeLuca et al., 2020). Both walking impairments and cognitive impairments worsen over time and expectedly become very pronounced in older pwMS. Thorough screening and assessment of pwMS across their symptoms are thus essential to provide them with the most optimal and personalized treatment plan (Skjerbaek et al., 2023).

The presence and severity of symptoms depend on the number and position of CNS lesions, ultimately leading to structural and functional changes. For example, optic neuritis, which is an inflammation of the optic nerve, causes vision problems. There is however a discrepancy between the extent of neurodegeneration and symptom presentation/severity. This has been argued to depend on the individual's "reserve capacity," meaning that compensatory mechanisms can fully/partly counteract symptom presentation/severity, as outlined extensively with cognitive reserve capacity (Sumowski et al., 2013).

20.4 Medical and Pharmacological Treatment

Over the past two decades, major advances have been made in the medical/pharmacological treatment (i.e., disease-modifying therapies) of MS primarily aimed at reducing relapse rates, brain and spinal cord lesions, as well as disability. Disease-modifying therapies suppress or modulate immune function and have anti-inflammatory effects mainly in relapsing MS and these are found in both oral, infused, and injection formats (Jakimovski et al., 2023). The first disease-modifying therapies, interferons, and glatiramer acetate, were discovered by chance and had modest effects. Animal models of MS showed that T-cells were important in MS, but T-cell-based treatments failed in relapsing-remitting MS. Strategies that blocked lymphocyte entry to CNS (natalizumab, S1P receptor modulators) were effective in MS and animal models. Newer models showed that B-cells were also important in MS. B-cell-depleting therapies (anti-CD20 antibodies) reduced relapses and progression in relapsing-remitting MS and in progressive MS. At this point, disease-modifying therapies therefore exist to both relapsing-remitting MS and to progressive MS forms and cover more than 25 FDA-approved treatments.

In addition to disease-modifying therapies, a number of symptomatic *medical* treatments exist targeting bowel and bladder dysfunction, depression, pain, spasticity, walking impairment, dizziness and vertigo, fatigue, and emotional problems.

20.5 Nonpharmacological Treatment

In addition to disease-modifying therapies and other medical treatments, neurorehabilitation is a pivotal treatment for pwMS. Neurorehabilitation overall aims to (1) elicit disease-modifying effects by targeting and counteracting the MS-induced neurodegeneration (i.e., structural and functional changes of the brain/CNS) as well as the underlying mechanisms, and (2) to alleviate symptoms and improve the quality of life (Figs. 20.1 and 20.2). Whilst this can be shown as *improvements* over shorter periods of time (weeks to months), which has been the main focus of most research studies, it will more likely manifest as better *preservation* over longer periods of time (years). Regarding the disease-modifying effects, this is believed to involve alterations across different brain/CNS tissues; the neuroglia (size and number), gray matter (formation of new synapses, axonal sprouting, dendritic branching), and white matter (remyelination, fiber density alterations) (Sîrbu et al., 2022). Neurorehabilitation has sometimes been labeled as an adjuvant therapy to disease-modifying therapies, although this seems erroneous as the former can elicit adaptations that the latter cannot, and vice versa. In most cases, pwMS will receive a mix of different neurorehabilitation modalities including physical rehabilitation and exercise along with behavioral and educational interventions (fatigue management programs, energy conservation interventions, mindfulness-based interventions, cognitive and psychological interventions). At certain facilities (e.g., rehabilitation hospitals), multidisciplinary rehabilitation is offered purposedly to address the complexity of MS (Boesen et al., 2018; Freeman, 2001).

Substantial evidence supports, that neurorehabilitation is an effective symptomatic treatment option (Amatya et al., 2019; Sîrbu et al., 2022), although it should be noted, that the primary focus of previous research has been on physical rehabilitation and exercise (see Fig. 20.2). To exemplify, physical rehabilitation can substantially improve motor/physical function (e.g., dexterity, muscle strength, balance, walking endurance, walking balance/coordination) (Amatya et al., 2019; Lamers et al., 2016; Sîrbu et al., 2022) and can reduce the severity and impact of fatigue (Amatya et al., 2019; Rooney et al., 2019), reduce pain (Amatya et al., 2019), reduce depression (Amatya et al., 2019), and improve quality of life (Amatya et al., 2019). Moreover, exercise – especially the modalities resistance training, aerobic training, and balance/coordination training – has been proven to be particularly potent in eliciting beneficial effects on the outcomes exemplified above (Dalgas et al., 2019) (see also Box 20.3).

As for counteracting and/or managing cognitive impairment, cognitive rehabilitation (memory rehabilitation in particular) has been proven quite effective in improving different cognitive domains such as verbal/visual/working memory,

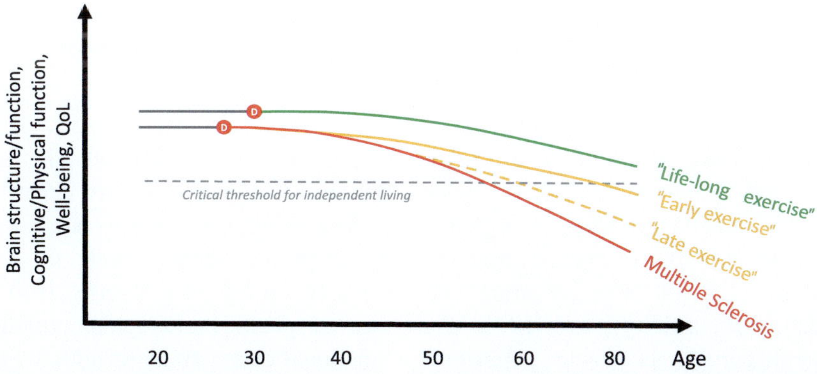

Fig. 20.1 Hypothetical conceptualization illustrating the proposed impact of having multiple sclerosis without engaging in regular exercise (red line) on various outcomes across the lifespan. In addition, the likely effects of starting exercise at later stages after being diagnosed with multiple sclerosis (orange dashed and solid lines), as well as the effects of engaging in regular lifelong exercise (green line), are illustrated. The MS diagnosis is denoted by "D"

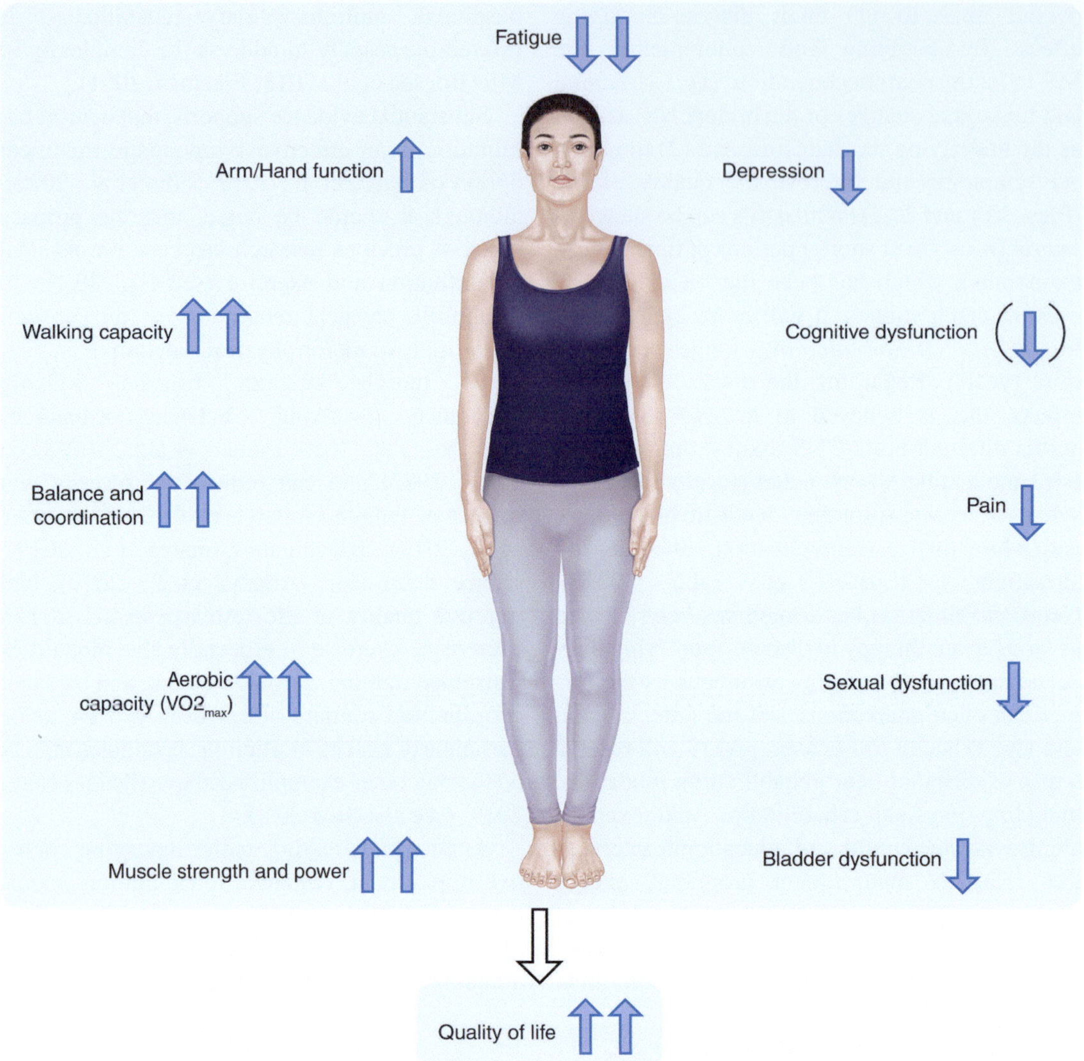

Fig. 20.2 Illustration of common symptoms and how exercise/physical rehabilitation affects these symptoms. Evidence exists to support substantial beneficial effects (two arrows), beneficial effects (one arrow), and somewhat uncertain beneficial effects (one arrow in brackets)

information processing speed, and executive function in pwMS (Chen et al., 2021; Taylor et al., 2021). Two main approaches of cognitive rehabilitation comprise the *restorative approach* involving modification of brain structure and function (i.e., neuroplasticity), as well as the *compensatory approach* involving behavioral strategies or environmental modifications designed to bypass cognitive impairments.

Regarding neuroplastic adaptations induced by cognitive rehabilitation in pwMS, some research studies have reported increased recruitment of specific brain regions as well as increased functional connectivity of brain region networks

(Chen et al., 2021; Sîrbu et al., 2022). The current evidence is nevertheless still sparse and somewhat inconclusive.

Box 20.3 The Effects of Exercise
Regarding neuroplasticity induced by exercise in pwMS, substantial evidence from animal studies has shown beneficial effects on the innate and adaptive immune system, reduced neuroinflammation (involving astrogliosis, microgliosis, macrophages infiltration), and beneficial effects on the neurotrophic environment (involving BDNF, GDNF, NGF, etc.), which ultimately promote remyelination (and reduce demyelination), axonal regeneration (and reduce axonal degeneration), synaptogenesis, and angiogenesis within the brain/CNS (Gentile et al., 2019; Guo et al., 2020). Moreover, these studies have reported a milder disease course with less accumulating clinical disability in those animals undergoing exercise. In contrast, substantially less evidence exists from human (pwMS) studies, where the limited evidence has primarily focused on brain/CNS morphology and function (Hvid et al., 2021; Sandroff et al., 2023; Tavazzi et al., 2021). Several exercise studies in pwMS have failed to report any improvements in systemic levels of pro/anti-inflammatory biomarkers (Dalgas et al., 2019), whereas systemic levels of BDNF (and potentially also other neurotrophic factors) can be increased (Diechmann et al., 2021). Whilst the latter may potentially translate into beneficial environmental changes as well as brain/CNS adaptations, limited evidence currently exists to support this. As for brain/CNS morphology (e.g., whole and regional brain volumes), existing evidence is sparse and inconclusive (Hvid et al., 2021; Sandroff et al., 2023; Tavazzi et al., 2021). To exemplify, the study by Riemenschneider and colleagues (designed to investigate the effects of exercise on brain morphology as the primary aim) failed to observe any changes in whole or regional brain volumes following 24 weeks of moderate-to-high intensity aerobic exercise in $n = 84$ newly diagnosed pwMS (Riemenschneider et al., 2022). Improvements were, however, observed in the microstructural integrity of important motor-related tracts and nuclei. As for brain/CNS function, existing evidence is also sparse yet supports that exercise have beneficial effects, especially in relation to functional and structural connectivity (assessed by fMRI during rest or active tasks) (Sandroff et al., 2023; Sîrbu et al., 2022; Tavazzi et al., 2021). This may especially affect important motor-related tracts and nuclei, which appear to depend on the exercise modality and specific motor tasks.

20.5.1 Current Knowledge Gaps and Future Directions

Whilst important information has been gained from existing neurorehabilitation studies involving pwMS, several knowledge gaps and limitations deserve to be mentioned. First, the quality of existing studies is generally poor, with most studies being too small, too short-lasting (at least for those investigating brain/CNS morphology), not designed to address neuroplastic adaptations (i.e., these outcomes are almost always secondary), and failing to properly address the translation from mechanisms to function. Second, many studies evaluating the symptomatic treatment potential of neurorehabilitation interventions are often limited by patients not having a well-defined clinical symptom at baseline (e.g., not being fatigued at study entry in a study evaluating if an intervention can reduce fatigue). These aspects must be considered when designing future neurorehabilitation research studies.

Lastly, the application of technologies to help advance the effects of neurorehabilitation will undoubtedly play a bigger role in the future. This can include tele-rehabilitation which can offer improved access to treatment options by reducing travel time and cost. Through this, long-term adherence to a healthier lifestyle may be improved. Moreover, it can include technologies to be used in treatment such as noninvasive brain stimulation (e.g., transcranial direct current stimulation or repetitive transcranial magnetic stimulation) targeting MS-induced neurodegeneration and/or symptoms (see Chap. 16).

Review Questions

- Why is it important to be aware of fatigue in people with MS?
- How can fatigue be addressed in persons with MS?

References

Amatya, B., Khan, F., & Galea, M. (2019). Rehabilitation for people with multiple sclerosis: An overview of Cochrane reviews. *Cochrane Database of Systematic Reviews, 1*, CD012732.

Boesen, F., Norgaard, M., Trenel, P., Rasmussen, P. V., Petersen, T., Lovendahl, B., & Sorensen, J. (2018). Longer term effectiveness of inpatient multidisciplinary rehabilitation on health-related quality of life in MS patients: A pragmatic randomized controlled trial—the Danish MS Hospitals Rehabilitation Study. *Multiple Sclerosis, 24*, 340–349.

Chen, M. H., Chiaravalloti, N. D., & DeLuca, J. (2021). Neurological update: Cognitive rehabilitation in multiple sclerosis. *Journal of Neurology, 268*, 4908–4914.

Compston, A., & Coles, A. (2008). Multiple sclerosis. *Lancet, 372*, 1502–1517.

Dalgas, U., Langeskov-Christensen, M., Stenager, E., Riemenschneider, M., & Hvid, L. G. (2019). Exercise as medicine in multiple sclerosis-time for a paradigm shift: Preventive, symptomatic, and disease-modifying aspects and perspectives. *Current Neurology and Neuroscience Reports, 19*, 88.

DeLuca, J., Chiaravalloti, N. D., & Sandroff, B. M. (2020). Treatment and management of cognitive dysfunction in patients with multiple sclerosis. *Nature Reviews. Neurology, 16*, 319–332.

Diechmann, M. D., Campbell, E., Coulter, E., Paul, L., Dalgas, U., & Hvid, L. G. (2021). Effects of exercise training on neurotrophic factors and subsequent neuroprotection in persons with multiple sclerosis-a systematic review and meta-analysis. *Brain Sciences, 11*(11), 1499.

Freeman, J. A. (2001). Improving mobility and functional independence in persons with multiple sclerosis. *Journal of Neurology, 248*, 255–259.

Gentile, A., Musella, A., De Vito, F., Rizzo, F. R., Fresegna, D., Bullitta, S., Vanni, V., Guadalupi, L., Stampanoni Bassi, M., Buttari, F., Centonze, D., & Mandolesi, G. (2019). Immunomodulatory Effects of Exercise in Experimental Multiple Sclerosis. *Frontiers in Immunology, 10*, 2197.

Guo, L. Y., Lozinski, B., & Yong, V. W. (2020). Exercise in multiple sclerosis and its models: Focus on the central nervous system outcomes. *Journal of Neuroscience Research, 98*, 509–523.

Hvid, L. G., Harwood, D. L., Eskildsen, S. F., & Dalgas, U. (2021). A critical systematic review of current evidence on the effects of physical exercise on whole/regional grey matter brain volume in populations at risk of neurodegeneration. *Sports Medicine, 51*(8), 1651–1671.

Jakimovski, D., Bittner, S., Zivadinov, R., Morrow, S. A., Benedict, R. H., Zipp, F., & Weinstock-Guttman, B. (2023). Multiple sclerosis. *Lancet, 403*(10422), 183–202.

Lamers, I., Maris, A., Severijns, D., Dielkens, W., Geurts, S., Van Wijmeersch, B., & Feys, P. (2016). Upper limb rehabilitation in people with multiple sclerosis: A systematic review. *Neurorehabilitation and Neural Repair, 30*, 773–793.

McGinley, M. P., Goldschmidt, C. H., & Rae-Grant, A. D. (2021). Diagnosis and treatment of multiple sclerosis: A review. *Journal of the American Medical Association, 325*, 765–779.

Riemenschneider, M., Hvid, L. G., Ringgaard, S., Nygaard, M. K. E., Eskildsen, S. F., Gaemelke, T., Magyari, M., Jensen, H. B., Nielsen, H. H., Kant, M., Falah, M., Petersen, T., Stenager, E., & Dalgas, U. (2022). Investigating the potential disease-modifying and neuroprotective efficacy of exercise therapy early in the disease course of multiple sclerosis: The Early Multiple Sclerosis Exercise Study (EMSES). *Multiple Sclerosis, 28*, 1620–1629.

Rooney, S., Moffat, F., Wood, L., & Paul, L. (2019). Effectiveness of fatigue management interventions in reducing severity and impact of fatigue in people with progressive multiple sclerosis: A systematic review. *International Journal of MS Care, 21*, 35–46.

Sandroff, B. M., Rafizadeh, C. M., & Motl, R. W. (2023). Neuroimaging technology in exercise neurorehabilitation research in persons with MS: A scoping review. *Sensors (Basel), 23*(9), 4530.

Sîrbu, C. A., Thompson, D. C., Plesa, F. C., Vasile, T. M., Jianu, D. C., Mitrica, M., Anghel, D., & Stefani, C. (2022). Neurorehabilitation in multiple sclerosis—a review of present approaches and future considerations. *Journal of Clinical Medicine, 11*(23), 7003.

Skjerbaek, A. G., Dalgas, U., Stenager, E., Boesen, F., & Hvid, L. G. (2023). The six spot step test is superior in detecting walking capacity impairments compared to short- and long-distance walk tests in persons with multiple sclerosis. *Multiple Sclerosis*

Journal Experimental, Translational and Clinical, 9, 20552173231218127.

Sumowski, J. F., Rocca, M. A., Leavitt, V. M., Riccitelli, G., Comi, G., DeLuca, J., & Filippi, M. (2013). Brain reserve and cognitive reserve in multiple sclerosis: What you've got and how you use it. *Neurology, 80*, 2186–2193.

Tavazzi, E., Cazzoli, M., Pirastru, A., Blasi, V., Rovaris, M., Bergsland, N., & Baglio, F. (2021). Neuroplasticity and motor rehabilitation in multiple sclerosis: A systematic review on MRI markers of functional and structural changes. *Frontiers in Neuroscience, 15*, 707675.

Taylor, L. A., Mhizha-Murira, J. R., Smith, L., Potter, K. J., Wong, D., Evangelou, N., Lincoln, N. B., & das Nair, R. (2021). Memory rehabilitation for people with multiple sclerosis. *Cochrane Database of Systematic Reviews, 10*, CD008754.

Thompson, A. J., Moccia, M., Amato, M. P., Calabresi, P. A., Finlayson, M., Hawton, A., Lublin, F. D., Marrie, R. A., Montalban, X., Panzara, M., Sormani, M. P., Strum, J., Vickrey, B. G., & Coetzee, T. (2023). Do the current MS clinical course descriptors need to change and if so how? A survey of the MS community. *Multiple Sclerosis, 29*, 1363–1372.

Walton, C., King, R., Rechtman, L., Kaye, W., Leray, E., Marrie, R. A., Robertson, N., La Rocca, N., Uitdehaag, B., van der Mei, I., Wallin, M., Helme, A., Angood Napier, C., Rijke, N., & Baneke, P. (2020). Rising prevalence of multiple sclerosis worldwide: Insights from the Atlas of MS, third edition. *Multiple Sclerosis, 26*, 1816–1821.

Parkinson's Disease

21

Martin Langeskov-Christense and Ulrik Dalgas

Abstract

Parkinson's disease is an irreversible and gradually progressing neurological condition that results in several motor and non-motor symptoms. Currently, there are no pharmaceutical substances capable of halting the progression or evolution of Parkinson's disease, and pharmacological treatments aimed at alleviating symptoms have limited efficacy on certain symptoms and frequently produce adverse effects. Consequently, non-pharmacological interventions with the potential to slow down or ameliorate the disease are of paramount importance. Exercise is a secure and pivotal component of the rehabilitation process for people with Parkinson's disease, and it is the most well-researched Parkinson rehabilitation intervention. Preliminary knowledge suggests that exercise can initiate neuroprotection and regeneration through various molecular pathways. These pathways involve the upregulation or control of neurotrophic factors that regulate or support different processes, enhancing neurogenesis, angiogenesis, dopamine transport, synaptic transmitter release, autophagy, neuronal sprouting, and mitochondrial function, while also reducing inflammation and cellular demise. However, people with Parkinson's face specific neuroplastic challenges related to their reduced dopaminergic response, which affects their motivation and reward-driven learning. To address these challenges, strategies like cueing and feedback can be helpful.

This chapter describes the prevalence, incidence, prognosis, and pathophysiology of Parkinson's disease. Characteristic motor and non-motor symptoms of the disease are presented, and treatment of many of these symptoms is discussed with a special focus on exercise as an intervention.

Keywords

Parkinson · Exercise therapy · (Neuro) Rehabilitation · Movement disorders · Rehabilitation strategies

M. Langeskov-Christense (✉)
Department of Clinical Medicine, Aarhus University, Aarhus, Denmark

Department of Neurology, Viborg Regional Hospital, Viborg, Denmark
e-mail: mach@clin.au.dk

U. Dalgas
Department of Public Health, Aarhus University, Aarhus, Denmark
e-mail: dalgas@ph.au.dk

Box 21.1 Case Story

Peter, diagnosed with Parkinson's disease 10 years ago, is experiencing the progressive nature of the disease with several debilitating motor and non-motor symptoms. He is primarily affected by two of the four core motor symptoms, namely bradykinesia (slowness of movement) and postural insta-

(continued)

J. B. Nielsen et al. (eds.), *Neuroplasticity-based Neurorehabilitation*,
https://doi.org/10.1007/978-3-031-81120-3_21

Box 21.1 (continued)
bility (balance impairment), and to a lesser extent tremor (rhythmic shaking) and rigidity (stiff or inflexible muscles). Postural instability affects Peter's gait, leading to increased physical inactivity and increasing social isolation. Additionally, the disorder is causing a broad range of non-motor symptoms, with the most disabling being pain and cognitive dysfunction.

Targeted exercises and activities have demonstrated their effectiveness in enhancing overall motor function through the improvement of muscle strength, cardiorespiratory fitness, balance, and coordination, thus mitigating the impacts of bradykinesia and postural instability, which in turn facilitate smoother movements. Also, engaging in exercise may help reduce pain perception through the release of endorphins or improved flexibility and mobility, but currently knowledge is lacking in this area. Lastly, various exercise modalities have been shown to improve cognition, although the literature is not consistent on this aspect. As Peter's learning potential and ability to initiate and sustain exercise are impaired due to reduced dopaminergic response, cueing and feedback may provide structure, guidance, and positive reinforcement, making exercise more engaging and effective.

21.1 Prevalence and Incidence of Parkinson's Disease

Parkinson's disease ranks as the second most prevalent neurodegenerative condition, following Alzheimer's disease (Tysnes & Storstein, 2017). Its prevalence typically ranges from 1 to 2 cases per 1000 individuals in population-based samples (Tysnes & Storstein, 2017), with varying reported incidence rates due to methodological variations. However, many studies frequently report an annual incidence ranging from 10 to over 20 cases per 100,000 person-years (Tysnes & Storstein, 2017). Presently, Parkinson's disease stands as the most rapidly growing neurological disorder, affecting over ten million individuals worldwide (Armstrong & Okun, 2020). Parkinson's disease is rarely diagnosed before the age of 50, but its prevalence and incidence progressively rise after the age of 60 (Tysnes & Storstein, 2017). Age is the primary risk factor for developing Parkinson's disease, and given the increasing life expectancy in developed nations, both its incidence and prevalence are anticipated to rise further in the coming years. Men are more frequently diagnosed with Parkinson's disease than women, with a male-to-female ratio of 1.5. Possible explanations for this gender difference include potential neuroprotective effects from estrogen in women, X-linked genetic factors, and a higher frequency of high-risk occupational exposures among men (Elbaz et al., 2016).

21.2 Prognosis

As there is currently no cure for Parkinson's disease, it is expected that the burden of both motor and non-motor symptoms will increase with age, while life expectancy decreases (Bloem et al., 2021; Elbaz et al., 2016). The average survival period following diagnosis varies, ranging from 8 to 20 years, depending on the specific characteristics of the Parkinson's disease condition (De Pablo-Fernández et al., 2019). People with Parkinson's disease most commonly face the same causes of death as those without the disease, including heart disease, stroke, and complications stemming from hip fractures (Bloem et al., 2021; Elbaz et al., 2016). Additionally, aspiration pneumonia stands as the leading Parkinson's disease-related symptom contributing to mortality (Armstrong & Okun, 2020). People with Parkinson's disease also face an elevated risk of developing cognitive impairment and dementia, with a relative risk ranging from 1.7 to 5.9 compared to individuals without the condition (Elbaz et al., 2016). A growing body of evidence suggests that the presence of dementia significantly impacts decreased life expectancy in Parkinson's disease (Elbaz et al., 2016).

21.3 Pathophysiology of Parkinson's Disease

The pathophysiology of Parkinson's disease is characterized by the progressive degeneration of dopaminergic neurons in primarily the substantia nigra. Dopamine, a neurotransmitter, plays a pivotal role in both the direct and indirect pathways of the basal ganglia, influencing motor and non-motor behaviors, cognition, and emotions (see also Chap. 5). Notably, the key pathological changes begin long before the onset of motor symptoms in Parkinson's disease. Furthermore, it is estimated that motor symptoms become noticeable when the loss of dopaminergic neurons exceeds 50%. In contrast to motor symptoms, non-motor symptoms arise from the progressive degeneration of other neuronal systems, including the cholinergic, noradrenergic, and serotonergic systems. This divergence explains why many non-motor symptoms do not respond well to dopamine-based medications (Armstrong & Okun, 2020).

Box 21.2 Pathogenesis

The pathophysiological hallmark of Parkinson's disease revolves around the presence of Lewy bodies, primarily composed of aggregated misfolded alpha-synuclein. Lewy bodies are named after Fritz Heinrich Lewy, the German doctor who first identified the abnormal deposits of protein within brain cells. Lewy bodies cause a range of symptoms, some of which are shared by dementia disease and some by Parkinson's disease. The precise cause of this aggregation remains unknown, but it is suggested that Lewy bodies initiate mitochondrial respiratory dysfunction, leading to an increase in reactive oxygen species and subsequent oxidative stress. This oxidative stress, in turn, promotes the aggregation of alpha-synuclein, creating a vicious cycle. Furthermore, a pro-inflammatory environment and exposure to environmental toxins contribute to this cycle. This complex interplay is believed to result in neurotoxicity, ultimately leading to the demise of primarily dopaminergic neurons within a brain subregion known as the substantia nigra pars compacta (Bloem et al., 2021).

21.3.1 Brain-First or Body-First Parkinson's Disease

Recent findings indicate that alpha-synuclein aggregation (see Box 21.2) can initiate through one of two distinct pathways: the brain-first or the body-first. The differentiation between these two subtypes of Parkinson's disease is primarily established based on the presence of rapid eye movement sleep behavior disorder during the prodromal phase of the disease (Borghammer & Van Den Berge, 2019; Horsager et al., 2020). Currently, it is believed that brain-first Parkinson's disease originates within the central nervous system, specifically in the limbic system, from where it extends to the olfactory bulb and subsequently progresses to the peripheral autonomic nervous system. Brain-first Parkinson's disease is characterized by dysfunction in nigrostriatal dopaminergic pathways before the peripheral autonomic nervous system is involved, resulting in a lack of rapid eye movement sleep behavior disorder symptoms during the prodromal phase (Borghammer & Van Den Berge, 2019). In contrast, body-first Parkinson's disease is typified by patients exhibiting rapid eye movement sleep behavior disorder symptoms during the prodromal phase. This subtype commences with pathological changes in the nerve terminals of the enteric nervous system (innervating the gastrointestinal tract) or the peripheral nervous system and then spreads through the vagus nerve to the central nervous system (Horsager et al., 2020). Animal studies have supported this hypothesis by demonstrating the propagation patterns of injected preformed alpha-synucleins from the duodenum to the celiac ganglion and, via the vagal nerve, to the medulla (Borghammer & Van Den Berge, 2019; Kim et al., 2019).

21.4 Symptoms

Parkinson's disease manifests a spectrum of both motor and non-motor symptoms (Armstrong & Okun, 2020), and Fig. 21.1 provides a general overview of its clinical symptoms and timeline. Non-motor symptoms exhibit considerable heterogeneity as they affect various organ systems in an individualized manner. During the pre-diagnosis or prodromal phase, non-motor symptoms encompass rapid eye movement sleep behavior disorder, impaired sense of smell, constipation, urinary dysfunction, orthostatic hypotension, excessive daytime sleepiness, and depression (Armstrong & Okun, 2020). These symptoms are not exclusive to Parkinson's disease, which may account for the extended prodromal phase experienced by some individuals (up to 20 years) (Bloem et al., 2021). Other factors contributing to this prolongation may include a lack of awareness of Parkinson's disease symptoms or feelings of embarrassment related to them (Armstrong & Okun, 2020). Following diagnosis, non-motor symptoms may involve pain, fatigue, cognitive impairment, and dementia. The definitive diagnosis of Parkinson's disease is established when motor symptoms, such as bradykinesia, tremors, and rigidity, become evident. In the later stages of Parkinson's disease, postural instability, gait difficulties, speech problems, and dysphagia may arise concurrently. Ultimately, complications arising from years of pharmacotherapy can lead to motor and non-motor fluctuations, dyskinesia, and psychosis.

21.5 Treatment

Currently, there is no available medical treatment that can provide a cure or effectively slow down the progression of Parkinson's disease. However, multiple treatment approaches exist to alleviate the burden of symptoms (Armstrong & Okun, 2020). Given the diverse nature of Parkinson's disease, it is crucial to tailor the treatment strategy individually and engage in a thorough discussion with the patient, weighing the risks and benefits.

Pharmacotherapy stands as a key pillar of treatment, with numerous drugs designed to mitigate the symptoms of Parkinson's disease. These drugs include levodopa, dopamine agonists, COMT inhibitors, and MAO-B inhibitors (Bloem et al., 2021). Among these, levodopa is the most effective and commonly used medication for enhancing mobility and motor skills (Bloem et al., 2021; Jankovic & Tan, 2020). Levodopa works by increasing the levels

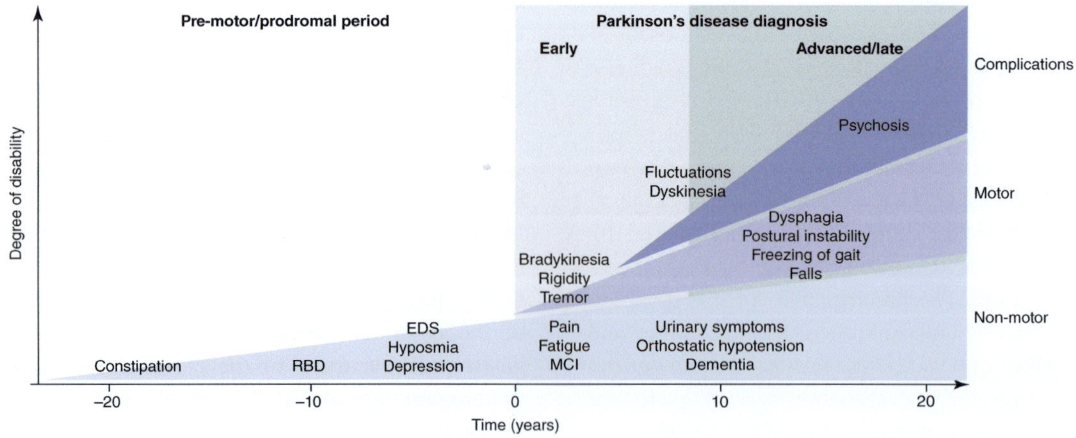

Fig. 21.1 Symptoms and degree of disability in persons with Parkinson's disease with respect to the time of diagnosis

of dopamine in the striatum. To enhance treatment efficacy, levodopa is often combined with MAO-B or COMT inhibitors, which reduce levodopa degradation and thus increase and prolong its effect in striatal dopaminergic neurotransmission. Nonetheless, it is frequent for individuals using levodopa to require an increased dose frequency due to the gradual decline of their response over time. Also, their short-duration response diminishes due to disease-related changes in brain physiology. Eventually, the brain loses its ability to store excess dopamine for later use, leading to side effects and the development of resistance to levodopa after several years of usage (Armstrong & Okun, 2020; Bloem et al., 2021). Therefore, it is vital to adopt a comprehensive approach that incorporates both pharmacological and non-pharmacological treatment strategies (Bloem et al., 2021).

An alternative treatment approach involves surgical procedures, particularly deep brain stimulation, which becomes especially pertinent for individuals with moderate or advanced-stage Parkinson's disease. Deep brain stimulation involves the surgical implantation of electrodes in specific brain regions, such as the subthalamic nucleus or globus pallidus, to modulate abnormal neuronal activity and alleviate motor symptoms. This group often experiences a diminished quality of life due to issues like fluctuating treatment responses, dyskinesia, or unresponsive symptoms despite levodopa use. Nevertheless, it's essential to acknowledge that surgical interventions carry a higher risk of (severe) adverse events when compared to conventional medical treatments (Jankovic & Tan, 2020).

A promising emerging non-pharmacological treatment avenue for Parkinson's disease revolves around exercise therapy. Recent reviews and meta-analyses (Gamborg et al., 2022) propose that endurance training may act as a disease modifyier, while resistance training improves quality of life. Of note, the disease-modifying potential is most often assessed with the Movement Disorder Society-Sponsored Revision of the Unified Parkinson's Disease Rating Scale (MDS-UPDRS) III score, which evaluates a person's motor function and is composed of several items that assess different aspects of motor performance, including tremor, rigidity, bradykinesia, and postural instability. Animal studies using Parkinson's disease models provide further support for the potential neuroprotective benefits of endurance training, reporting reduced alpha-synuclein aggregation and improved motor and cognitive function following an endurance training intervention (Zhou et al., 2017). Animal studies also suggest that exercise promotes neuroprotection and regeneration through various molecular processes, with neurotrophic factors playing a pivotal role. For example, treadmill running in rodent Parkinson's disease models boosts neurotrophin levels in the brain, leading to enhanced neurogenesis, angiogenesis, dopamine transport, synaptic function, and more (Langeskov-Christensen et al., 2024). These changes strengthen neural networks, improving motor and cognitive function. Additionally, human studies involving individuals with Parkinson's disease have demonstrated elevated levels of brain-derived neurotrophic factors after an exercise program (Langeskov-Christensen et al., 2024). Further research reports increased brain activity in the basal ganglia and motor cortex (Duchesne et al., 2016; Shah et al., 2016), as well as improved dopaminergic signaling following exercise in Parkinson's disease patients (Langeskov-Christensen et al., 2024). Intriguingly, aerobic exercise has also led to increased functional connectivity within cortico-striatal and fronto-parietal networks while simultaneously reducing global brain atrophy in people with Parkinson's disease (Johansson et al., 2021).

Cumulatively, the current body of literature suggests that intensive exercise may have the capacity to attenuate or even reverse the neurodegenerative processes associated with Parkinson's disease. However, though this is highly plausible, the evidence underlying such effects is less robust and needs further support in future well-designed trials.

21.6 Perspectives for Clinical Practice

Several studies offer some substantiation for a potential disease-modifying impact of exercise in Parkinson's disease (for review please see

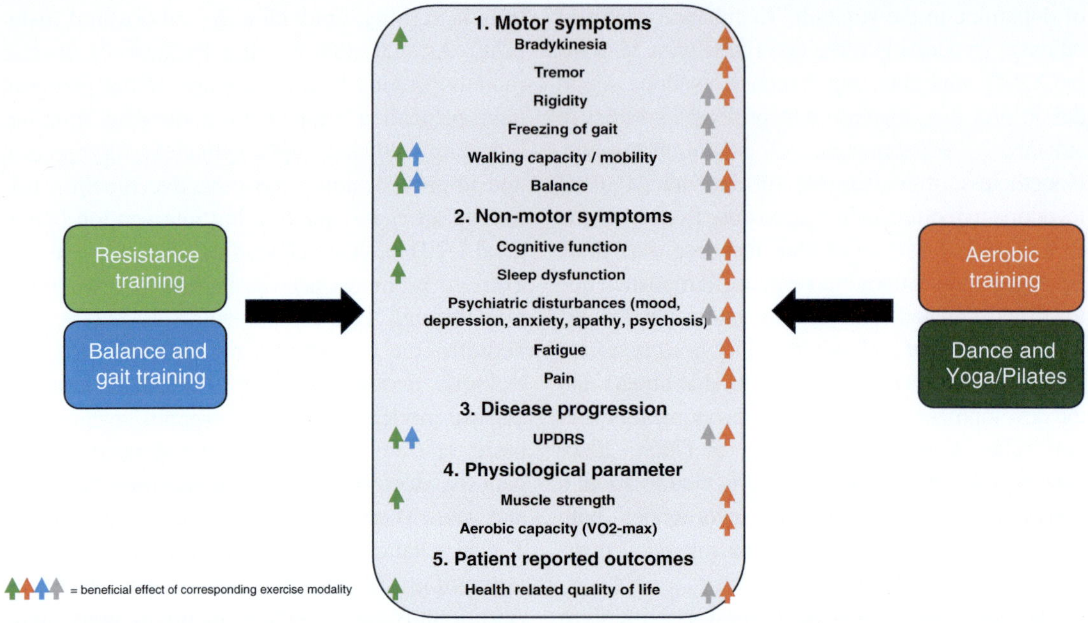

Fig. 21.2 Documented effects of different exercise modalities on selected outcomes of relevance to persons with Parkinson's disease. A colored arrow corresponding to an intervention's box color indicates existing evidence supports a beneficial effect on the respective outcome

Langeskov-Christensen et al., 2024). These studies summarize potential mechanisms of action, encompassing functional or anatomical changes and molecular pathways. To effectively use exercise as rehabilitative medicine for Parkinson's disease, a deeper understanding is needed of how exercise alleviates symptoms and potentially modifies the disease. Recent research reveals Parkinson's disease affects multiple body systems (Horsager et al., 2020), including potential effects on the recently suggested gut-muscle-brain axis (Morella et al., 2023), suggesting that exercise's diverse effects on various tissues and systems may underlie its benefits in Parkinson's disease.

While most evidence comes from animal studies, research in people with Parkinson's disease supports exercise's potential benefits. Neurotrophic factors, such as brain-derived neurotrophic factor and glial-derived neurotrophic factor, have been a focus, but their effects are inconsistent (Langeskov-Christensen et al., 2024). Non-invasive brain imaging techniques, like PET and MRI scans, show promise in revealing exercise-induced changes in brain function, such as increased dopamine D2 receptors following endurance training (Fisher et al., 2013).

Although these findings are encouraging, comprehensive and definitive insights into the underlying mechanisms are still incomplete. Nevertheless, when considering the consistent observations in Parkinson's disease animal models and the overall impact of exercise on clinical scores (MDS-UPDRS) in individuals with Parkinson's disease, it suggests that exercise may have a preventive effect on factors influencing disease progression. Consequently, the existing body of knowledge supports exercise as a potentially safe, cost-effective, and readily accessible therapy with disease-modifying potential in Parkinson's disease. Whereas evidence for a disease-modifying effect is less robust, albeit highly plausible, convincing evidence suggests that exercise offers symptomatic alleviation in Parkinson's disease. This is visualized in Fig. 21.2, showing positive effects of different exercise modalities on several outcomes. Interestingly, all forms of exercise modalities result in enhancements in walking capacity, postural stability/balance, and the (MDS)-UPDRS-III score. Except for balance and gait exercises, all other exercise modalities also improve cognition, sleep disturbances, and quality of life. Considering the information presented above, it becomes evident that participating in any form of exercise yields significant benefits for individuals with Parkinson's disease. This knowledge is crucial for both people with Parkinson's disease, who may be unable to perform specific types of exercise due to impairments or lack of motivation (as there are alternative, potentially more motivating options that are effective), and for healthcare providers who prescribe exercise. Nevertheless, considering the diversity of Parkinson's disease presentations, it is advisable to prioritize specific exercise therapy objectives and task-specific interventions in addition to general exercise programs, which is consistent with PD exercise guidelines (Keus et al., 2014; Osborne et al., 2022). This approach is essential for tailoring interventions targeting the unique challenges faced by individuals with Parkinson's disease. In this context, fundamental exercise modalities such as aerobic exercise, resistance training, and balance and gait exercises can enhance aerobic capacity, muscle strength, and postural stability/balance, respectively. It is important to note that muscle weakness holds significant implications since it contributes to issues like postural instability, gait problems, bradykinesia, and the potential for falls (Gamborg et al., 2023). On the other hand, aerobic capacity serves as a robust indicator of health and performance in both healthy individuals and clinical populations (Thrue et al., 2023). Together, the summarized effects of exercise in Fig. 21.2 clearly show that exercise has favorable effects in Parkinson's disease and may induce a postponement of clinical disability.

Lastly, however, it should be acknowledged that people with Parkinson's disease face several neuroplastic challenges when it comes to exercise due to the reduced dopaminergic response in their brains. Dopamine plays a crucial role in the brain's reward system, motivation, and learning. Reduced dopamine levels in the basal ganglia, a brain region responsible for initiating and maintaining motor routines, can make it challenging for individuals to start and stick with exercise routines. Also, reduced dopaminergic response can diminish the sense of pleasure and reinforcement that typically comes from physical activity. To address these challenges, strategies like cueing and feedback can be helpful. Cueing involves using external or internal prompts to facilitate movement. External cues, such as auditory or visual cues (e.g., metronome beats, lines on the floor, or rhythmic music), can help stimulate motor patterns and overcome freezing episodes. These cues provide timing and spatial reference for movements and can improve gait and balance. Feedback is also essential for people with Parkinson's to improve their motor skills and ensure they are performing exercises correctly. It helps individuals understand their performance and make necessary adjustments. Feedback can be visual, auditory, or tactile and can come from physical therapists, fitness trainers, or wearable devices. It reinforces proper movement patterns and can enhance self-efficacy. Collectively, this provides structure, guidance, and positive reinforcement, making exercise more engaging and effective. Additionally, support and encouragement from healthcare professionals and caregivers can further motivate individuals with Parkinson's to maintain an active lifestyle.

Review Questions

- Why is it important to be aware of cognitive deficits and/or decreased motivation, and how can it be addressed?
- What type of exercise would you recommend to persons with Parkinson's disease having one or more of the four core symptoms?
- Discuss if exercise should be used as *prevention* by building reserve capacity and thereby prolonging the time until critical thresholds are reached or if it should focus on *symptomatic treatment* of existing symptoms or both.

References

Armstrong, M. J., & Okun, M. S. (2020). Diagnosis and treatment of Parkinson disease: A review. *JAMA, 323*(6), 548–560. https://doi.org/10.1001/jama.2019.22360

Bloem, B. R., Okun, M. S., & Klein, C. (2021). Parkinson's disease. *Lancet, 397*(10291), 2284–2303. https://doi.org/10.1016/S0140-6736(21)00218-X

Borghammer, P., & Van Den Berge, N. (2019). Brain-first versus gut-first Parkinson's disease: A hypothesis. *Journal of Parkinson's Disease, 9*(s2), S281–S295. https://doi.org/10.3233/JPD-191721

De Pablo-Fernández, E., Lees, A. J., Holton, J. L., & Warner, T. T. (2019). Prognosis and neuropathologic correlation of clinical subtypes of Parkinson disease. *JAMA Neurology, 76*(4), 470–479. https://doi.org/10.1001/jamaneurol.2018.4377

Duchesne, C., Gheysen, F., Bore, A., Albouy, G., Nadeau, A., Robillard, M. E., Bobeuf, F., Lafontaine, A. L., Lungu, O., Bherer, L., & Doyon, J. (2016). Influence of aerobic exercise training on the neural correlates of motor learning in Parkinson's disease individuals. *NeuroImage Clinical, 12*(C), 559–569. https://doi.org/10.1016/j.nicl.2016.09.011

Elbaz, A., Carcaillon, L., Kab, S., & Moisan, F. (2016). Epidemiology of Parkinson's disease. *Revue Neurologique, 172*(1), 14–26. https://doi.org/10.1016/j.neurol.2015.09.012

Fisher, B. E., Li, Q., Nacca, A., Salem, G. J., Song, J., Yip, J., Hui, J. S., Jakowec, M. W., & Petzinger, G. M. (2013). Treadmill exercise elevates striatal dopamine D2 receptor binding potential in patients with early Parkinson's disease. *Neuroreport, 24*(10), 509–514. https://doi.org/10.1097/WNR.0b013e328361dc13

Gamborg, M., Hvid, L. G., Dalgas, U., & Langeskov-Christensen, M. (2022). Parkinson's disease and intensive exercise therapy—An updated systematic review and meta-analysis. *Acta Neurologica Scandinavica, 145*(5), 504–528.

Gamborg, M., Hvid, L. G., Thrue, C., Johansson, S., Franzen, E., Dalgas, U., & Langeskov-Christensen, M. (2023). Muscle strength and power in people with Parkinson disease: A systematic review and meta-analysis. *Journal of Neurologic Physical Therapy, 47*(1), 3–15. https://doi.org/10.1097/NPT.0000000000000421

Horsager, J., Andersen, K. B., Knudsen, K., Skjaerbaek, C., Fedorova, T. D., Okkels, N., Schaeffer, E., Bonkat, S. K., Geday, J., Otto, M., Sommerauer, M., Danielsen, E. H., Bech, E., Kraft, J., Munk, O. L., Hansen, S. D., Pavese, N., Goder, R., Brooks, D. J., Berg, D., & Borghammer, P. (2020). Brain-first versus body-first Parkinson's disease: A multimodal imaging case-control study. *Brain, 143*(10), 3077–3088. https://doi.org/10.1093/brain/awaa238

Jankovic, J., & Tan, E. K. (2020). Parkinson's disease: Etiopathogenesis and treatment. *Journal of Neurology, Neurosurgery and Psychiatry, 91*(8), 795–808. https://doi.org/10.1136/jnnp-2019-322338

Johansson, M. E., Cameron, I. G. M., van der Kolk, N. M., De Vries, N. M., Klimars, E., Toni, I., Bloem, B. R., & Helmich, R. C. (2021). Aerobic exercise alters brain function and structure in Parkinson's disease a randomized controlled trial. *Annals of Neurology, 91*(2), 203–216. https://doi.org/10.1002/ana.26291

Keus, S. H. J. M. M., Graziano, M., et al. (2014). *European physiotherapy guideline for Parkinson's disease*. KNGF/ParkinsonNet.

Kim, S., Kwon, S.-H., Kam, T.-I., Panicker, N., Karuppagounder, S. S., Lee, S., Lee, J. H., Kim, W. R., Kook, M., Foss, C. A., Shen, C., Lee, H., Kulkarni, S., Pasricha, P. J., Lee, G., Pomper, M. G., Dawson, V. L., Dawson, T. M., & Ko, H. S. (2019). Transneuronal propagation of pathologic α-Synuclein from the gut to the brain models Parkinson's disease. *Neuron (Cambridge, Mass), 103*(4), 627–641.e627. https://doi.org/10.1016/j.neuron.2019.05.035

Langeskov-Christensen, M., Franzen, E., Grondahl Hvid, L., & Dalgas, U. (2024). Exercise as medicine in Parkinson's disease. *Journal of Neurology, Neurosurgery, and Psychiatry, 95*(11), 1077–1088. https://doi.org/10.1136/jnnp-2023-332974

Morella, I., Negro, M., Dossena, M., Brambilla, R., & D'Antona, G. (2023). Gut-muscle-brain axis: Molecular mechanisms in neurodegenerative disorders and potential therapeutic efficacy of probiotic supplementation coupled with exercise. *Neuropharmacology, 240*, 109718. https://doi.org/10.1016/j.neuropharm.2023.109718

Osborne, J. A., Botkin, R., Colon-Semenza, C., DeAngelis, T. R., Gallardo, O. G., Kosakowski, H., Martello, J., Pradhan, S., Rafferty, M., Readinger, J. L., Whitt, A. L., & Ellis, T. D. (2022). Physical therapist management of Parkinson disease: A clinical practice guideline from the American Physical Therapy Association. *Physical Therapy, 102*(4), pzab302. https://doi.org/10.1093/ptj/pzab302

Shah, C., Beall, E. B., Frankemolle, A. M. M., Penko, A., Phillips, M. D., Lowe, M. J., & Alberts, J. L. (2016). Exercise therapy for Parkinson's disease: Pedaling rate is related to changes in motor connectivity. *Brain Connectivity, 6*(1), 25–36. https://doi.org/10.1089/brain.2014.0328

Thrue, C., Hvid, L. G., Gamborg, M., Dawes, H., Dalgas, U., & Langeskov-Christensen, M. (2023). Aerobic capacity in persons with Parkinson's disease: A systematic review. *Disability and Rehabilitation, 45*(15), 2409–2421. https://doi.org/10.1080/09638288.2022.2094480

Tysnes, O.-B., & Storstein, A. (2017). Epidemiology of Parkinson's disease. *Journal of Neural Transmission, 124*(8), 901–905. https://doi.org/10.1007/s00702-017-1686-y

Zhou, W., Barkow, J. C., & Freed, C. R. (2017). Running wheel exercise reduces alpha-synuclein aggregation and improves motor and cognitive function in a transgenic mouse model of Parkinson's disease. *PLoS One, 12*, e0190160.

Dementia

22

Laila Øksnebjerg

Abstract

There is increasing focus on the potential of rehabilitation for people living with dementia. This partly reflects a paradigm shift, moving away from a narrow focus on decline and deficits caused by dementia diseases and towards a greater emphasis on interventions, e.g. rehabilitation, and positive approaches to promote capacity and quality of life despite living with dementia. It also reflects the growing evidence that both the risk of getting a dementia disease and the time of onset and progression can be influenced by a complex set of potentially modifiable factors, including biological, lifestyle, and psychosocial aspects. This chapter presents various approaches to rehabilitation for people with dementia and discusses the challenges that need to be considered. First, the most common dementia diseases are presented, and the move towards a multifactorial and bio-psychosocial understanding of dementia is discussed. Various examples of rehabilitation methods are presented, and psychosocial and cognition-focused interventions, complementary to rehabilitation, are introduced. Finally, overarching factors that challenge such interventions are discussed, including progression of symptoms, reduced symptom awareness, and challenges related to involving family caregivers.

L. Øksnebjerg (✉)
Department of Psychology, University of Copenhagen, Copenhagen, Denmark
e-mail: laoe@psy.ku.dk; laila@curax.dk

Keywords

Dementia · Cognition · Rehabilitation · Alzheimer's disease · Treatment

Box 22.1 Case Story
Eric is 73 years old; he and his wife Ann are both former schoolteachers. They have close relationships with their two sons, daughters-in-law, and four grandchildren, who all live close by. Eric and Ann enjoy various hobbies and activities, some together and some individually, and having an active and independent lifestyle is important for them. Eric enjoys riding his bike around the countryside, and he likes cooking. Together, they enjoy singing in a local church choir and often take care of their grandchildren. During the last 2 years Ann has become increasingly concerned about Eric's memory. He often seems confused about dates and times for various activities; he repeats questions and forgets things they have talked about. She has also noticed that he generally cooks simple meals and often forgets to buy some of the ingredients needed. Eric does not deny these symptoms, but he finds Ann exaggerating the problems. He is referred to a memory clinic, where he is diagnosed with early-stage Alzheimer's disease. After receiving this diagnosis, a community

(continued)

J. B. Nielsen et al. (eds.), *Neuroplasticity-based Neurorehabilitation*,
https://doi.org/10.1007/978-3-031-81120-3_22

Box 22.1 (continued)
dementia care worker pays a visit to Eric and Ann, and she introduces them to various kinds of support and activities for people with dementia and family caregivers. Eric does not want to take part in any of these; he is satisfied with the activities he already has. Ann expresses her concern that Eric might lose his way when going on bike rides alone, and she is frustrated that he often forgets about shared and individual activities. When she is out on her own, he often calls her, asking where she is, because he has forgotten what she has told him earlier on. The dementia care worker introduces Eric and Ann to various ways of coping with these challenges. She introduces the idea of Eric using a watch with GPS so Ann can locate him if he should lose his way. She also introduces a short program of rehabilitation in their home, where Eric is introduced to strategies and tools to support memory and structure when shopping for and cooking meals, enabling him to continue his activities as independently as possible.

22.1 Dementia Diseases: Frequency and Characteristics

The term *dementia* is an umbrella term for a range of brain diseases, characterised by a collection of symptoms, also known as a syndrome. These symptoms include cognitive dysfunction, along with psychological and behavioural symptoms, sometimes referred to as neuropsychiatric symptoms. For a person to be diagnosed with dementia, these symptoms must be at a level where they significantly affect daily life. It is beyond the scope of this chapter to give a detailed presentation of the many diseases that can cause dementia. An overview of the most common disease that causes dementia is presented in Fig. 22.1, and the four most common dementia diseases are presented in Box 22.2.

It is estimated that worldwide more than 55 million people live with dementia, and the number is expected to almost double every 20 years, reaching more than 150 million in 2050 (ADI, 2022). This large increase in the prevalence of dementia is caused by the fast-growing number of elderly people. But, contrary to previous

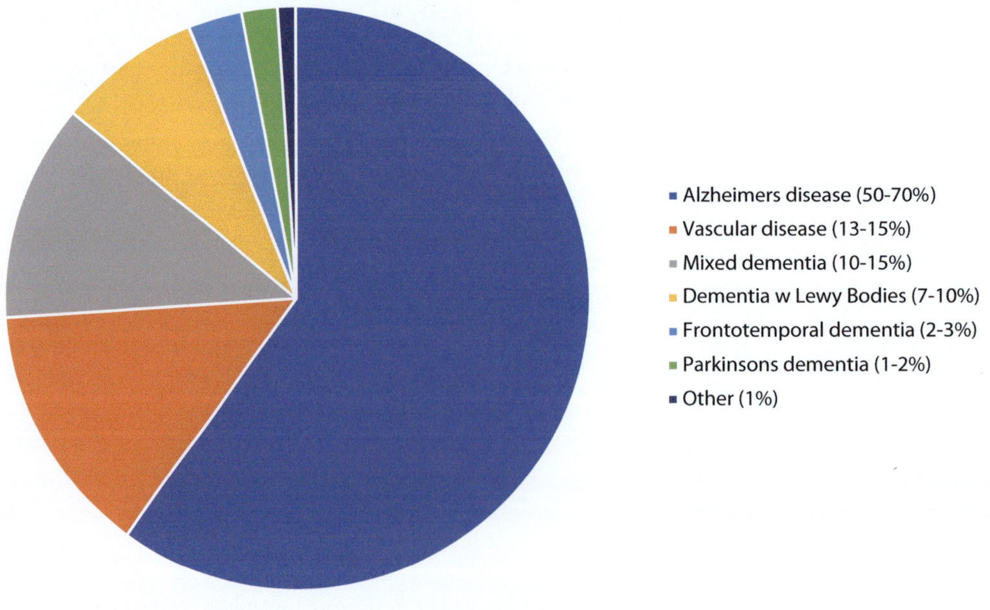

Fig. 22.1 Subtypes of dementia

beliefs, dementia is not caused by ageing, and the term "senile dementia" is obsolete. Dementia is always caused by a disease, and dementia diseases most often affect older people, but it can also affect younger people. It is estimated that worldwide 3.9 million people under the age of 65 live with young onset dementia (Hendriks et al., 2021). In rare cases, people in their 30s are diagnosed with a dementia disease, and prevalence gradually increases with age (ibid.). People with early-onset dementia generally suffer from the same diseases and symptoms as people who are diagnosed later in life, but the frequency of various dementia diseases differs due to genetic risk components. E.g. frontotemporal dementia is relatively more frequent in this subgroup. Moreover, their situation is often marked by other psychosocial and socioeconomic circumstances compared to the older group.

22.1.1 The Most Common Causes of Dementia

Most dementia diseases are neurodegenerative, leading to progressive cognitive and functional decline. As illustrated in Fig. 22.1, Alzheimer's disease (AD) is the most common neurodegenerative dementia disease, estimated to account for 50–70% of all cases. Vascular dementia (VaD) is the second most common cause of dementia, but it is not considered a neurodegenerative dementia disease. VaD is an umbrella term covering a group of conditions where vascular neuropathology causes dementia symptoms. Furthermore, a large proportion of people living with dementia have a mixed form, with both AD and VaD pathology. The risk of this mixed condition significantly increases for people in their 80s or older. Lewy body dementia (DLB) is another neurodegenerative dementia disease, estimated to account for around 7% of all dementia cases, but the prevalence of this disease is debated and might be underdiagnosed in clinical practice. Additionally, frontotemporal dementia (FTD) is estimated to account for approximately 3% of all dementia cases. Characteristics of these four most common causes of dementia are presented in the box below.

Box 22.2 The Most Common Diseases that Cause Dementia

Alzheimer's Disease

Alzheimer's disease (AD) is caused by a slowly progressing cascade of neuropathological processes that are still only partly uncovered. The earliest sign of AD pathology is characterised by deposits of beta-amyloid between the brain's cells. It is a naturally occurring protein, but in AD it is not sufficiently broken down and removed from the brain. Instead, it aggregates in clusters between nerve cells, where it affects communication between the cells, reduces energy metabolism, and leads to inflammatory changes. The next step of neuronal damage is caused by neurofibrillary tangles, tau protein, which accumulate inside nerve cells. Normally, tau stabilises nerve cells, but when it accumulates inside the cells, it is a sign of damage. As AD pathology progresses, neurones stop functioning, they lose connections with other neurones, and they die. In AD these disease processes are most predominant in parts of the brain involved in memory, including the entorhinal cortex and hippocampus. As the disease progresses, other areas in the cerebral cortex are gradually affected, and eventually most of the brain is affected by these neurodegenerative processes.

Hence, at the stage where a person is diagnosed with early-stage AD, the most prominent symptom is often severe memory problems, especially learning and recalling new episodic memories, but other aspects of memory, e.g. prospective memory and semantic memory, will also be reduced. Other cognitive domains, such as language, visuospatial functions, and executive functions, are also, to some degree,

(continued)

Box 22.2 (continued)

affected. More rarely, early AD is marked by other cognitive symptoms than amnesia in early stages. For instance, cases where visuoperceptual and visuospatial deficits are predominant, also known as posterior cognitive atrophy, or cases of primary progressive aphasia, where AD can be the underlying aetiology. These subvariants are seen more often in young-onset dementia. AD can also progress as a behavioural variant.

Vascular Dementia

Vascular dementia (VaD) is caused by decreased blood flow causing damage to brain tissue. A range of conditions that can cause VaD, including blood clots, bleedings, small vessel disease, causing lesions in the brain's white matter, or by inadequate supply of oxygen to the brain caused by anoxia or hypoxia. Due to the great variations in vascular pathology, and hence variation in size and location of the affected areas, the symptoms of VaD are quite heterogeneous. Reduction of processing speed, attention, and executive dysfunction are often predominant symptoms, reflecting subcortical vascular lesions. Memory is also often affected, but mostly secondary to reduced attention and executive functions, affecting the ability to retrieve stored memory. VaD can of course also be accompanied by other neurological symptoms, e.g. sensory disturbance, impaired balance, urinary problems, etc., depending on the size and location of vascular damages. If preventive treatment of cardiovascular risk factors is successful, VaD will potentially not progress.

Lewy Body Dementia

Lewy body dementia (DLB) is characterised by both cognitive and motor symptoms, with either simultaneous onset or within 1-year onset of motor symptoms. DLB has pathology and symptoms in common with both AD and Parkinson's disease (PD) (see Chap. 21). It is characterised by so-called Lewy bodies, consisting of the proteins alpha-synuclein and ubiquitin, which are intertwined with abnormally phosphorylated neurofilament protein accumulated inside the brain cells. These Lewy bodies are found in deep brain structures in both PD and DLB and are involved in motor symptoms. And in early-stage DLB, and some cases of later-stage PD, they are also found in cortical areas involved in cognitive functions. It is not known why these Lewy bodies accumulate in the cells and why the cells degenerate as a result. There is also a significant overlap between AD and DLB, not only in symptoms but also in pathological changes. Around half of people with DLB will also have AD-related changes in their brains. Cognitive symptoms in DLB are characterised by reduced attention and visuospatial, executive, and memory dysfunction. People with DLB often have less impairment of delayed recognition memory, compared with people with AD, indicating that memory problems in DLB can be due to impaired retrieval. Visual hallucinations and fluctuation in cognitive impairment are also characteristic symptoms in DLB.

Frontotemporal Dementia

In fronto-temporal dementia (FTD), neurodegeneration also occurs due to an abnormal protein buildup in the brain, but in contrast to AD and DLB, there are several different disease mechanisms that can lead to FTD symptoms, and it is not within the scope of this chapter to give a detailed overview of these. The proteins most often involved in FTD are TDP-43 (TAR DNA binding protein 43) and a variety of tau pathologies. There is no clear-cut correlation between pathology and symptoms and disease progression in FTD. Clinically, FTD can be classified into three variants. The most common type is the behavioural variant, which is characterised by progres-

(continued)

Box 22.2 (continued)

sive behavioural and executive deficits. More rare variants are progressive non-fluent aphasia, characterised by progressive deficits in speech, grammar, and word output, and the subtype semantic-variant FTD, characterised by progressive disorder of semantic knowledge. Not all cases can, however, be clearly defined in one of these variants, and as the disease progresses, symptoms often occur across these three disease variants. In some cases, FTD progresses as motor neurone disease or atypical parkinsonian disorder.

MCI

When discussing dementia, it is also important to be familiar with the condition Mild Cognitive Impairment (MCI). MCI is characterised by subjective and objective cognitive symptoms beyond what can be expected as age-related changes, but compared with a person who is diagnosed with dementia, the cognitive symptoms are less severe in MCI, and abilities in everyday life are not reduced to the same degree. The condition covers a spectrum of symptoms. Reduced memory is often a prominent symptom, known as the amnestic variant of MCI. But various cognitive domains can be affected, e.g. language or visuospatial functions, known as non-amnestic variants, and the condition can also involve multiple cognitive domains. The prevalence of MCI is estimated to be between 15% and 20% in people who are 60 years and older, and the annual rate at which MCI progresses to dementia varies between 8% and 15% per year. Even though symptoms are less predominant, people living with MCI have marked cognitive symptoms and can benefit from interventions to support cognitive functions and everyday functional ability, e.g. rehabilitation.

22.1.2 Pharmaceutical Treatment

There is no cure for any neurodegenerative dementia disease. Currently approved drugs can, to some extent, alleviate symptoms and slow progression. Two classes of medicines approved for clinical use are acetylcholine receptor inhibitors and N-methyl-D-aspartate receptor inhibitors, prescribed to people with AD, DLB, and, in some cases, VaD; however, it is not within the scope of this chapter to give a detailed description of pharmaceutical treatment for dementia diseases. For many years, many resources have been allocated to this line of research without success until recently. Currently, there are promising perspectives regarding disease-modifying agents for AD. However, there is also increased acknowledgement that the future of successful dementia interventions lies in a combination of disease prevention, tailored pharmaceutical treatment, and individualised non-pharmaceutical/psychosocial interventions, e.g. rehabilitation and related interventions, as described in this chapter.

22.1.3 The Progressive Nature of Dementia Diseases

Besides seeing dementia from an etiological perspective, it is also essential to have the progressive nature of most of the diseases in mind when understanding life with dementia. The three stages—mild, moderate, and severe—are often used to describe the degree to which dementia symptoms affect functional ability. As illustrated in Fig. 22.2, moving from a mild stage, where the person is marked by the disease but generally able to manage with some level of support, to a moderate stage, where many everyday activities can be managed when support is provided, and into a severe stage, where 24-h care is essential. The stages are generally equivalent to disease progression from an early, middle, and late stage. These

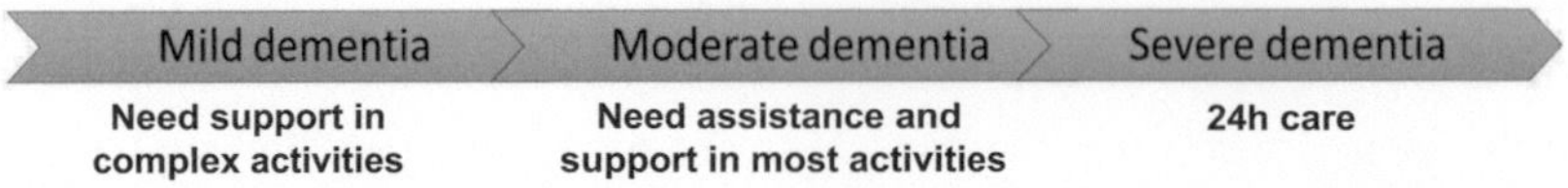

Fig. 22.2 The three stages—mild, moderate, and severe dementia—are useful when describing the level of dementia symptoms and how it influences functional ability in everyday life, including the need for support from others

stages, though general, can guide our understanding of a person's capacity and needs when planning interventions.

22.2 Moving Towards a Multifactorial and Bio-Psychosocial Understanding of Dementia

The understanding of dementia has evolved significantly over the last century. The word dementia derives from Latin for "loss of mind," but there is a strong movement away from this stigmatising focus on decline and deficits towards a more positive coping approach.[1] This paradigm shift reflects a growing public and political awareness on ethics, human rights, and inclusion of people living with dementia, and it both calls for and facilitates a greater focus on interventions to reinforce capacity, reduce symptoms, and promote quality of life. The paradigm shift is, however, also influenced by increasing evidence that dementia diseases not only reflect neuropathological processes but are influenced by a range of risk and protective factors, e.g. education, hypertension, hearing impairment, smoking, obesity, depression, physical activity, diabetes, social contact, excessive alcohol consumption, traumatic brain injury, and air pollution (Livingston et al., 2020). During a person's life course, these factors affect cognitive reserve and trigger the development of neuropathology, and hence influence the risk for developing dementia (ibid.). Consequently, to fully comprehend the many factors influencing whether a person develops a dementia disease, and when and how a disease progresses, it is essential to move beyond purely focusing on neurodegenerative factors and instead explore the complex interactions between biological, socioeconomic, lifestyle, social, and psychological factors and how these can be addressed in tailored interventions to reduce the negative consequences of the diseases and promote capacity, quality of life, and other positive outcomes (Vernooij-Dassen et al., 2021).

22.3 Rehabilitation, Psychosocial, and Cognitive Interventions for People with Dementia

Within the field of dementia, the term "rehabilitation" is used to describe a variety of interventions that differ in terms of the context in which they are offered and the specific methods used. Terms such as reablement, restorative care, or tertiary prevention are sometimes used synonymously. Rehabilitation for people with dementia includes home and community rehabilitation, cognitive rehabilitation, and rehabilitation programs in nursing home settings. In addition, this chapter includes other psychosocial and cognition-focused interventions, which are not regarded as rehabilitation per se, but are complementary to rehabilitation since they target similar goals, e.g. improvement on specific cognitive or more general functional abilities, e.g. cognitive training and cognitive stimulation therapy. Moreover, physical training is also discussed in this context. Most of these interventions are

[1] The term "dementia" is also criticised from a diagnostic perspective, and more disease-specific concepts have been requested. This has led to changes in the latest edition of the American classification system DSM-5, where the term "dementia" is replaced with the term "major neurocognitive disorder," followed by various subtype diagnoses, based on aetiology, and with the term "mild cognitive disorders" covering MCI. In the most recent version of the World Health Organisation's (WHO) diagnostic classification, ICD 11, the term dementia is still used, with various subtypes based on aetiology, and MCI is covered by the term "mild neurocognitive disorder."

applied individually, but some are applied in small group settings.

22.3.1 Home- and Community-Based Rehabilitation Methods

Home and community are often the main settings for rehabilitation interventions for people with dementia, since they enable a holistic approach to a person's needs, habits, and everyday activities, and direct involvement of family and other supporters, which is often essential to rehabilitation for people with dementia. As in the case with Eric, where his wife Ann was involved in both defining the aims and the rehabilitation interventions. Together, they were introduced to coping strategies and tools, e.g. the watch with GPS, enabling Ann to locate Eric if he lost his way. It also promotes the transfer of the rehabilitation intervention when rehabilitation strategies, tools, etc., are implemented directly in everyday life. Transferring the outcome of a rehabilitation intervention to daily life is a well-known challenge of rehabilitation in general.

Home- and community-based rehabilitation interventions have been investigated in various study designs, including occupational therapy rehabilitation programs for people with mild to moderate dementia and their caregivers (Wenborn et al., 2021). Another approach is goal-directed cognitive rehabilitation, a method developed for people living with cognitive impairment caused by brain injury and adapted to people with mild-to-moderate dementia (Clare et al., 2019). Such methods could involve training of compensatory strategies, tailored methods for learning or relearning, adaptation to the environment, and various supportive tools, including assistive technology. In the case with Eric, part of the rehabilitation program was to implement strategies and tools to support memory and structure when shopping for and cooking meals. This could be an individualised set of instructions on how to prepare a set of favourite meals. It could consist of tailored shopping lists and recipes, highly structured, with photos and time intervals, to support him through the whole process of having ideas of what to cook, shopping, and preparing meals.

Studies of such rehabilitation interventions show varied evidence, reflecting both variation in intervention methods, study design, and outcome measures. A Cochrane review of six cognitive rehabilitation randomised controlled trials with people with mild to moderate dementia showed significant changes in participant's and family caregiver's ratings of attaining individual goals for rehabilitation, both post-intervention and at follow-up, and a tendency towards positive effects on measures of attention and quality of life (Kudlicka et al., 2023).

Rehabilitation methods can also be applied in group-based programs, for instance, as part of a self-management group program. A group setting gives unique opportunities for peer support, psychoeducation, support, and sharing the experiences of life with dementia and how to apply coping strategies and supportive tools in daily life. The feasibility and positive benefits of such group interventions have been demonstrated in pilot studies (Øksnebjerg et al., 2020).

Most rehabilitation programs are applied to people with mild-to-moderate dementia, who have some ability to compensate for dementia symptoms, often with support from family members. However, rehabilitation methods can also be adapted for people living with a more severe stage of dementia, e.g. in a nursing home setting, where care professionals take a function-focused rehabilitation approach to support and care to optimise a person's functional abilities and participation in activities (Resnick et al., 2021). In Eric's case, at a more advanced stage of his disease, the intervention could be to support him in participating in activities related to bike rides and cooking, adapted to the level of support he would be needing. E.g. going on by-side tandem bike rides with staff or being involved in small-scale activities related to cooking.

22.3.2 Cognitive Training Interventions

The aim of cognitive training is to strengthen specific cognitive functions through guided systematic training of these functions, e.g. attention, mental speed, or memory. Cognitive training can be applied under various conditions and in various formats, e.g. through mental exercises, paper-and-pencil tasks, or in a digital format. It is applied across many conditions where people have reduced cognitive functions, e.g. due to brain injury, psychiatric conditions, or developmental disorders, and it is also, to some extent, used in the field of dementia. The effect of cognitive training is, however, questioned. Studies often find evidence for a training effect; participants are often able to improve their performance on specific and related tasks, but cognitive training is criticised for the general lack of evidence that the effects of cognitive training can be transferred to a more general level of cognitive function and to everyday activities.

It can, however, be relevant to offer tailored training of specific cognitive functions to individuals with rare forms of dementia, e.g. primary progressive aphasia, semantic dementia, or posterior cortical atrophy (Cadório et al., 2017; Roca et al., 2010). In such cases, training of specific cognitive functions would normally be highly individualised and be part of an overall rehabilitation approach also involving compensatory strategies, use of assistive technologies or other tools, psychoeducation, etc. (ibid.)

Cognitive training is also discussed in relation to cognitive reserve and in relation to MCI. Studies generally indicate that training improves cognitive performance in the domain trained, but there is no convincing evidence that cognitive training can prevent or delay cognitive decline or dementia (Gates et al., 2019). This field of research is, however, generally marked by low quality of evidence (ibid.).

22.3.3 Cognitive Stimulation Therapy

Cognitive Stimulation Therapy (CST) is a manualized and structured form of "mental exercise" developed specifically for people with dementia. It is delivered by trained staff to a small group of people with dementia for around 45 minutes twice weekly. Various cognitive abilities, such as memory, communication, and executive functions, are stimulated through a range of activities involving, e.g. reminiscence, games, music, physical activity, and creative activities (Spector et al., 2003). CST differs from other approaches, such as cognitive training and cognitive rehabilitation, by its broad cognitive focus and social elements, aiming to improve both participant's general cognitive function, quality of life, and mood. The rationale of CST is that stimulation of multiple brain functions can support, maintain, and strengthen the brain's plastic network and thereby maintain and enhance the general functional ability of people with dementia. Functional and structural mechanisms of cognitive stimulation have been explored in pilot studies using functional MRI (Liu et al., 2021). Though preliminary and limited, these studies suggest that cognitive stimulation maintains or perhaps enhances brain reserve both structurally and functionally by increased connectivity despite an overall decline in the volume of grey matter (ibid.). In the case with Eric, CST could be a feasible intervention in the mild to moderate stage of his disease, as a supplement to continuing his other activities.

Studies on the effect of CST generally show clinically relevant improvements in measures of cognitive ability, and, with some variation, studies also show improvement in communication, social interaction, quality of life, mood, and behavioural symptoms in people with mild to moderate dementia (Woods et al., 2023). CST was developed as a group-based intervention, and it has also been investigated as an individual intervention, and with less convincing results, probably due to factors related to variations in fidelity and dose (ibid.).

22.3.4 Physical Exercise

It is well established that physical exercise lowers the risk of developing dementia, but physical exercise is also considered an important intervention to reduce dementia symptoms. Numerous scientific studies have been conducted on physical activity and exercise in people with MCI or dementia, mainly AD or VaD, and there is great variation in interventions and design within this field of research. Generally, studies indicate a potential benefit on both cognitive and neuropsychiatric symptoms (Demurtas et al., 2020). The mechanisms behind these potential positive effects are not fully understood, and it is outside the scope of this chapter to give an overview of this extensive field of research (see Sect. 15.5.1). Apart from having disease-modifying potential, studies also show that exercise can benefit activities of daily living skills for people with dementia or MCI, especially multicomponent exercise programs that also include cognitive, physical, and multitasking exercises (Begde et al., 2022).

22.4 Challenges Related to Rehabilitation for People with Dementia

There are a range of factors that can influence both the feasibility and effect of rehabilitation and related interventions, and these are necessary to consider when planning interventions. These include, e.g. the progressive nature of the disease, reduced awareness of symptoms, and the need to involve and gain support from family caregivers.

22.4.1 Dementia Diseases: Progress and Symptoms Changes

Due to the progressive nature of neurodegenerative dementia diseases, a person's symptoms, and the way they influence capacity and ability, constantly change, and it can influence a rehabilitation process in many ways. Consequently, the specific methods, or tools applied, need to be adapted, or the person needs more direct support from a caregiver to be able to carry on with the activity. In most cases, as a disease progresses, it will change the person's capacity to an extent where the rehabilitation intervention is no longer possible or relevant. Hence, rehabilitation interventions for people constantly have to be tailored to current individual needs, and a successful outcome of a rehabilitation process is rarely stationary over a long period of time. Interventions will need to be repeated, adapted, and changed throughout the course of the disease.

22.4.2 Reduced Symptom Awareness

Reduced awareness of symptoms (anosognosia) is a well-known symptom across neurological diseases, and it is a predominant neuropsychiatric symptom in dementia diseases, associated with disease aetiology and stage. It is most often marked in people with moderate and severe dementia, but it can also be a significant symptom in the early stage of a dementia disease, e.g. in the behavioural variant of FTD, reduced symptom awareness is among the earliest symptoms.

Reduced awareness, of course, has a great influence on which psychosocial interventions are suitable for a person with dementia and how the person can engage in an intervention. For instance, in home- and community-based rehabilitation interventions, it is essential that the person has some insight into symptoms and how they influence daily life to be able to engage in the rehabilitation process. Whereas symptom awareness is not essential in rehabilitation methods based on professionals' approaches to activities and care.

Since reduced symptom awareness is a neuropsychiatric symptom, it should not be seen as a psychological reaction or defence, which can be subject to "treatment." However, to promote rehabilitation and related interventions, it is essential to address whether the person with dementia has been offered information about the disease, symptoms, and how to cope with these and ensure that this knowledge has been communicated in a way that complies with the person's cognitive resources. Self-management group programs, applied to people with MCI or early-stage dementia, can be a fruitful setting to promote such psychoeducation.

22.4.3 Involving Caregivers

Compared to other chronic diseases, rehabilitation and related interventions for people with dementia often necessitate direct involvement and collaboration with family caregivers or other supporters. Often the intervention even relies on it. Collaborating with caregivers often plays a crucial role in whether rehabilitative methods and tools are transferred and integrated into daily life and continue to be used. It is particularly important to involve caregivers if the methods and tools bring about significant changes or require active participation from caregivers. This may include situations where new technology or other tools are part of the intervention, and caregivers are involved in supporting and assisting using these, as in the case with Eric and Ann, where the watch with GPS was introduced. The involvement of caregivers is, of course, more essential with disease progression. Often it will be caregivers who observe if methods or tools need to be adjusted and if the rehabilitation approach needs major adjustments, or is no longer applicable.

Involving family caregivers is not always straightforward, however. It is important to consider their capacity and resources to participate in interventions since they are often considerably burdened by the caregiver situation. Moreover, many people with dementia live alone, and this, of course, poses significant challenges on how rehabilitation methods can be applied.

Review Questions

- What disease-related factors need to be considered when planning rehabilitation for people with dementia, and what implications do they have?
- How can theories and methods of rehabilitation for people with dementia be related to knowledge about risk and protective factors for developing a dementia disease?
- What are the major challenges when applying rehabilitation to people with dementia, and how can these challenges be approached?

References

ADI. (2022). *Numbers of people with dementia around the world*. https://www.alzint.org/u/numbers-people-with-dementia-2017.pdf

Begde, A., Jain, M., Hogervorst, E., & Wilcockson, T. (2022). Does physical exercise improve the capacity for independent living in people with dementia or mild cognitive impairment: An overview of systematic reviews and meta-analyses. *Aging & Mental Health, 26*(12), 2317–2327. https://doi.org/10.1080/13607863.2021.2019192

Cadório, I., Lousada, M., Martins, P., & Figueiredo, D. (2017). Generalization and maintenance of treatment gains in primary progressive aphasia (PPA): A systematic review. *International Journal of Language & Communication Disorders, 52*(5), 543–560.

Clare, L., Kudlicka, A., Oyebode, J. R., Jones, R. W., Bayer, A., Leroi, I., et al. (2019). Individual goal-oriented cognitive rehabilitation to improve everyday functioning for people with early-stage dementia: a multicentre randomised controlled trial (the GREAT trial). *International Journal of Geriatric Psychiatry, 34*(5), 709–721. https://doi.org/10.1002/gps.5076

Demurtas, J., Schoene, D., Torbahn, G., Marengoni, A., Grande, G., Zou, L., et al. (2020). Physical activity and exercise in mild cognitive impairment and dementia: An umbrella review of intervention and observational studies. *Journal of the American Medical Directors Association, 21*(10), 1415–1422.

Gates, N. J., Vernooij, R. W., Di Nisio, M., Karim, S., March, E., Martínez, G., et al. (2019). Computerised cognitive training for preventing dementia in people with mild cognitive impairment. *Cochrane Database of Systematic Reviews, 3*(3), CD012279. https://doi.org/10.1002/14651858.cd012279.pub2

Hendriks, S., Peetoom, K., Bakker, C., Van Der Flier, W. M., Papma, J. M., Koopmans, R., et al. (2021). Global prevalence of young-onset dementia. *JAMA Neurology, 78*(9), 1080. https://doi.org/10.1001/jamaneurol.2021.2161

Kudlicka, A., Martyr, A., Bahar-Fuchs, A., Sabates, J., Woods, B., & Clare, L. (2023). Cognitive rehabilitation for people with mild to moderate dementia. *Cochrane Database of Systematic Reviews, 6*, CD013388. https://doi.org/10.1002/14651858.CD013388.pub2

Liu, T., Spector, A., Mograbi, D. C., Cheung, G., & Wong, G. H. Y. (2021). Changes in default mode network connectivity in resting-state fMRI in people with mild dementia receiving cognitive stimulation therapy. *Brain Sciences, 11*(9), 1137.

Livingston, G., Huntley, J., Sommerlad, A., Ames, D., Ballard, C., Banerjee, S., et al. (2020). Dementia prevention, intervention, and care: 2020 report of the Lancet Commission. *The Lancet, 396*(10248), 413–446. https://doi.org/10.1016/s0140-6736(20)30367-6

Øksnebjerg, L., Woods, B., Vilsen, C. R., Ruth, K., Gustafsson, M., Ringkøbing, S. P., et al. (2020). Self-management and cognitive rehabilitation in early stage dementia—Merging methods to promote coping and adoption of assistive technology. A pilot study. *Aging and Mental Health, 24*(11), 1894–1903. https://doi.org/10.1080/13607863.2019.1625302

Resnick, B., Boltz, M., Galik, E., Fix, S., Holmes, S., Zhu, S., et al. (2021). Testing the implementation of function-focused care in assisted living settings. *Journal of the American Medical Directors Association, 22*(8), 1706–1713.e1. https://doi.org/10.1016/j.jamda.2020.09.026

Roca, M., Gleichgerrcht, E., Torralva, T., & Manes, F. (2010). Cognitive rehabilitation in posterior cortical atrophy. *Neuropsychological Rehabilitation, 20*(4), 528–540.

Spector, A., Thorgrimsen, L., Woods, B., Royan, L., Davies, S., Butterworth, M., et al. (2003). Efficacy of an evidence-based cognitive stimulation therapy programme for people with dementia. *British Journal of Psychiatry, 183*(3), 248–254. https://doi.org/10.1192/bjp.183.3.248

Vernooij-Dassen, M., Moniz-Cook, E., Verhey, F., Chattat, R., Woods, B., Meiland, F., et al. (2021). Bridging the divide between biomedical and psychosocial approaches in dementia research: The 2019 INTERDEM manifesto. *Aging & Mental Health, 25*(2), 206–212. https://doi.org/10.1080/13607863.2019.1693968

Wenborn, J., O'Keeffe, A. G., Mountain, G., Moniz-Cook, E., King, M., Omar, R. Z., et al. (2021). Community Occupational Therapy for people with dementia and family carers (COTiD-UK) versus treatment as usual (Valuing Active Life in Dementia [VALID]) study: A single-blind, randomised controlled trial. *PLoS Medicine, 18*(1), e1003433. https://doi.org/10.1371/journal.pmed.1003433

Woods, B., Rai, H. K., Elliott, E., Aguirre, E., Orrell, M., & Spector, A. (2023). Cognitive stimulation to improve cognitive functioning in people with dementia. *Cochrane Database of Systematic Reviews, 1*, CD005562. https://doi.org/10.1002/14651858.CD005562.pub3

Traumatic Brain Injury

23

Skye McDonald

Abstract

Severe traumatic brain injuries (TBI) can occur across the lifespan but are especially common among young adults and can lead to lifelong disabilities. This chapter introduces a young man, Liam, who has experienced such a TBI leaving him with mild cognitive problems and some significant interpersonal difficulties after discharge from rehabilitation. Using Liam as an example, the prevalence, incidence, and neuropathology of severe TBI will be described, as well as some special issues with respect to rehabilitation. Remediation needs to be tailored to the recovery trajectory with different approaches at different times in the recovery process. Common problems with self-awareness, anxiety, depression, and fatigue can also interfere with motivation to engage in the rehabilitation process and need to be factored in when tailoring treatment. The chapter considers the use of restorative approaches and some of the constraints on this type of approach as well as occasions when more compensatory approaches may be better. In doing so, consideration is given to the current levels of evidence and practice guidelines that have recently been published. The chapter concludes with a brief discussion of potential areas of future treatment research and a consideration of the problems that beset rehabilitation research in this field.

Keywords

Traumatic brain injury · Rehabilitation · Self-awareness · Depression · Restoration · Compensation

Box 23.1 Case Story

At 20 years of age, Liam was involved in a head-on collision as a passenger in a car that careered off a country road, hitting a tree. The driver and other passenger were both killed. Liam sustained a severe traumatic brain injury (TBI). He was taken to hospital unconscious and required intubation. An MRI scan revealed multiple small haemorrhages in both frontal lobes. He gradually regained consciousness 2 weeks later and was transferred to a brain injury rehabilitation unit. He remained agitated and confused for a further 12 weeks with no memories for that time and with ongoing difficulties complying with therapy requirements. For example, although he needed physiotherapy to avoid painful contractures and limb spasticity resulting from the brain injury, his tolerance for uncomfortable or protracted exercises was very low. He gradually became more oriented in time and place and more cooperative although he had limited insight into the extent of his difficul-

(continued)

S. McDonald (✉)
UNSW Psychology, Sydney, NSW, Australia
e-mail: s.mcdonald@unsw.edu.au

J. B. Nielsen et al. (eds.), *Neuroplasticity-based Neurorehabilitation*,
https://doi.org/10.1007/978-3-031-81120-3_23

Box 23.1 (continued)
ties, arguing that he would be fine if he could just go home and resume his job as a plumber.

When Liam was first assessed by a neuropsychologist at 4 months post-injury, he demonstrated very poor attention, impulse control, problem-solving, and ability to learn and recall information. These cognitive abilities all improved markedly at 7 months and even more so at 10 months coming close to normal limits although he retained mild difficulties with learning and retaining verbal information and with problem-solving. He was also noted to have impaired ability to recognise facial emotions. He was discharged at 10 months post-injury with very little physical limitations and only mild cognitive impairments. His family was initially relieved that he had regained consciousness, and his survival was assured. However, they started to remark on the fact that he was often rude and insensitive to others, even when they were visibly distressed, and was very egocentric. He would make lewd jokes and talk about topics (such as seeing sex workers) that were embarrassing and not appropriate for the context. They described him as a sensitive, rather introverted young man before the injury. Initially, they attributed the changes in his behaviour to the stress of being in hospital and expressed their belief that he would be much better at home. However, after discharge, it became apparent that the behavioural issues were ongoing.

23.1 Incidence and Prevalence of TBI

Liam's presentation is typical of a severe TBI and, indeed, it is not uncommon. The annual incidence of traumatic brain injury (TBI) has been estimated to be ten million people worldwide (Hyder et al., 2007). The vast majority of TBIs are in the mild category also known as concussion. For these, the person is unlikely to experience ongoing effects (although a minority will have continuing symptoms and repeated injuries may have cumulative, devastating effects). While the incidence for moderate or severe TBI is far lower (estimated as 12–20 per 100,000 people per annum) (Tate et al., 1998), most people who experience severe injuries will experience ongoing disability and reduced participation. Furthermore, the prevalence of such injuries (i.e., number of people who will experience a severe TBI in their lifetime) is far greater. For example, in Finland it was estimated that 269 per 100,000 people would experience a moderate to severe injury by the age of 34 (Winqvist et al., 2007). While one can experience a significant TBI at any age, in Western countries young adults (18–25 years) and especially males (2:1), like Liam, are disproportionately affected.

23.2 Pathophysiology

At the time of impact, acceleration-deceleration forces distort, stretch, compress, and rotate brain tissue including grey and white matter and blood vessels. This leads to contusions (bruising), micro-bleeds, diffuse axonal injury including micro-lesions in white matter tracts and shearing of white-grey matter junctions. Further damage may occur due to direct impact, contra-coup injuries (due to ricochet effects), and skull fractures. Although damage can occur anywhere in the brain, there is a tendency for damage to be concentrated in the medial and ventral areas of the frontal and temporal lobes due to the brain scraping against the bony surfaces of the skull floor. The corpus callosum is also particularly vulnerable. The immediate and protracted sequelae of TBI are complex as axons swell and biochemical cascades compromise brain function further. Wallerian degeneration of surrounding tissue can continue to occur months after the initial injury (Bigler & Maxwell, 2011).

Because of this complex neuropathology, every person with a severe TBI is different. However, it is common for patients to have reduced information processing efficiency (possibly reflecting axonal disruption) as well as poor new learning and difficulties with drive (inflexibility) and control (disinhibition) (Tate et al., 1991), most likely due to damage to medial temporal and dorsolateral frontal lobes. Deficits in interpersonal skills are also common. There may be a loss of social cognition characterised by a loss of empathy and impairments in gauging what other people are feeling and thinking. There may also be problems with emotion regulation such as apathy, disinhibition, anger, and irritability. Problems with both social cognition and emotion regulation have been associated with overlapping distributed neural networks that include orbitomedial prefrontal regions and the temporal lobes (McDonald et al., 2023). Thus, the profile of impairments experienced by Liam, including mild learning and problem-solving deficits and problems with social functioning, is typical of the deficits seen although the pattern and pervasiveness of his difficulties are by no means universal.

23.3 Challenges Related to Rehabilitation Following TBI

23.3.1 Timing of Rehabilitation

The timing of rehabilitation needs to be carefully considered following TBI. Liam was unconscious for 2 weeks, during which time interaction for the purposes of therapy was essentially not possible (although there has been some research on working with minimally conscious patients). During the following 12 weeks, he was in a transient state referred to as post-traumatic amnesia (PTA), since during this time patients do not lay down new conscious memories. This period is also characterised by disorientation, confusion, possible agitation and delirium, behaviour change, and very little capacity to attend to tasks, all of which limits the kind of rehabilitation that can take place. While some therapy (such as physiotherapy in Liam's case) is necessary, the session length, intensity, and location need to be flexibly adapted in view of the level of agitation, fatigue, and cognitive impairment the patient is experiencing (Ponsford et al., 2023a). There is also evidence that activities of daily living can begin to be reinstated during this period without adding to agitation. Given the cognitive impairments people with PTA experience, techniques such as errorless learning (whereby the patient is prevented from making mistakes while learning) and a focus on procedural (implicit) learning are recommended (Ponsford et al., 2023a).

Once PTA has resolved, more conventional approaches to rehabilitation can commence. Rehabilitation needs to be designed to cater for the individual's specific constellation of weaknesses while building on and exploiting their strengths. It is critical that the patient is motivated to engage with rehabilitation for this to be effective. However, the patient's insight and motivation will be influenced by both neurogenic factors, i.e., conditions arising from the structural brain damage and psychogenic factors, i.e., pre-existing psychological and cultural factors and psychological adjustment to the injury. Consequently, while some rehabilitation is effective immediately after PTA has resolved, other aspects of rehabilitation, e.g., social and interpersonal skills, may be better addressed once the patient has returned home and has had the opportunity to understand what and where their problems might be when resuming everyday activities. This also gives the clinician the opportunity to learn more about the patient's socio-cultural context so as to tailor therapy to their personal needs and circumstances.

23.3.2 Changes in Self-Awareness

To adjust to life with a TBI, Liam needs to have a realistic understanding of how his abilities may have changed and how he may need to adapt his behaviour accordingly. In the acute stages of rehabilitation, the patient often over-estimates his abilities (such as Liam believing he would be fine provided he could just go home and resume work) and this can create a challenge for engaging with rehabilitation due to lack of motivation and the setting of goals. Self-awareness often improves once the patient is discharged home, has re-commenced everyday tasks, and can appreciate, for themselves, their strengths and limitations. This is not, however, always the case with a large proportion of people continuing to have impaired self-awareness long term. The alternative scenario is where the patient is overly focused on acquired deficits, and this is frequently associated with depression and anxiety (Ownsworth et al., 2007). Metacognitive skills training (MST) has proven efficacy for improving self-awareness. MST involves providing structured opportunities for the patient to perform everyday tasks and to get feedback on the errors they make (or by observing the therapist make errors) and is endorsed as a practice standard for treating deficits in self-awareness (Jeffay et al., 2023).

23.3.3 Depression, Anxiety, and Fatigue

About a third of people with TBI experience clinical levels of depression and/or anxiety. Fatigue and sleep disturbances are also common (Alway et al., 2016; Ponsford et al., 2012). Depression and anxiety predict reduced independence in activities of daily living, lower participation, increased physical disability, and poorer quality of life and need, therefore, to be a target of rehabilitation. Cognitive-behavioural therapies (CBT) are the treatment of choice for depression and anxiety. CBT encompasses psychoeducation and cognitive restructuring to help the patient think differently about situations and to problem solve solutions, graded exposure to difficult situations, and a focus on positive behaviours and relaxation techniques. While conventional wisdom has assumed that CBT is too "cognitive" for people with cognitive impairments, CBT can be successful if adapted, such as increased repetition, written aids, a focus on behaviour rather than thoughts and homework (Hodgson et al., 2005).

23.4 Practical Use

Issues with timing of rehabilitation, the impact of changes to self-awareness, mood disorders, and fatigue, as well as a myriad of other concerns including pain, substance use, and medication effects all need to be factored into any rehabilitation effort (Ponsford et al., 2023b). Along with these considerations, developing a collaborative remediation programme that has the patient and their goals at the centre is pivotal to any success. Within this context, there is a range of treatment approaches that have been used, including techniques aimed at restoration, compensation, and/or environmental support. The choice of approach is guided by the functional goals of the patient along with a consideration of the severity and type of difficulties being experienced.

23.4.1 Restoration of Lost Skills

Restoration techniques based on neuroplasticity principles assume that if target processes are repetitively activated, synaptic connections will increase. Functional recovery along with expansion of cortical activation has been seen in many motor, perceptual, and cognitive abilities following such targeted, repetitive, graduated practice (Bornhofen & McDonald, 2008). Bottom-up approaches focus on simple processes. So, for example, to retrain Liam's emotion perception abilities he might undergo regular training to focus on and interpret the shape of the eyes in a facial expression, then move on to the mouth, the whole face and so on. Explicit reinforcement, cueing, feedback, role-plays, modelling, and games are all techniques that can introduce variety and interest and thus enhance motivation during such repetitive practice. Top-down techniques are often used to complement these bottom-up exercises by providing strategies that help focus attention on the requisite process, e.g., Liam may be prompted to learn and apply the acronym WSTC "**W**hat am I trying to do?" What **S**trategy should I use?" **T**ry it out, **C**heck how it went (**C**ongratulate myself for trying) when faced with a social setting. Other kinds of social cognitive impairments, such as an incapacity to understand the viewpoint of others, can also be improved. For example, Liam could be encouraged to practise seeing an ambiguous situation (e.g., having a shopping bag knocked to the floor by a passerby) from a range of different perspectives (blaming the passerby, blaming self, relaxed perspective) (Cassel et al., 2020).

Restorative techniques such as these have sufficient evidence in TBI to form part of recommended practice standards for executive function, memory, and social cognition (Jeffay et al., 2023; Togher et al., 2023; Velikonja et al., 2023). However, it is important to note that simple, decontextualised drills, e.g., on a computer, are not recommended for any cognitive skill. Throughout the research for interventions, the evidence strongly favours client-centred goal setting, a focus on everyday tasks and individualising therapy within the patient's socio-cultural context. The type of intervention selected depends on the severity of injury and breadth of cognitive impairments experienced. For example, some cognitive memory strategies are only possible if the patient retains reasonable executive ability.

23.4.2 Compensation and/or Environmental Support

In many cases, restoration may not be realistic due to the nature or severity of impairments, and/or co-existing problems. In these cases, environmental changes or other compensatory devices (such as mobile phone reminders) may be more practical. A related and powerful approach is to modify the environment to enhance functioning. Modifications can be physical (e.g., putting up checklists in Liam's workplace to remind him of what to do) or social. For example, communication partner training can train people around Liam to provide support and structure to facilitate social interactions (Togher et al., 2023).

23.4.3 New Approaches

There is increasing interest in finding new methods to enhance rehabilitation following TBI and some hold clear promise. For example, virtual reality platforms have potential, providing the opportunity for enriched virtual settings within which to practise skills. There is also already good evidence that music therapy has efficacy in improving executive processes (Jeffay et al., 2023). On the other hand, despite initial excitement about transcortical magnetic stimulation, there is no evidence for its efficacy to date (Jeffay et al., 2023; Ponsford et al., 2023b; Velikonja et al., 2023).

One of the major problems for finding good evidence for new rehabilitation techniques is that every person with TBI is different leading to high heterogeneity in group comparison trials. Relatedly, the number of patients who may be sufficiently similar to undertake a treatment trial in a given location for a given skill is usually small, reducing the power of the trial to identify treatment effects. Methods other than randomised controlled trials, such as single case experimental designs (Tate et al., 2019), may be one way forward although these also hold significant challenges. Despite these problems, there is now sufficient evidence to produce clinical practice guidelines for the use of clinical interventions in TBI. The latest guidelines (2023) identified significant advances since the original set in 2014, and this is a positive trend, holding promise for future, better treatments for this most disabling condition.

Review Questions

- Should rehabilitation commence during post-traumatic amnesia?
- What are the drawbacks of decontextualised computer exercises to retrain lost skills?
- When would environmental compensatory techniques be preferable to retraining?

References

Alway, Y., Gould, K. R., Johnston, L., McKenzie, D., & Ponsford, J. (2016). A prospective examination of Axis I psychiatric disorders in the first 5 years following moderate to severe traumatic brain injury. *Psychological Medicine, 46*(6), 1331–1341.

Bigler, E. D., & Maxwell, W. L. (2011). Neuroimaging and neuropathology of TBI. *NeuroRehabilitation, 28*(2), 63–74.

Bornhofen, C., & McDonald, S. (2008). Emotion perception deficits following traumatic brain injury: A review of the evidence and rationale for intervention. *Journal of the International Neuropsychological Society, 14*(4), 511–525.

Cassel, A., McDonald, S., & Kelly, M. (2020). Establishing 'proof of concept' for a social cognition group treatment program (SIFT IT) after traumatic brain injury: Two case studies. *Brain Injury, 34*(13–14), 1781–1793.

Hodgson, J., McDonald, S., Tate, R. L., & Gertler, P. (2005). A randomised controlled trial of a cognitive-behavioural therapy program for managing social anxiety after acquired brain injury. *Brain Impairment, 6*, 169–180.

Hyder, A. A., Wunderlich, C. A., Puvanachandra, P., Gururaj, G., & Kobusingye, O. C. (2007). The impact of traumatic brain injuries: A global perspective. *NeuroRehabilitation, 22*(5), 341–353.

Jeffay, E., Ponsford, J., Harnett, A., Janzen, S., Patsakos, E., Douglas, J., et al. (2023). INCOG 2.0 guidelines for cognitive rehabilitation following traumatic brain injury, part III: Executive functions. *Journal of Head Trauma Rehabilitation, 38*(1), 52–64.

McDonald, S., Wearne, T., & Kelly, M. (2023). Calling on clinicians to get social and emotional. *The Clinical Neuropsychologist, 37*(3), 506–544.

Ownsworth, T. L., Fleming, J., Strong, J., Radel, M., Chan, W., & Clare, L. (2007). Awareness typologies, long-term emotional adjustment and psychosocial outcomes following acquired brain injury. *Neuropsychological Rehabilitation, 17*, 129–150.

Ponsford, J. L., Ziino, C., Parcell, D. L., Shekleton, J. A., Roper, M., Redman, J. R., et al. (2012). Fatigue and sleep disturbance following traumatic brain injury—Their nature, causes, and potential treatments. *The Journal of Head Trauma Rehabilitation, 27*(3), 224–233.

Ponsford, J., Trevena-Peters, J., Janzen, S., Harnett, A., Marshall, S., Patsakos, E., et al. (2023a). INCOG 2.0 guidelines for cognitive rehabilitation following traumatic brain injury, part I: Posttraumatic amnesia. *Journal of Head Trauma Rehabilitation, 38*(1), 24–37.

Ponsford, J., Velikonja, D., Janzen, S., Harnett, A., McIntyre, A., Wiseman-Hakes, C., et al. (2023b). INCOG 2.0 guidelines for cognitive rehabilitation following traumatic brain injury, part II: Attention and information processing speed. *Journal of Head Trauma Rehabilitation, 38*(1), 38–51.

Tate, R. L., Fenelon, B., Manning, M., & Hunter, M. (1991). Patterns of neuropsychological impairment after severe blunt head injury. *Journal of Nervous and Mental Disease, 179*(3), 117–126.

Tate, R. L., McDonald, S., & Lulham, J. M. (1998). Incidence of hospital-treated traumatic brain injury in an Australian community. *Australian and New Zealand Journal of Public Health, 22*(4), 419–423.

Tate, R. L., Perdices, M., Rosenkoetter, U., McDonald, S., Togher, L., Shadish, W., et al. (2019). Reprint of "The Single-Case Reporting Guideline In BEhavioural Interventions (SCRIBE) 2016: Explanation and Elaboration". *Pratiques Psychologiques, 25*(2), 119–151.

Togher, L., Douglas, J., Turkstra, L. S., Welch-West, P., Janzen, S., Harnett, A., et al. (2023). INCOG 2.0 guidelines for cognitive rehabilitation following traumatic brain injury, part IV: Cognitive-communication and social cognition disorders. *Journal of Head Trauma Rehabilitation, 38*(1), 65–82.

Velikonja, D., Ponsford, J., Janzen, S., Harnett, A., Patsakos, E., Kennedy, M., et al. (2023). INCOG 2.0 guidelines for cognitive rehabilitation following traumatic brain injury, part V: Memory. *Journal of Head Trauma Rehabilitation, 38*(1), 83–102.

Winqvist, S., Lehtilahti, M., Jokelainen, J., Luukinen, H., & Hillbom, M. (2007). Traumatic brain injuries in children and young adults: A birth cohort study from northern Finland. *Neuroepidemiology, 29*(1–2), 136–142.

Concussion

24

Michael J. Grey

Abstract

Concussion is classified as a mild traumatic brain injury. However, despite this nomenclature it is a significant health concern that has complex and inadequately understood pathology. Concussions are prevalent across all ages and walks of life, with a variety of causes ranging from sports and recreational activities to workplace accidents and falls among the elderly. This chapter explores the multifaceted nature of concussions addressing the complexities associated with its diagnosis and management. The chapter also explores the significant recent progress made in developing return-to-activity protocols for athletes returning to sport and for children returning to school, stressing the necessity of adopting these protocols in broader contexts, such as the workplace. An argument is made for the need for a conservative and personalised approach in treatment following evidence-based protocols for return to activity that allow the brain to heal itself.

Keywords

Mild traumatic brain injury (mTBI) · Sport-related concussion (SRC) · Postconcussion syndrome (PCS) · Graded return to activity

M. J. Grey (✉)
School of Sport, Exercise and Health Sciences
National Centre for Sport and Exercise Medicine,
Loughborough University, Leicestershire, UK
e-mail: M.J.Grey@lboro.ac.uk

Box 24.1 Case Study

Freya, a 20-year-old university student and avid handball player, was participating in a competitive match for her top-tier university club. During a particularly intense segment of the match, she was struck in the head by an opposing player's elbow during an attempt to score. Freya reported feeling disoriented and dizzy immediately after the incident, with a headache developing rapidly. She was removed from the match by her coach. The next day, Freya could not attend classes and was advised to go to the hospital for a thorough evaluation. Neuroimaging, including CT and MRI scans, was normal, showing no structural damage. Freya was discharged with a diagnosis of concussion. Despite following a cautious and structured protocol for return to study and sport, Freya's symptoms persisted for 3 weeks; significantly impacting her daily life, her ability to engage fully in her studies, and she could not continue playing handball. Freya was referred for vestibular rehabilitation therapy to address concerns with her balance and dizziness. Over several weeks, Freya engaged in this therapy under the guidance of a specialist physiotherapist, gradually experiencing a reduction in her symptoms. Whilst her assignments and exams were deferred, she was ultimately able to return to full-time classes and to finish the handball season, winning the final tournament with her team.

J. B. Nielsen et al. (eds.), *Neuroplasticity-based Neurorehabilitation*,
https://doi.org/10.1007/978-3-031-81120-3_24

24.1 Introduction

Concussion is classified as a mild traumatic brain injury (mTBI). TBI itself is often described as a silent epidemic affecting millions of people each year worldwide (Goldstein, 1990) (see Chap. 23). mTBI represents the vast majority of these cases (75–90%), and despite the nomenclature, it is a significant public health concern due to their frequency, potential for long-term negative life consequences, and prevalence in sports, recreational activities, and accidents (Voss et al., 2015). Spontaneous resolution occurs in most patients within 7 days, yet 15–30% will develop postconcussion syndrome (PCS; e.g., Moore & Sandsmark, 2023). The delays in return to school, work, recreational, and social activities caused by PCS can deeply impact the individual's quality of life and have major long-term negative life consequences. The societal burden extends beyond the affected individual to families, healthcare systems, and communities at large. The economic costs associated with medical care, rehabilitation, and lost productivity are substantial.

The majority of research in this field has focussed on sport-related concussion (SRC), and this has emerged as an area of significant concern (e.g., Patricios et al., 2023). However, this research has predominantly targeted adult males, whilst research involving children, older adults, and females has been notably scarcer. Despite this, concussion is observed across all ages and walks of life with a variety of causes and consequences. In school-age children, for example, concussions occur frequently due to falls and playground accidents, contributing to cognitive impairments and challenges in academic performance. In the workplace, they result from accidents particularly in the construction, manufacturing, and transportation industries, leading to lost workdays and long-term occupational challenges. Among the elderly, falls are the leading cause of concussions, with such injuries increasing the risk of further falls and prolonged hospital stays.

In many sports, the incidence rate of SRC offers a quantitative measure that provides a snapshot of the current state of concussions in sports, allowing for the monitoring of trends over time. Furthermore, sport governing bodies have leveraged these rates to inform rule changes aimed at SRC reduction. One of the primary strategies has been the modification of rules to reduce high-risk behaviours. It is common in competitive sport for athletes not to report symptoms due to fear of being removed from play, lack of awareness, or perceived pressure from coaches or teammates. Similar lack of reporting is common in schools and the workplace due to fear of missing studies or work and lack of understanding of the potential serious consequences associated with a so-called minor injury.

24.2 Pathophysiology

Concussion is defined as a transient disturbance of brain function resulting from biomechanical forces applied to the head or body, causing the brain to undergo rapid acceleration and deceleration within the skull (e.g., Patricios et al., 2023). These forces lead to shear, strain, and compression injuries to neuron cell bodies and axons. Central to the pathophysiology is a sudden and temporary disruption of brain function due to a transient neurometabolic cascade initiated by this mechanical insult, leading to a flood of excitatory neurotransmitters, altered neurochemistry, and neuroinflammation (Howell & Southard, 2021; Romeu-Mejia et al., 2019) (see Box 24.2).

Second impact syndrome is a rare but potentially fatal condition, observed primarily in chil-

Box 24.2 Metabolic Cascade Following Concussive Brain Injury

Following the mechanical insult, a sudden release of neurotransmitters creates dysregulation of ionic homeostasis, notably characterised by a significant influx of calcium ions into the cells, producing an ionic imbalance that disrupts cellular communication. Elevated intracellular calcium can then foster a series of deleterious pathways including mitochondrial dysfunction and apoptosis, further exacerbating neuronal damage. Excessive release of excitatory

(continued)

Box 24.2 (continued)
neurotransmitters, most notably glutamate, coupled with a reduction in cerebral blood flow, leads to an energy supply-demand mismatch, a state referred to as "neurometabolic energy crisis." This hypermetabolic period is followed by a phase of relative glucose hypometabolism that can last for 5 to 10 days post-injury, and this is a state where both glucose metabolism and brain blood flow are lower than normal.

Concurrent with the influx of calcium ions, there is a decline in inhibitory neurotransmitters, contributing to an imbalanced neuronal firing pattern. An immune response is also triggered resulting in the release of pro-inflammatory cytokines and chemokines. Microglia then become activated, releasing inflammatory mediators that further contribute to cellular damage and excitotoxicity. Following the neurometabolic cascade, the insult can also produce axonal damage resulting a disruption of the axonal transport system, axonal swelling, and ultimately disconnection. Concussion is also marked by alterations in the blood-brain barrier permeability that can further stimulate inflammatory responses and potentially lead to secondary brain injury.

dren, that occurs when a second head injury is sustained before the brain is fully recovered (Romeu-Mejia et al., 2019). The neurometabolic energy crisis prohibits the brain from responding to the damage produced by the second insult. This results in rapid brain swelling and a sudden increase in intracranial pressure which can be fatal.

24.3 Concussion Signs Symptoms and Diagnosis

The neurometabolic cascade produces an array of transient, and predominantly reversible symptoms, which can span cognitive, physical, emotional, and sleep dimensions (Fig. 24.1). Importantly, individual variations and the severity of the injury play a key role in the clinical manifestation of concussion. Whilst recovery is expected in most cases, a growing body of literature reveals that repeated brain trauma can lead to prolonged symptoms and increase the risk of chronic neurodegenerative diseases.

In the acute phase following a concussion, the most common symptom is headache. Dizziness follows closely, and there is also a notable presence of balance disorders during this period. In contrast with a widely held belief among the public, it is important to note that only about 10% of individuals experiencing a concussion lose consciousness. Other symptoms that might manifest include nausea, vomiting, and sleep disturbances, although these can sometimes be non-specific and overlap with other health issues. Physical symptoms can be accompanied by emotional and behavioural changes such as irritability and anxiety. The duration of acute symptoms can vary from a few days to a few weeks, and most people recover fully within a week.

However, a significant concern is that 15–30% of people who experience concussion have symptoms that persist for months, a phenomenon known as postconcussion syndrome (PCS; Babcock et al., 2013). PCS symptoms can persist for weeks to months following the initial injury. Individuals in this phase commonly report persistent post-traumatic headache and dizziness, akin to the acute phase, but they also face complex issues including insomnia, exercise intolerance, and cognitive intolerance. Psychological symptoms such as depressed mood, irritability, and anxiety become more pronounced, coupled with cognitive problems involving memory loss, poor concentration, and problem-solving difficulties. Fatigue (Box 9.5), noise, and light sensitivity are additional concerns. A notable aspect of PCS is the involvement of vestibular functions, influencing symptoms like dizziness and balance issues. Whilst the symptoms in the PCS phase are an extension of those in the acute phase, they tend to be more severe and prolonged, requiring comprehensive management and ample recovery time. PCS can result in significant delays for return to school, work, recreational, and social activities,

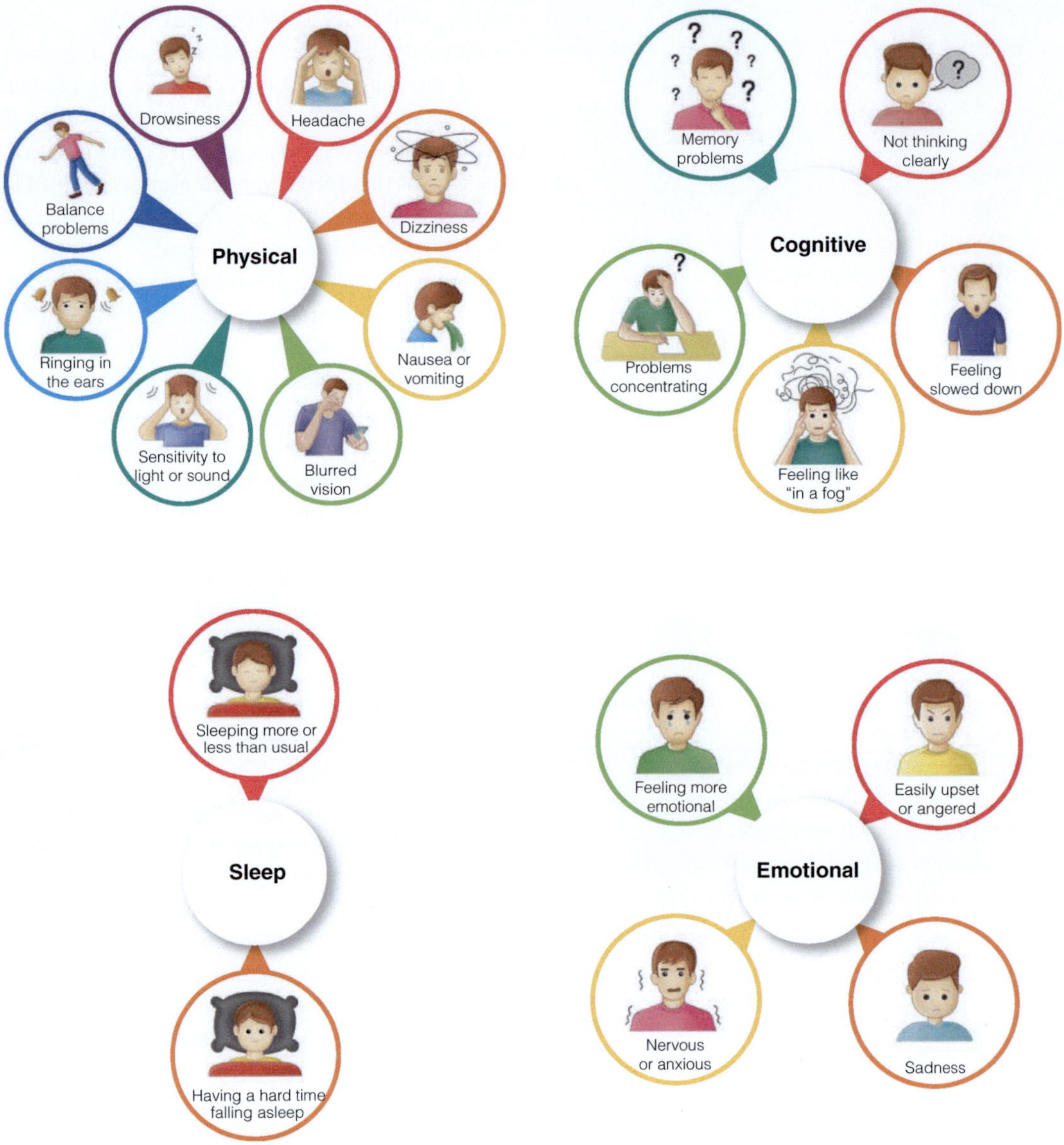
Physical
Drowsiness
Headache
Dizziness
Balance problems
Ringing in the ears
Sensitivity to light or sound
Blurred vision
Nausea or vomiting
Cognitive
Memory problems
Not thinking clearly
Problems concentrating
Feeling like "in a fog"
Feeling slowed down
Sleep
Sleeping more or less than usual
Having a hard time falling asleep
Emotional
Feeling more emotional
Easily upset or angered
Nervous or anxious
Sadness

Fig. 24.1 Concussion symptoms. The symptoms of a concussion, grouped into four domains: cognitive, physical, emotional, and sleep are illustrated with some of the most common symptoms

and this can deeply impact the quality of life and have major long-term negative life consequences.

Diagnosing concussions is not a trivial process, and it presents some difficult challenges. The symptoms illustrated in Fig. 24.1 can be quite subtle and do not always present immediately after the injury but can be delayed hours to days following injury. Individuals might under-report their symptoms due to unawareness of the severity of their condition, or because they feel compelled by internal or external pressure to resume normal activity (i.e., return to school, sport, and/or work). Compounding these issues is a lack of objective diagnostic tests, which means that healthcare providers often must rely on the affected individual's self-reported symptoms and a physical examination to make a diagnosis. As a result, the diagnosis ideally should be made by a healthcare provider who is familiar with the individual and has specific expertise in recognising and evaluating concussions.

Graded symptom checklists offer an objective method to assess a range of symptoms and to track the severity of those symptoms over time through serial evaluation. However, there is limited validation available for these standardised assessment tools, which means relying solely on them can potentially miss some cases or not fully capture the extent of an individual's symptoms.

A variety of tools have been designed for the initial clinical assessment of concussion, both in the clinic/hospital and at the sideline in the case of SRC. The Glasgow Comma Scale (see Box 12.3) is commonly used for TBI but is much less useful for all but the more serious concussions. The Acute Concussion Evaluation (ACE) is an evidence-based structured clinical interview designed to assist healthcare providers in the assessment and triage of children and adolescents (ages 3 to 18 years). One of the more common assessments for SRC is the Sport Concussion Assessment Tool 6 (SCAT6), which provides a structured framework for the initial assessment of a suspected concussion, including checking symptoms, cognitive evaluation, and balance tests. However, the sensitivity, specificity, validity, and reliability of these types of screening tools vary significantly depending on age, culture factors, and settings. Whilst not practical outside of higher level sport, the use of pre-season baseline assessments improves the efficacy of SRC screening tools. Importantly, neuroimaging is reserved for cases where there is a suspicion of intracerebral bleeding, and is not currently suitable for use in the diagnosis of concussions.

24.4 Special Considerations for Age and Sex

As noted above, there is a dearth of research involving children, older adults, and females. Nevertheless, even in the absence of extensive literature for these demographic groups, there are particular issues concerning concussion that warrant attention.

24.4.1 Children

Children are at a higher risk of concussion than are adults (Yeates et al., 2023). One of the most significant factors is the greater head-to-body ratio in children compared to adults, making them more top-heavy and increasing the likelihood of head impact during falls or collisions. The neck musculature in children is also generally weaker, providing less support compared with adults. A child's head will therefore accelerate more compared with an adult's head following a similar direct or indirect force, thereby increasing the risk of brain injury. The developing brain of a child is more susceptible to injury. Neural connections are still forming, and the mechanical insult can disrupt this crucial developmental process. Furthermore, children have higher cerebral blood flow, which can exacerbate brain swelling following an injury, thus putting children at greater risk of second impact syndrome than adults. Children also experience PCS to a greater extent than do adults (Babcock et al., 2013).

Behavioural factors also contribute to the increased risk of concussion in children. Risk-taking behaviour is more common in children, especially adolescents, making them more likely to engage in activities that can result in head injuries. Lack of skill or experience in sports and physical activities also makes children more vulnerable to injury. Moreover, younger children may not be fully aware of the dangers around them, making them more susceptible to accidents that could result in a concussion. Another layer of complexity is added by the fact that children, particularly young children, are not able to articulate their symptoms well, leading to delayed diagnosis and treatment.

24.4.2 Older People

Concussion in older adults presents a unique set of challenges that differ from those faced by younger populations (Elias et al., 2024). The outcomes of concussion in older adults are influenced by a variety of psychological and physiological factors. One of the most pressing concerns is the long-term impact of concussion on the ageing brain. The brain's sensitivity to TBI varies across one's lifetime, and outcomes are generally worse for severe TBIs occurring in early childhood or after the age of 40. This suggests that older adults may be more susceptible to the long-term consequences of concussion, including a lower threshold for subsequent concussions and more severe symptoms.

The concept of cognitive reserve is particularly relevant here. This is the concept that individuals with a greater number of neurons, more intricate neuronal connections, and a stronger neurological framework can afford to lose a certain degree of cognitive function before presenting with clinically significant deficits. Cognitive reserve tends to diminish as one ages, and the rate of this reduction can vary by a range of factors including biology, behaviour, and environmental conditions. Younger adults typically have a robust cognitive reserve, and this may partially explain why they initially display fewer cognitive and motor impairments following a concussion compared with older people.

Frailty is a variable that adversely impacts psychological well-being in elderly. Furthermore, pre-existing health conditions also have a role in shaping the recovery path, particularly for those who do not fully recover or continue to show cognitive dysfunction postconcussion. Comorbidities such as cancer or dementia are significant predictors of concussion outcomes, and their presence often results in the exclusion of older adults from key research trials, potentially skewing the data.

24.4.3 Sex Differences

Female athletes are not only more likely to sustain a concussion but also to face more severe repercussions than are male athletes (Walshe et al., 2022). Women participating in contact sports have higher rates of concussion than men. For example, in women's ice hockey, where body-checking is prohibited (unlike in the men's game), the rates of concussion are almost equivalent to those in the male version of the sport. Female athletes also tend to experience higher symptom scores, slower reaction times, greater cognitive decline, and longer times for returning to play compared with males who play similar sports (Rizzone & Ackerman, 2021).

Whilst considerably more research is required to understand sex differences associated with concussion, these differences have been suggested to be attributed to a combination of anatomical, behavioural, and physiological factors. As discussed above for children, females tend to have narrower neck girth and comparatively reduced neck strength, making them more susceptible to greater head-neck acceleration during impacts. Additionally, females are generally more forthcoming in reporting their concussion-related symptoms.

Gonadal hormones, particularly progesterone and oestrogen, are known to have neuroprotective and reparative effects on the central nervous system. Given that women generally have higher circulating levels of progesterone and oestrogen compared to men, it might be assumed that women would experience better outcomes following TBI or concussion. However, the situation is more nuanced, and these hormones could account for the greater susceptibility and worse outcomes in women compared to men (Levin et al., 2021). For example, the levels of gonadal hormones fluctuate throughout a woman's life, affecting the body's response to concussion. Normal cycling females, who have regular fluctuations of these hormones, have been suggested to exhibit better outcomes compared to males and females lacking sex hormones (e.g., due to ovariectomy). Furthermore, the hormonal cycles themselves have been correlated with variability in outcomes, making women more susceptible at certain times. Women aged 30–39 are most susceptible to experiencing symptoms after sustaining a brain injury. As hormone levels begin to decline years before menopause, women aged 35–49 are found to be most vulnerable to post-concussion symptoms. This age-related variability in hormone levels could contribute to the greater effect of concussion in women. Finally, progesterone and oestrogen have complex actions that extend beyond neuroprotection, interacting with various neurotransmitters, influencing inflammation, and modulating cellular metabolism, among other effects. These multifaceted roles could contribute to the complexity of concussion outcomes in women. See also Box 24.3 for a discussion on mechanisms affecting neuroplasticity following concussion.

Box 24.3 Neuroplasticity and Concussion

Neuroplasticity is a particularly understudied area of concussion and mTBI research. However, TBI research in animal models is relevant to neuroplasticity (Albensi & Janigro, 2003). Rodent models for TBI include controlled cortical impact, fluid percussion injury, and weight drop models in addition to more recent genetic models. In larger mammals, blast injury and rotational and acceleration models have been utilised.

Animal models have demonstrated that TBI attenuates long-term potentiation (LTP), particularly in the hippocampus, thus leading to impairments in learning and memory (see Chap. 6). This attenuation is not merely a transient phenomenon, as excitatory post-synaptic potentials (EPSPs) are significantly reduced in injured animals 2–3 h post-injury. The reduction in EPSPs leads to reduced excitatory signalling and therefore reduced LTP. Suppressed population spikes observed in brain injured animals shows a long-lasting impact on synaptic strength and plasticity. The impact of TBI on long-term depression (LTD) is more variable and is more affected by the severity of the injury, the specific brain regions affected, and the time elapsed since the injury.

Both LTP and LTD are affected by the disruption of glutamate receptor activation. Disruptions in glutamate receptor activation could, therefore, have a cascading effect on both LTP and LTD. Furthermore, TBI-induced disruptions in calcium homeostasis have a broad impact on synaptic plasticity. Finally, because TBI affects GABA-mediated inhibition, the balance between excitatory and inhibitory signals is disrupted, thus decreasing the effective functioning of both LTP and LTD.

The hyperexcitability associated with TBI is prevalent in inhibitory neurons, particularly in the dentate hilus. This compromises the inhibitory control of dentate granule cells, leading to increased neural excitability, susceptibility to seizures, and excitotoxic damage. GABAergic mediated inhibition is notably affected, as evidenced by a decrease in the frequency of inhibitory post-synaptic currents observed in numerous studies.

On the other hand, synaptic depression represents a reduction in synaptic strength, which can be paradoxical when considered alongside hyperexcitability. This complexity suggests that the effects of TBI on neural function are both time—and region-dependent. Whilst hyperexcitability may be more prevalent in certain neural circuits, synaptic depression could manifest in others. Both phenomena have significant implications for synaptic plasticity, affecting both LTP and LTD, and by extension, cognitive functions such as learning and memory.

24.5 Treatment

24.5.1 Graded Return to Activity

The treatment of concussion is a complex and evolving field, often requiring a multidisciplinary approach involving both pharmacological and non-pharmacological interventions. The cornerstone of treatment is a symptom-guided protocol with a structured and graded approach to return to normal activity, allowing the brain to recover from the initial metabolic cascade and subsequent repair processes. Graded return-to-activity protocols have largely been developed for return to play (RTP) and return to study (RTS) in sport and education, respectively (Dichiaro et al., 2023; Patricios et al., 2023). Whilst protocols are available for return to work (RTW), they are less well-known and have received much less attention in the literature (Cancelliere et al., 2014).

The protocols are designed to ensure the individual is symptom-free and fully recovered before returning to full-time study or work, and to competition in the case of athletes. This minimises risk of further injury or extensive delays in returning full-time activity. The process is incremental, with each step challenging the individual progressively, ensuring a gradual return to activity. The protocols have distinct stages, each with their own set of activities and guidelines. The primary principle underlying the protocols is that the individual should only progress to the next stage if symptoms are both mild and short-lasting. If symptoms worsen, the individual should revert to the previous stage. Irrespective of the activity (i.e., return to school, work, or sport), *the first stage* involves physical and cognitive rest for 24 (adults) to 48 (children) hours. During this period, any activity that could potentially exacerbate symptoms, such as exercise, screen time, and mobile phone use, should be avoided. If tolerated, 20–30 min of reading or other light cognitive tasks may be carried out at home. This initial stage serves as a foundational period for recovery, allowing the brain to heal without any additional stressors. Full cognitive and physical rest beyond this initial 24–48 h inhibits efficient recovery. However, progressing too quickly through the next stages will slow recovery. The next stages are then specific to the activity to which the individual wishes to return (RTP, RTS, and/or RTW); however, in all cases, symptoms should be monitored—and ideally diaried—and activities should not be increased to the point of cognitive or physical fatigue (see Fig. 24.2).

The next stage in the graded return-to-activity protocol involves light aerobic exercise such as walking or regular chores in the house, with the objective of slightly elevate the heart rate, albeit not to the levels experienced during sport-specific activities. Cognitive demand is increased through activities such as reading, and limited phone or computer work. Some work (e.g., email) or light school work can be attempted, but television and computer games should be limited. More challenging study or work tasks should be avoided. Importantly, no resistance training is permitted at this stage.

In the third stage, the individual can begin to engage in activities away from the home. Ideally, this will include part-time school or work with accommodations. Light resistance training may be introduced at this stage. Sport-specific exercises that do not involve any head impact can be started in order to reintroduce sport-specific motor skills whilst maintaining a low risk of further brain injury. This should progress to more complex, non-contact training drills; increasing the individual's physical and cognitive load, in preparation for more sport-specific activities.

The objective of *the fourth stage* is to get the individual back to full-time school or work. After receiving medical clearance, athletes can begin the final stage, where they begin full-contact practice sessions. This is a crucial step to regain confidence and for coaching staff to assess return to play readiness. The individual should be closely monitored for any symptoms.

The final stage, which is specific to sport, is return to full game play, and this should only be attempted after the individual has successfully been back to full-time school or work. Even at this stage, the individual should continue to be monitored during and after the game to ensure that no symptoms reappear.

Specific for RTS, after the initial 24–48 h of rest, the student can begin light study as tolerated followed by return to school for partial days, initially avoiding more cognitively demanding subjects. During this phase, academic accommodations should be implemented. These can range from providing the student with study notes in advance, to offering extended test-taking time, or even modifying the classroom environment to reduce sensory stimuli that could exacerbate symptoms, such as bright lights or loud noises. As the student tolerates increased cognitive load without symptom recurrence, they may transition to attending school full-time but with continued academic accommodations. The focus then shifts to catching up on missed coursework and assessments.

For student athletes, the RTS protocol should be meticulously coordinated with RTP. These

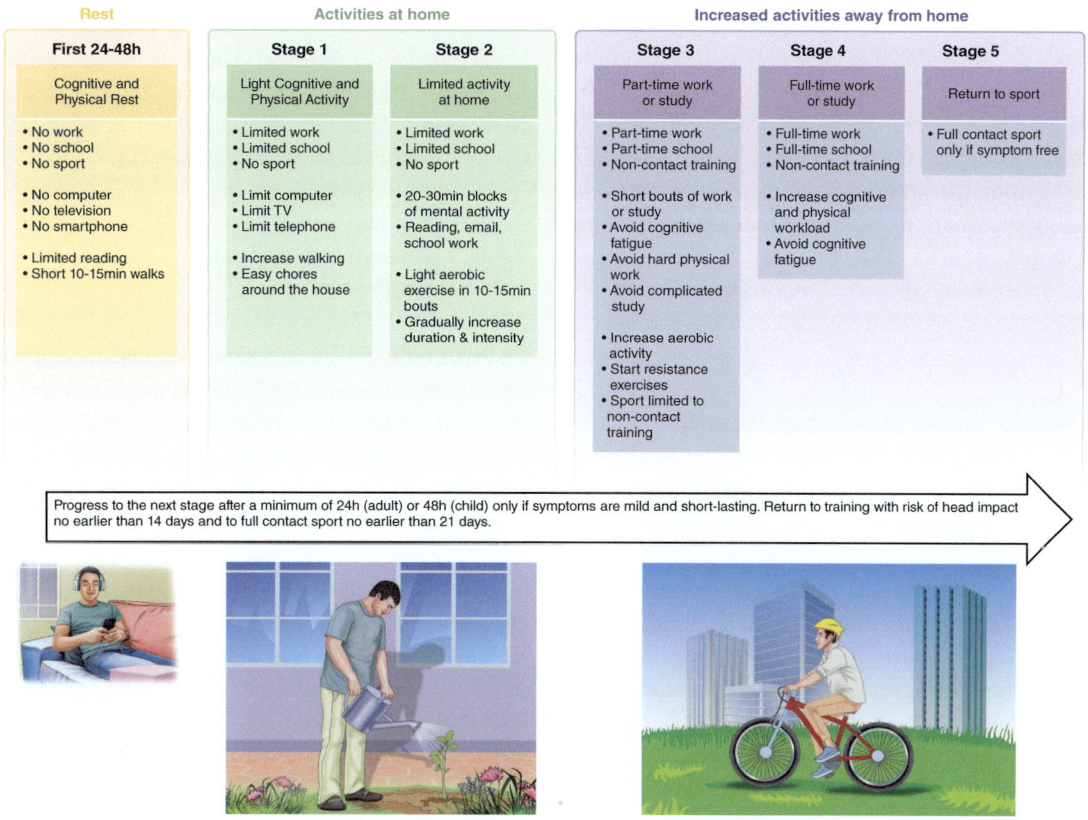

Fig. 24.2 Graded return to activity. Following concussion, a gradual stepwise return-to-activity protocol should be followed to enable an efficient and safe return to school, sport, and/or work. After an initial short period of rest, the individual should progress through each stage of activity. Progression to the next stage should only be made when symptoms are both mild and short-lasting. Sport should only be resumed after the individual has progressed to full-time school or work. Individuals with symptoms that continue beyond 28 days should seek medical advice from their doctor

individuals must successfully complete the RTS protocol before being cleared for full athletic participation to ensure exertional activities that can exacerbate cognitive symptoms do not delay academic reintegration. The entire process must be individualised and adjusted based on ongoing assessments and feedback from the injured student, healthcare providers, and educators.

Return to work protocols are considerably less well developed than are RTP and RTS protocols (Cancelliere et al., 2014). However, like the RTP and RTS protocols, RTW should involve a plan that outlines the stages of the RTW process, starting with less demanding tasks and shorter work hours. The plan should be tailored to the individual's job requirements and symptoms, to include part-time work or work from home where possible. Employers should be prepared to make reasonable accommodations to facilitate the employee's return to work, including modifying tasks, providing additional breaks, or altering the work environment to minimise sensory overload. Tasks assigned should be less cognitively and physically demanding, thus allowing the individual to adapt to the work environment again without overwhelming them. If symptoms do not worsen, the individual can gradually take on more hours and more complex tasks.

To evaluate exercise tolerance, various assessments such as the Buffalo Concussion Treadmill Test (BCTT)—a validated assessment tool—can be used to assess the severity of postconcussion symptoms and to guide the rehabilitation process (Patricios et al., 2023;

Wilber et al., 2021). The participant walks or jogs on a treadmill whilst the incline is gradually increased. The speed remains constant, but the incline increases by 1% every minute. The test continues until the participant reaches a symptom threshold, meaning they experience an exacerbation of their concussion-related symptoms. The time or level at which symptoms are exacerbated is recorded and used as a measure of exercise tolerance.

24.5.2 Vestibular Rehabilitation

Given that symptoms like dizziness, nausea, and vertigo frequently occur after a concussion and are especially prevalent in individuals with PCS, vestibular rehabilitation is often a recommended treatment (Yeates et al., 2023). It can be employed for patients with acute concussion following an initial rest period; however, it is most frequently utilised for patients with PCS. The therapy comprises a range of specialised exercises and activities designed to enhance balance, spatial awareness, and eye coordination. The treatment strategy embraces an “active, expose-recover” methodology, in which patients undergo activities that trigger symptoms within a controlled setting, followed by designated recovery intervals. The ultimate objective is to diminish both the severity and frequency of symptoms over an extended period.

As an example, balance retraining is frequently used in people with PCS, with an aim of maintaining stability, reducing the risk of falls and improving confidence in daily activities. Balance retraining progressively challenges the brain by adjusting the afferent flow of proprioceptive and vestibulo-ocular information. It might begin by asking the patient to stand on one leg, with the other foot lifted slightly off the ground for as long as possible. This might be performed with the patient next to a stable surface that they can hold or touch. As performance increases and symptoms are reduced, the exercise can be conducted with the eyes closed to increase the challenge. The exercise can be made more difficult still by standing on foam to introduce more instability. Balance retraining can be progressed further by integrating vestibulo-ocular reflex training, whereby head movements are added to the single leg stance exercise. These exercises should follow the principles of neuroplasticity by being challenging, yet achievable and repeating them frequently without exacerbating symptoms.

24.5.3 Pharmacological Interventions

Pharmacological interventions for the treatment of concussion primarily focus on symptom management rather than reversing the underlying injury. Analgesics such as acetaminophen and NSAIDs like ibuprofen are commonly used for pain relief. Antidepressants, particularly SSRIs, may be prescribed for mood disturbances, whilst antinausea medications like ondansetron can control nausea and vomiting. In some cases, sleep aids such as zolpidem may be used for insomnia. Stimulant medications such as methylphenidate are sometimes used for persistent attention and concentration issues, although they are generally considered second—or third-line options. In all cases, pharmacological treatment should be individualised based on the predominant signs and symptoms and can include some symptom-specific pharmacological therapies.

24.5.4 Future Directions

There has been an exponential increase in the published literature on concussion over the last decade. The number of concussions seen in emergency departments is increasing, largely due to heightened awareness and media exposure. Reducing exposure to sport-related concussions via rule changes in sport, particularly among children, and monitoring repetitive impacts are currently the best strategies to mitigate this silent epidemic. The pathophysiology of concussion is complex, and evidence-based biomarkers and diagnostic techniques are still lacking. Neuroimaging is not yet able to significantly contribute to a clinician’s diagnosis, but rapid progress is being made in this area. Future research should focus on identifying reliable cognitive and physical biomarkers and improving neuroimaging techniques to facilitate early and accurate diagnosis. Significant strides have been made in developing return-to-activity protocols for athletes returning to sport and for children returning to school. However, the adoption of these protocols outside of elite sports remains limited. There is an urgent need for better evidence-based return to work protocols and public education to ensure their implementation. Further research is necessary to understand the specific needs and responses to concussion in different demographic groups, including children, older adults, and females. These groups experience concussion differently due to physiological, anatomical, and hormonal factors, and tailored treatment and recovery protocols are essential. Moreover, a deeper understanding of the pathophysiology associated with postconcussion syndrome will be crucial. Exploring neuroplasticity and its impact on recovery could open new avenues for the treatment of persistent postconcussion symptoms. Enhanced knowledge of pathophysiology and biomarkers, particularly concerning recovery, will improve the efficiency and safety of return-to-activity protocols. Ultimately, a combination of advanced research, better diagnostic tools, tailored treatment protocols, and widespread public education is essential to address the complexities of concussion and its long-term effects.

Review Questions

- What are the difficulties associated with concussion diagnosis?
- What are the major features of a graded return-to-activity protocol?

References

Albensi, B. C., & Janigro, D. (2003). Traumatic brain injury and its effects on synaptic plasticity. *Brain Injury, 17*(8), 653–663.

Babcock, L., Byczkowski, T., Wade, S. L., Ho, M., Mookerjee, S., & Bazarian, J. J. (2013). Predicting postconcussion syndrome after mild traumatic brain injury in children and adolescents who present to the emergency department. *JAMA Pediatrics, 167*(2), 156–161. https://doi.org/10.1001/jamapediatrics.2013.434

Cancelliere, C., Kristman, V. L., Cassidy, J. D., Hincapie, C. A., Cote, P., Boyle, E., et al. (2014). Systematic review of return to work after mild traumatic brain injury: Results of the International Collaboration on Mild Traumatic Brain Injury Prognosis. *Archives of Physical Medicine and Rehabilitation, 95*(3 Suppl), S201–S209.

Dichiaro, M., Baker, D., & Tlustos, S. J. (2023). Return to learn after traumatic brain injury. *Pediatric Clinics of North America, 70*(3), 445–460.

Elias, J., Sutherland, E., & Kennedy, E. (2024). Concussion management in older people: A scoping review. *The Journal of Head Trauma Rehabilitation, 39*(4), 293–303.

Goldstein, M. (1990). Traumatic brain injury: A silent epidemic. *Annals of Neurology, 27*(3), 327.

Howell, D. R., & Southard, J. (2021). The molecular pathophysiology of concussion. *Clinics in Sports Medicine, 40*(1), 39–51.

Levin, H. S., Temkin, N. R., Barber, J., Nelson, L. D., Robertson, C., Brennan, J., et al. (2021). Association of sex and age with mild traumatic brain injury-related symptoms: A TRACK-TBI study. *JAMA Network Open, 4*(4), e213046.

Moore, M., & Sandsmark, D. K. (2023). Clinical updates in mild traumatic brain injury (concussion). *Neuroimaging Clinics of North America, 33*(2), 271–278.

Patricios, J. S., Schneider, K. J., Dvorak, J., Ahmed, O. H., Blauwet, C., Cantu, R. C., et al. (2023). Consensus statement on concussion in sport: The 6th International Conference on Concussion in Sport-Amsterdam, October 2022. *British Journal of Sports Medicine, 57*(11), 695–711.

Rizzone, K. H., & Ackerman, K. E. (2021). Female athlete and sports-related concussions. *Clinics in Sports Medicine, 40*(1), 133–145.

Romeu-Mejia, R., Giza, C. C., & Goldman, J. T. (2019). Concussion pathophysiology and injury biomechanics. *Current Reviews in Musculoskeletal Medicine, 12*(2), 105–116.

Voss, J. D., Connolly, J., Schwab, K. A., & Scher, A. I. (2015). Update on the epidemiology of concussion/mild traumatic brain injury. *Current Pain and Headache Reports, 19*(7), 32.

Walshe, A., Daly, E., & Ryan, L. (2022). Epidemiology of sport-related concussion rates in female contact/collision sport: A systematic review. *BMJ Open Sport & Exercise Medicine, 8*(3), e001346.

Wilber, C. G., Leddy, J. J., Bezherano, I., Bromley, L., Edwards, A. E., Willer, B. S., & Haider, M. N. (2021). Rehabilitation of concussion and persistent postconcussive symptoms. *Seminars in Neurology, 41*(2), 124–131.

Yeates, K. O., Raisanen, A. M., Premji, Z., Debert, C. T., Fremont, P., Hinds, S., et al. (2023). What tests and measures accurately diagnose persisting post-concussive symptoms in children, adolescents and adults following sport-related concussion? A systematic review. *British Journal of Sports Medicine, 57*(12), 780–788.

Afterword: Future Directions

25

Jens Bo Nielsen, Jakob Lorentzen, Rasmus Feld Frisk, and Lisbeth Højkjær Larsen

Abstract

Neurorehabilitation may evolve through a deeper understanding of neuroplasticity, the brain's adaptability, which drives innovative interventions. Multi-center adaptive clinical trials offer a dynamic platform to evaluate interventions globally with real-time implementation of the currently best performing therapy. Bridging basic neuroscience with clinical practice offers the potential for targeted therapies that optimize recovery mechanisms. Personalized medicine provides possibilities of developing interventions based on genetic, biological, and psychosocial factors, while wearable technologies expand therapy beyond clinical settings. Challenges include demographic shifts and resource constraints, which require equitable access to sustainable funding. Collaboration among stakeholders is crucial for accelerating evidence-based practice and has the potential to revolutionize neurorehabilitation. By employing adaptive trials, integrating neuroscience, and utilizing wearable technology, the future of neurorehabilitation holds the potential to significantly enhance recovery for neurological populations worldwide.

Keywords

Neuroplasticity · Adaptive trials · Wearable technology · Personalized medicine · Evidence-based practice

Box 25.1 Case Story

In the year 2050, neurorehabilitation had reached unprecedented heights, offering tailored solutions for individuals with brain injuries. Sarah, a 32-year-old software engineer, suffered a severe traumatic brain injury (TBI) when her fully self-driving car avoids a deer on the road and drives into a tree instead.

Immediately after the accident, the emergency responders used advanced neuroimaging techniques to assess the extent of her brain injury. Within hours, a multidisciplinary team of neurologists, neurosurgeons, and rehabilitation specialists collaborated to develop a personalized neurorehabilitation plan for Sarah.

She underwent neural stimulation therapy, where non-invasive brain stimulation techniques were used to promote neuroplasticity and accelerate her recovery. Virtual reality simulations helped her relearn cognitive tasks and improve her memory and attention span.

As Sarah progressed in her rehabilitation, wearable devices became integral to her daily life. Smart sensors embedded in

(continued)

J. B. Nielsen (✉) · J. Lorentzen · R. F. Frisk
L. H. Larsen
Department of Neuroscience, University of Copenhagen, Copenhagen, Denmark
e-mail: jbnielsen@sund.ku.dk; jlorentzen@sund.ku.dk; frisk@sund.ku.dk; lihl@sund.ku.dk

J. B. Nielsen et al. (eds.), *Neuroplasticity-based Neurorehabilitation*,
https://doi.org/10.1007/978-3-031-81120-3_25

Box 25.1 (continued)
her clothing monitored her movements and provided real-time feedback on her posture and gait. A personalized rehabilitation app tracked her progress and adjusted her exercises accordingly, ensuring optimal recovery.

Furthermore, Sarah participated in multicenter adaptive clinical trials, where novel interventions were evaluated in real-time based on her response and outcomes. These trials not only advanced evidence-based practice but also contributed to the collective knowledge of neurorehabilitation.

Sarah's rehabilitation extended beyond the clinic. Tele-rehabilitation sessions allowed her to receive therapy remotely, ensuring continuity of care. Additionally, community-based support programs facilitated her reintegration into society and promoted social engagement, which played a crucial role in her recovery.

After months of intensive neurorehabilitation, Sarah made remarkable progress. While challenges remained, she regained independence and resumed her career as a software engineer, thanks to the comprehensive and personalized approach to neurorehabilitation in the year 2050.

25.1 Introduction

This book has outlined several crucial neurobiological concepts essential as a framework for clinical practice aimed at enhancing function recovery in neurological populations. The book has aimed to emphasize the malleability of the nervous system—neuroplasticity, wherein microcircuits and neural network connectivity undergo structural changes with experience, leading to lasting alterations in network structure and activity. Understanding this phenomenon is crucial for guiding neurorehabilitation programs to achieve optimal goals and outcomes for patients. This chapter will expand on this knowledge and explore future possibilities for optimizing neurorehabilitation and enhancing function recovery in neurological populations. Despite the challenges posed by the lack of evidence for many therapeutic interventions and the limitations of small-scale traditional randomized controlled trials (RCTs), there are numerous promising developments underway. These offer ample reasons for optimism, suggesting that the field will significantly enhance the treatment of neurological populations in the years ahead.

25.2 Bridging Science and Practice: Insights from Basic Neuroscience

In recent years, there has been a significant rise in the understanding of the function of the nervous system and its response to injury, thanks to the introduction of innovative techniques. These methods have facilitated an integrated understanding, spanning from the molecular and cellular levels to integrative behavioral aspects. Insights are emerging into how specific neurons and neural circuits generate behaviors and how these circuits undergo reorganization after injuries. Undoubtedly, this knowledge will continue to expand in the future, offering new insights that inform clinical practice and provide basic understanding of the effectiveness of interventions. Additionally, it will delineate interventions that are less likely to be effective or may even contradict the current understanding of nervous system function. It is crucial to enhance the transfer of knowledge from basic science to clinical practice to ensure that clinicians possess up-to-date information. Relying on outdated knowledge for decision-making regarding therapy implementation or costly clinical trials must be avoided. This necessitates ongoing lifelong learning and access to the latest research. Close collaboration between basic neuroscientists, clinical neurologists, and therapists is essential for this. Such collaboration can be facilitated by prioritizing translational efforts and creating platforms where researchers and clinicians from various disciplines can interact. Exchanging knowledge will promote mutual inspiration and idea generation as a crucial objective for future strategic planning within the healthcare sector.

Ongoing exploration of various emerging technologies holds clinical promise for both the near and distant future. Stem cell research, for instance, presents significant potential in developing therapeutic interventions aimed at replacing damaged neural tissue with precursor cells, potentially facilitating functional recovery. While fetal dopaminergic neurons have been investigated as a treatment for Parkinson's disease, the therapy has not yet been introduced as a routine clinical application. Similarly, stem cell therapy for spinal cord injury has demonstrated promising outcomes in animal studies but has yielded variable results in human clinical trials, casting doubts on its efficacy. Ongoing trials are also investigating the potential role of stem cell therapy in other neurological disorders like multiple sclerosis and cerebral palsy; however, it is premature to determine its suitability for these conditions. Crucial for advancing these efforts is obtaining more knowledge on the function of relevant neurons and neural circuits, as well as on the behavior, function, growth, and differentiation of stem cells, through ongoing basic neuroscience research.

Brain-computer interfaces (BCIs) have witnessed rapid expansion in recent years and offer promising prospects for restoring function in individuals with brain injuries. While there are encouraging reports of successful BCI in clinical trials, their integration into routine clinical practice remains premature. Achieving this requires a multidisciplinary approach involving collaboration among basic neuroscientists, engineers, computer scientists, neurologists, and therapists.

Advancements have also been made in modifying the function of specific neurons within animal nervous systems by introducing specific genes into neuronal DNA using retrovirus or herpes virus vectors. Such modifications hold potential for gene substitution in individuals with genetic neurological disorders and may also prompt specific cells to undertake functions like injury repair or facilitating establishment of new connections. In the future, it may be feasible to manipulate gene activity to recreate an embryonic-like environment within the central nervous system, conducive to neural growth, potentially surpassing the limitations of the adult nervous system. However, this requires a much better understanding of the factors that regulate axonal growth and establishment of connectivity in the developing and mature nervous system than what is available today.

Deep brain stimulation has proven to be an effective therapy for many Parkinson's disease patients who no longer respond to Levodopa treatment. Additionally, spinal cord stimulation using implanted epidural electrodes is emerging as a potential treatment for individuals with spinal cord injuries. Technological advancements in the development of more sophisticated electrodes and other stimulation modalities (such as optogenetic stimulation) must coincide with new insights from basic neuroscience into the functioning of various circuits in different regions of the nervous system.

25.3 Neuroplasticity: What Lies Ahead?

This book aims to illustrate how current knowledge of neurobiology and neuroplasticity can provide a framework for neurorehabilitation. This knowledge not only guides interventions but also provides objective measures of functionally relevant changes in the nervous system. These measures can be used alongside clinical outcome measures to document intervention effectiveness. As the understanding of neurobiology and neuroplasticity advances, the focus can shift toward therapies with strong theoretical support, while reevaluating those lacking support. Importantly, this knowledge allows clinical trials to concentrate on therapies with the highest likelihood of efficacy, ensuring that human and economic resources, as well as valuable patient time, are not wasted on treatments unlikely to be effective.

In recent years, the understanding of neurobiology and neuroplasticity has grown substantially, yet much remains to be discovered, particularly in developing new interventions to aid recovery for individuals with brain and spinal cord injuries. The insights gained into the molecular and cellular mechanisms of neuroplasticity, learning, and memory now pave the way for new pharmacological therapies. These pharmacological therapies can directly influence the intracellular and intercellular signaling pathways involved, potentially enhancing both learning and memory. This advancement holds significant promise not only for dementia treatment but also for improving motor and cognitive learning and memory in neurorehabilitation.

Future neurorehabilitation will likely include combined therapies where training is paired with targeted pharmacological treatments that enhance the signaling processes involved in plasticity. Understanding that structural changes in the nervous system are driven by intracellular signaling to the nucleus, gene expression modification, synaptic material production, and the establishment of new nerve cell connections opens up the possibility of modifying gene expression to facilitate plastic changes and functional recovery. As knowledge about gene expression regulation expands, new opportunities are emerging to directly modify how DNA responds to training and other interventions.

Epigenetic mechanisms largely regulate the opening and closing of sensitive periods during development or following injuries. One such mechanism involves the extent to which DNA is twisted around histones, affecting the availability of binding sites for gene transcription factors. Pharmacological agents targeting histone deacetylase, which controls DNA twisting around histones, might be used to regulate this process, potentially opening sensitive periods that enhance the efficacy of training and learning interventions. Another example involves proteins in the nervous system, such as Nogo proteins, which inhibit axon growth and the formation of new connections in the adult nervous system. Antibodies against Nogo proteins may facilitate the recovery of functional connectivity following injury.

25.4 Multi-Center Adaptive Clinical Trials: Advancing Evidence-Based Practice

Convincing evidence about which therapies are effective and which are not is vital for improving clinical neurorehabilitation. This ensures that all patients receive the most efficient treatment and that resources are not wasted on ineffective therapies. Clinical studies are essential, but the field is currently plagued by too many small, poorly designed studies. This is evident from numerous systematic reviews that have failed to draw definitive conclusions about the effectiveness of interventions.

There is an urgent need for a transformative approach. The increasing globalization and ease of communication promise future collaborative efforts in multi-center networks, which can coordinate studies of sufficient scale. Through international consensus and guidelines, these collaborative networks can ensure the use of unified, objective outcome measures, enabling proper evaluation of new and existing therapies. Addressing legislative, data protection (GDPR), and other issues related to different traditions and the need for individual sites to showcase their capabilities will be crucial for establishing these international collaborations. While challenging and time-consuming, this approach is necessary. Paradoxically, the experiences from the COVID-19 pandemic may have facilitated this international collaboration and provided ways to overcome obstacles.

Unfortunately, traditional randomized controlled trials (RCTs) are lengthy and resource-intensive, especially in an international collaborative network setting. New approaches, such as Bayesian statistical methods, should be considered. Adaptive clinical trials based on a Bayesian framework allow clinical practice to evolve as new data from international multi-site collaborations are collected. This approach enables continuous updates to clinical practice based on the most effective interventions from global multi-treatment trials. In essence, it allows the best therapies to prevail. Adaptive clinical trial networks have been established to guide clinical practice in numerous diseases and will likely also play an important role in future neurorehabilitation.

25.5 Personalized Neurorehabilitation: A Precision Approach

Personalized neurorehabilitation tailors interventions to individuals based on their distinct genetic composition, biological markers, and psychosocial characteristics. This personalized approach holds great promise in optimizing treatment outcomes by targeting specific pathways and mechanisms underlying the condition. Genomic advances enable clinicians to identify genetic predispositions to neurological conditions, allowing for the customization of rehabilitation strategies. For instance, in stroke rehabilitation, genetic testing can pinpoint variants associated with motor recovery, guiding therapists in designing tailored interventions to maximize outcomes. Moreover, neuroimaging techniques provide valuable insights into the brain's structural and functional connectivity. Functional magnetic resonance imaging (fMRI) and diffusion tensor imaging (DTI) help identify areas of brain damage and assess white matter integrity, guiding the selection of interventions aimed at promoting neuroplasticity and functional recovery. Consideration of psychosocial factors is also crucial in personalized neurorehabilitation. Understanding a patient's personality traits, motivation levels, and social support network informs the development of rehabilitation plans tailored to their unique needs. For instance, individuals with high motivation may benefit from intensive rehabilitation programs, while those with limited social support may require additional resources to facilitate their recovery.

25.6 Empowering Patients with Technology: From Clinic to Home

While centralized neurorehabilitation ensures that highly qualified therapists, doctors, and nurses provide the best possible care for patients, the rising costs of health care will inevitably limit how much and for how long individual countries can offer such services to every patient. Eventually, patients must transition from centralized rehabilitation units to their homes, where they will rely on more localized services or, potentially, no services at all.

It is crucial that this transition from a centralized clinical setting to a local home environment, and increasingly into daily activities, proceeds smoothly. A comprehensive plan is needed to guarantee continued support with clear goals that bridge the central and local settings. This requires close coordination between authorities and a unified plan to ensure continuity of care.

New technologies can significantly enhance communication and ensure that an overarching plan is consistently followed throughout rehabilitation, from centralized to local settings. Electronic healthcare platforms, where information is easily accessible and follows the patient regardless of location, have already been implemented in many countries. Advances in Internet connectivity and portable electronic devices will further simplify and reduce the cost of this coordination, enabling implementation in other countries. These technological advances will also facilitate data sharing and global coordination of neurorehabilitation research, making it more effective.

Wearable technologies integrated with mobile Internet-connected devices will allow direct communication with patients, enabling therapists and doctors to supervise the neurorehabilitation process more efficiently than through physical contact alone. Training programs can be delivered daily to patients via Internet-enabled technologies, with progression decisions based on feedback from wearable sensors and other devices. This may also improve the adherence of the rehabilitation, where the patients themself are empowered to maintain the active role in their rehabilitation programs.

Ultimately, a significant portion of the training program may be managed using artificial intelligence, which can draw on global knowledge to create the most effective training regimen for patients with specific characteristics. AI also can facilitate training progression decisions based on data from wearable sensors and other inputs, ensuring quick and appropriate optimization of the rehabilitation process. This will not replace therapists and doctors but will constitute tools that may facilitate their decision-making and help ensure that all healthcare professionals can offer the best possible neurorehabilitation to each patient. AI connected to a vast database of knowledge from ongoing adaptive clinical trials and all published scientific data will be a powerful tool for doctors and therapists in the future.

25.7 Training in Everyday Life: A Paradigm Shift in Rehabilitation

One important message from both basic scientific studies on motor learning and neuroplasticity and clinical studies on neurorehabilitation is that improvement and recovery of function can continue for many months and years with ongoing training and learning. There is a cost-benefit issue to consider, both in terms of healthcare resources and the patient's time and priorities, compared to the improvement in function that can be achieved at any given time after injury. Evidence suggests that most functional recovery occurs within the subacute phase following brain injury, while functional gains in the chronic phase require significantly more effort and time.

It is up to the individual patient to evaluate whether the time and effort invested in training are worthwhile compared to the functional gains achieved. In most countries, the financial means of the individual patient also determine whether it is possible to pay for continued training by specialized therapists for several years after injury. Despite these concerns, there is no doubt that functional improvements can still be achieved years after injury, although not as dramatically as in the initial months. The key factor is how much training the patient can incorporate into their daily routine and how many hours can be dedicated to neurorehabilitation. This poses a challenge when the goal for both the patient and society is to return to a normal life, including resuming work.

The obvious solution is to integrate training into daily life, making it a seamless part of the patient's activities at home or work. The integration of wearable devices into everyday life represents a paradigm shift in neurorehabilitation, blurring the lines between therapy and daily activities. By embedding rehabilitation exercises into routine tasks and environments, wearable devices facilitate continuous engagement and promote neuroplasticity through enriched environmental stimulation. Technologies such as augmented reality-based rehabilitation games and immersive virtual reality environments can enhance motivation, engagement, and outcomes. These relatively inexpensive approaches, which are not perceived as time-consuming but are integrated into what the patient wants or needs to do, offer significant future possibilities for improving function in the chronic stage following brain injury.

25.8 Future Challenges: Navigating Resource Constraints and Demographic Shifts

Despite the promise of innovation, neurorehabilitation faces significant challenges on the horizon. Demographic shifts, including an aging population and rising incidence of neurological disorders, will place increasing demands on healthcare systems and rehabilitation services. Ensuring equal access to neurorehabilitation across diverse populations and geographic regions will require innovative solutions that address resource constraints, workforce shortages, and disparities in care delivery. Moreover, navigating the complexities of healthcare financing and reimbursement models will be essential to sustainably fund neurorehabilitation services and support ongoing research and development efforts. Global collaboration is essential to addressing these issues. To achieve this, judicial, cultural, and traditional challenges must be resolved. Additionally, securing individual rights and personal data, as outlined by regulations like GDPR, is crucial when collaborating across borders. A balance must be struck between protecting these rights and advancing research for the well-being of all mankind. This necessitates prioritizing global interests over local and national concerns, enabling researchers and clinicians worldwide to work together without administrative and legislative barriers that focus on national security rather than the greater good of humanity. The feasibility of such collaboration is demonstrated by the contributions of authors from 14 different countries, representing all aspects of the field of neurorehabilitation, featured in this book.

Review Questions

- How does neuroplasticity contribute to advancements in neurorehabilitation?
- What are the benefits of multi-center adaptive clinical trials in evaluating interventions for neurorehabilitation?
- How are wearable technologies revolutionizing the delivery of neurorehabilitation interventions, and what impact do they have on patient engagement and outcomes?

Correction to: Neurorehabilitation Technologies

Andrew J. T. Stevenson, Erika G. Spaich,
Prithvi Ravi Kantan, Lisbeth Højkjær Larsen,
Jakob Lorentzen, and Thomas Sinkjær

Correction to:
Chapter 16 in : J. B. Nielsen et al. (eds.), *Neuroplasticity-based Neurorehabilitation*, https://doi.org/10.1007/978-3-031-81120-3_16

Dr. Prithvi Ravi Kantan's affiliation was incorrect. It has been updated in this corrected version.

The updated version of this chapter can be found at https://doi.org/10.1007/978-3-031-81120-3_16

J. B. Nielsen et al. (eds.), *Neuroplasticity-based Neurorehabilitation*,
https://doi.org/10.1007/978-3-031-81120-3_26

FSC
www.fsc.org
MIX
Papier aus verantwortungsvollen Quellen
Paper from responsible sources
FSC® C105338

If you have any concerns about our products,
you can contact us on
ProductSafety@springernature.com

In case Publisher is established outside the EU,
the EU authorized representative is:
Springer Nature Customer Service Center GmbH
Europaplatz 3, 69115 Heidelberg, Germany

Printed by Libri Plureos GmbH
in Hamburg, Germany